vital skincare

NATURAL HEALTHY SKIN IN JUST 5 MINUTES A DAY

Laura Pardoe

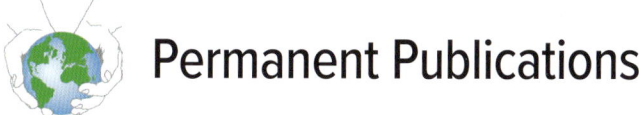
Permanent Publications

Published by
Permanent Publications
Hyden House Ltd
The Sustainability Centre
East Meon
Hampshire GU32 1HR
United Kingdom
Tel: 01730 823 311
          International code: +44 (0)
Email: enquiries@permaculture.co.uk
Web: www.permanentpublications.co.uk

Distributed in the USA by
Chelsea Green Publishing Company, PO Box 428, White River Junction, VT 05001
www.chelseagreen.com

© 2018 Laura Pardoe
The right of Laura Pardoe to be identified as the author of this work has been asserted by her in accordance with the Copyrights, Designs and Patents Act 1998

Principal photography by Richard Adams, additional images supplied by the author

Designed by Two Plus George Limited, www.TwoPlusGeorge.co.uk

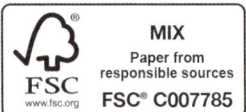

Printed in the UK by Bell & Bain, Thornliebank, Glasgow

All paper from FSC certified mixed sources.
The Forest Stewardship Council (FSC) is a non-profit international organisation established to promote the responsible management of the world's forests. Products carrying the FSC label are independently certified to assure consumers that they come from forests that are managed to meet the social, economic and ecological needs of present and future generations.

British Library Cataloguing-in-Publication Data
A catalogue record for this book is available from the British Library

ISBN 978 1 85623 322 4

All rights reserved. No part of this publication may be reproduced, stored in a retrieval system, rebound or transmitted in any form or by any means, electronic, mechanical, photocopying, recording or otherwise, without the prior permission of Hyden House Limited.

Disclaimer
The Author and Publisher shall not be liable in the event of damages in connection with, or arising out of the information offered here. Everyone has their own unique skin. Enjoy learning about your skin, its needs and the herbs and oils that can help it, while taking care to act with caution to identify any sensitivities you may have.

Foreword

Your vital guide to naturally great skin

Skin is your interface with the world and your foundation to looking good and feeling great. You notice it; others notice it. It is vital for your sense of wellbeing and self-confidence. That means it's worth investing in your skin, getting to know it and looking after it. It's the vital undergarment you wear every day of your life.

Choosing natural options makes sense for you and the environment, but where should you start among the vast range of products and ingredients? How do you know what's really good or bad and what will work best for your skin? What are the vital necessities for a simple approach that doesn't cost the earth?

Here you can find the best way to care for your skin – the vital approaches to suit your skin, your lifestyle, your values and your budget. You've got to be able to tick all those boxes to make it sustainable, enjoyable and authentic – and just how you want to be. Your skin presents you to the world: let it show your best and true self.

Start by getting to know your skin, befriending it. Understanding how your skin works, what it needs and the amazing way it's looking after you means you can make the right supportive interventions at the right time. Listen to your skin to make informed choices to your vital self-care.

Life is different every day; from the things you do, the environment you're in and the way you feel. So your skin has different requirements each day. Focus simply on what's vital today to keep your skincare easy and effective. Select plant-based ingredients that suit your skin to benefit from their vitality on a daily basis and connect with nature's grounding life force.

When you fall in love with your skin, listen to it and work with it, you feel a boost to your confidence and happiness that can impact every day for the rest of your life. Look after your skin and let your true vitality shine through.

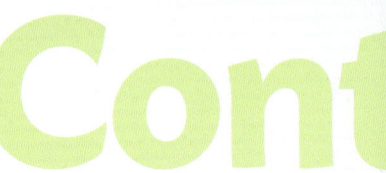

| Introduction | vii |

Part 1: Vital Skin

1. In Praise of Skin — 1
2. Why it is Vital to Look after your Skin — 7
3. How Skin Works — 11
   - Skin's layers — 13
   - The lymph system — 15
   - Essential fatty acids, oxygen, water — 16

Part 2: Vital Products

4. From Handmade to Off-the-shelf and Back Again — 19
5. Vital Products 1: The Vital Choices you make in Selecting Skincare — 25
6. Blending Your Own — 31
   - What will blending your own do for you? — 32
   - So why aren't we all doing it? — 36
7. Vital Products 2: Which Products are Vital to You? — 39
   - Your skincare personality — 40
   - Transitioning — 46
   - Patch testing — 48

Part 3: Vital Skincare

8. Vital Skincare: Simple as 1, 2, 3 — 51
   - Three determinants that make your skin what it is — 52
   - Three simple practices — 56
   - Time for action — 58
9. Cleansing — 59
   - Why we need to cleanse — 60
     1. Oil cleansing — 61
     2. Oil and water cleansing — 64
     3. Soap — 71
     4. Clay cleansers — 72
     5. Oat cleansers — 75
     6. Cleansing masks — 75
     7. Steam cleansing — 76
     8. Cleansing water — 76
   - Toners — 77
     1. Rebalancing the pH of your skin — 77
     2. Hydrating your skin — 78
     3. Conditioning skin — 78
   - When to cleanse; tips for using cleansers — 81
10. Exfoliating — 83
    - Physical exfoliation — 84

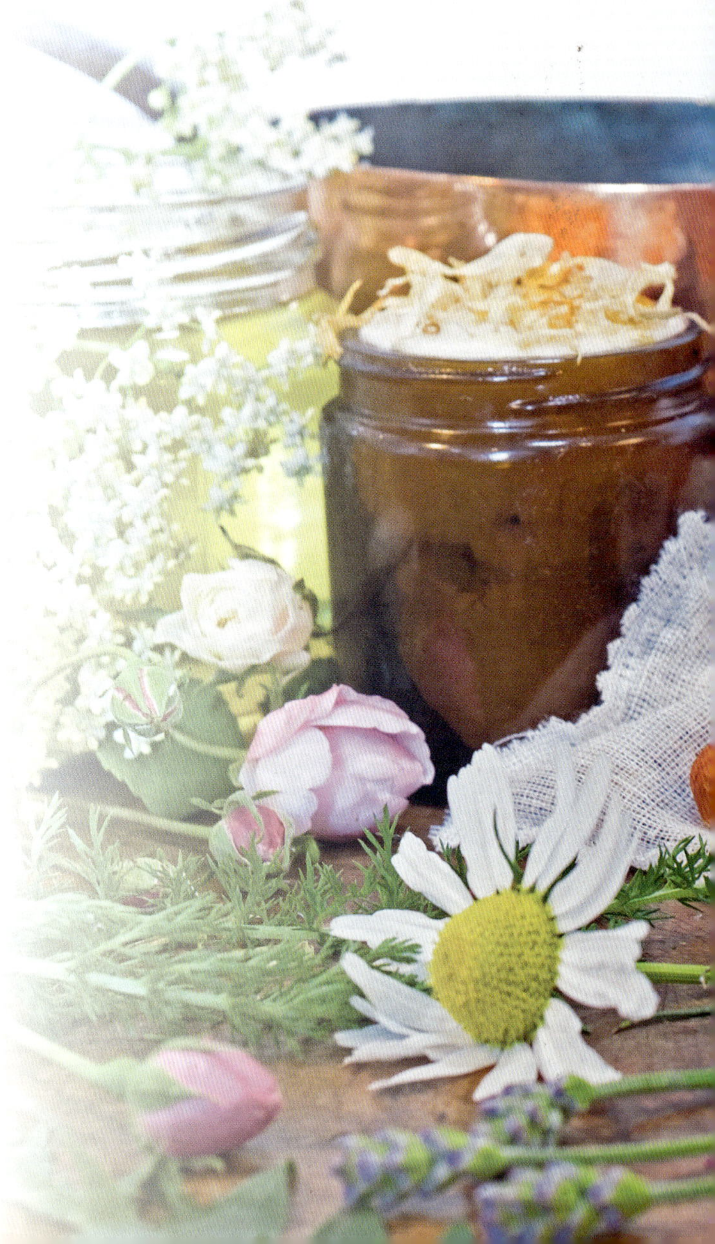

Chemical exfoliation	91
When to exfoliate; after exfoliating	98

11. Moisturising — 99

Why use moisturisers?	100
When to moisturise	100
What do moisturisers do?	101
How to moisturise when …	106
Moisturising in your teens and twenties …	108
Moisturising in your thirties, forties and fifties …	110
Moisturising forevermore …	114
Product form	116
Benefit of combining; some moisturising tips	120

Part 4: Vital Techniques

12. Learn to Blend like a Pro — 123

Kit and caboodle	124

Part 5: Vitality

13. Powerhouse Seed Oils — 133

14. Flower Power — 139

How to add flower power	140
Gathering herbs	144
Storing herbs	145
Essential power	146

15. Our Closest Herbs — 147

Spring – wild herbs	148
Blackberry, Chickweed, Cleavers, Comfrey, Dandelion, Horsetail, Nettles	
Spring – garden herbs	156
Bay, Houseleek, Lady's mantle, Lemon balm, Parsley, Raspberry leaf, Rosemary	
Summer – wild herbs	166
Chamomile, Elderflower, Horsechestnut, Limeflower, Marshmallow, Red clover, St John's Wort	
Summer – garden herbs	174
Borage, Calendula, Honeysuckle, Lavender, Pelargonium, Rose, Yarrow	

16. Little Rituals – Reflecting on your Skincare — 183

Ingredient Suppliers	187
References	187
Skincare Recipes: Summary and Index	188
General Index	192
Praise for this book	196

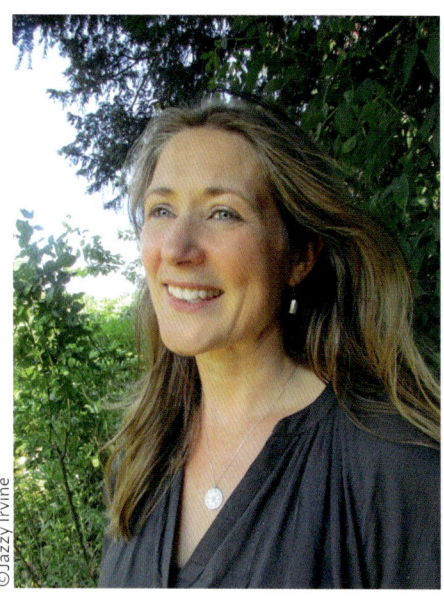
©Jazzy Irvine

DEDICATION

For Isabel and Jasmine, may you always be happy in your own skin.

Laura is a plantswoman and natural skincare formulator. Growing up in Birmingham, she valued the seasonal indicators provided by garden and wasteland plants. Interested in people and our interrelationships with the world around us, past, present and future, she read archaeology and anthropology at Cambridge and developed a career in marketing and insight. A decade working with National Trust reinforced her awareness of the importance of nature in our daily lives and inspired the creation of her artisanal brand, Field Fresh Skincare. Now living in the Cotswolds, her time is shared between family, hedgerows, garden, workshops, desk and lab as she blends traditional and modern approaches to bring the skincare benefits of temperate plants to all.

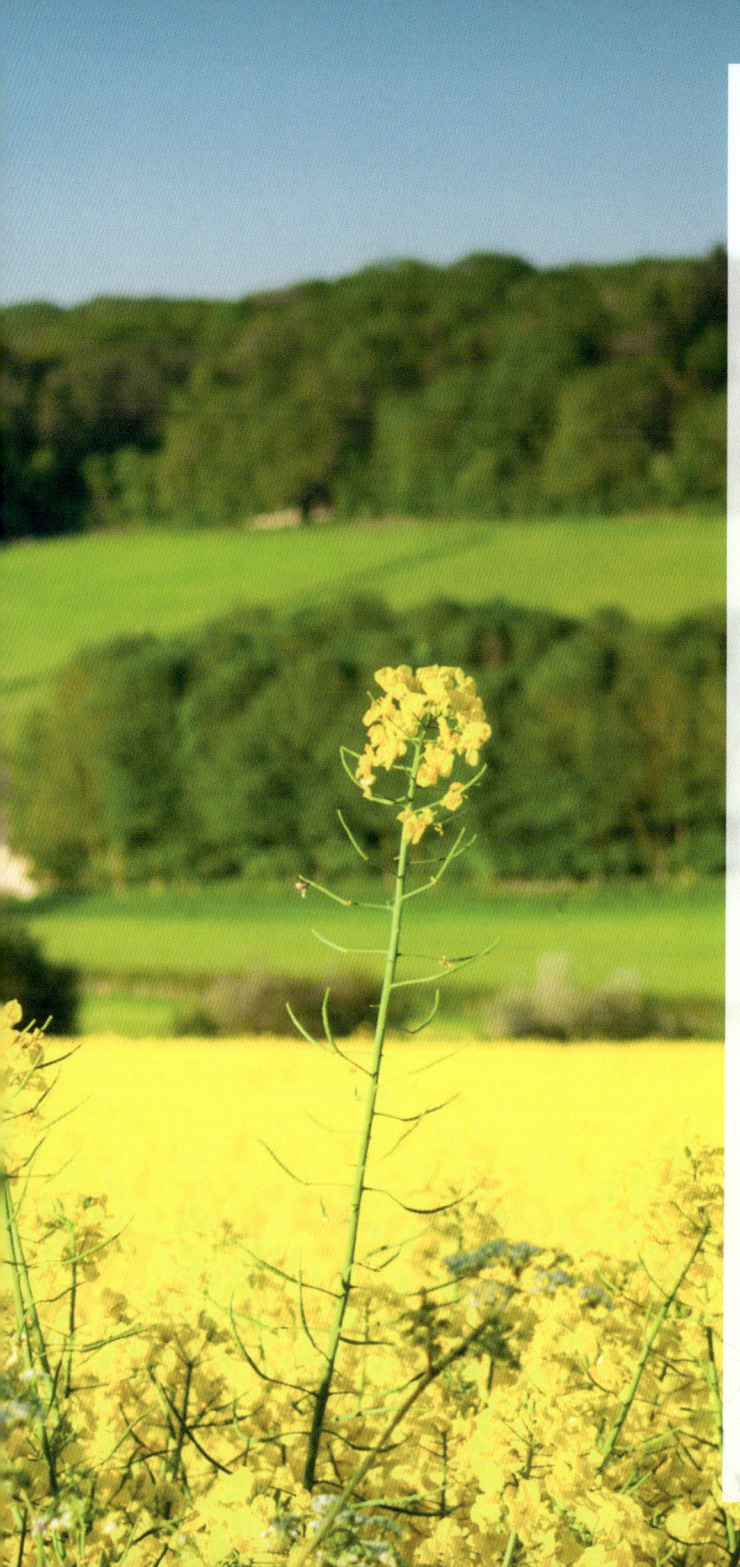

Introduction

Your skin is amazing.

You may not feel that every day (yet), but your skin does its amazing work every day. This book will help you love and appreciate your skin by understanding the fantastic ways it looks after you, inspiring you to think about how you look after it. You're in it together, after all.

By working with your skin and its natural processes, by helping your skin do what it does best, you will have that amazing skin feeling every day. You'll notice it and so will the people around you.

What you learn here, and the habits you can adopt, are a lifetime gift to yourself. Great skin can give you confidence in a way no clothes, makeup or accessories ever can. Any time invested in enhancing your skin will pay back many-fold – in your comfort, happiness and confidence. It's the ultimate statement of health and vitality. Great skin never goes out of fashion, so get the basics right.

You may already have a skincare regime you adhere to, or you may never have thought about how to look after your skin. You may have tried many different products, or be an advocate of just one. You may be blessed with trouble-free skin, or suffer from outbreaks, soreness or dry skin. You're here now and reading this, so you are taking an interest in your skin and that gives you the power to have great skin.

I'll explain: think of how people thrive when you show interest in them, get to know them well, understand their needs, create a supportive environment for them and let them work with their own strengths in their own way. Skin is just the same. It's a living thing after all. Your great skin will be a result of you observing and understanding and then providing the support it needs.

This may differ from traditional wisdom about skincare routines (we'll come to the power of routines later). It means if you're doing the same thing day-in, day-out, you probably need to think again. It doesn't mean using lots of different products and complicating life, but quite the opposite. In general you'll find less is best, as the simpler you can make your skincare, the more effective and reliable it can be. The key is knowing which interventions to make when; that's what this book can help you with.

This book can give you the confidence to do what's right for your skin, regardless of hype and persuasive product messaging. You are the person who knows your skin best – you live with it every day.

You also know your lifestyle, how you need to operate and what you are and are not prepared to change or compromise on. You know the things that are important to you and so you can reflect these in the choices you make. It's your personal brand and you can live it authentically with an honesty that engenders confidence.

So, for example, if you love animals you can choose to put effort into seeking out products that haven't been tested on animals. If you're not sure, ask. Of course, some brands may not be upfront with the information, but you'll find out in a few clicks. Once you get curious and you inform your choices, you build the inner confidence of knowing that the choices you make are right for you, and made for the right reasons.

Similarly, if you take care to select healthy foods to eat, it makes sense to look for skincare with healthy ingredients, as what you put on your skin is absorbed into your body and impacts in a similar way to food. With the right ingredients, you can turn your skincare from having a negative impact on your body (if you're using synthetic products) to having a positive impact by using skincare with natural ingredients that boost your health and vitality. It's amazing the difference this makes.

You might also have a preference to buy and use locally produced food and products to support the local economy and feel more connected to your local area. Connection is a very important emotion giving us strength and hope in our lives. You can connect better with your local environment by using ingredients in your skincare derived from plants and flowers that grow in the same environmet. These will have a better affinity with your skin.

We see this with food too. 'Superfoods' are never out of the news with new potential being found in berries, seeds and compounds. But we don't all respond to them in the same way. Someone living in a temperate climate may be more likely to feel the positive effect of eating blueberries than goji berries. Utilise the things that grow around you; your body will respond better to it and you'll feel more in touch with the world outside your window.

Skin has a natural empathy with pure plant preparations, something French beauty experts have always appreciated. There is science in this – plants contain phytohormones, which are substances similar to human hormones. It's when our hormones kick in as teenagers that skin problems can erupt, so it's clear the significant effect hormones have on our skin. The phytohormones from plants have real potential to help us.

Ultimately, the more confident you are about the choices you make, and the reasons you're making them, the happier you'll be. Your contentment will shine through, adding radiance to your appearance. Follow what you believe in, and be able to qualify and substantiate your beliefs with sound reasoning, knowing the clear benefits. Taking time to really think about what skincare you're using, and why, is a lifetime's investment that will keep you looking good and feeling great throughout the years to come.

As current predictions suggest that we've the potential to live a lot longer than previous generations, there could be a great payback for investing some time now.

This book provides you context within which you can make your own judgements and decisions. You have to be comfortable with whatever you do. Go beyond celebrity endorsements, paid promotions and experts expounding; view statistics and trends with caution – all these are based on mass assessments and generalisations across a broad spectrum of people. Focus instead on a unit of one – you – you need to find what's right for you. Because when you're happy, your skin's happy and, typically, when your skin's happy, you're happy. It's way more than skin deep.

The caring world you want starts with self-care. When you know how to look after yourself and practice it daily, you are fit (physically and mentally) and able (practically and knowledgeably) to look after others. The ripple effect can begin.

It all starts with what you think. Work with your own truths and change your practices to be meaningful to you. You'll be able to maintain that change because it fits your values and beliefs, and it's right for you.

There's so much to gain looking after our skin. There are ways to do it that are more kind to your body and to the environment. Once you know what you're about, your daily practice needn't take much time. If you need your skincare to be swift, you can still get great results. If you love the indulgence of lavishing time on beauty, enjoy it consciously to care for your mind, body and soul.

There is so much in life that we regard as normal, not thinking to question it. But in many areas, we're starting to re-evaluate some common assumptions. For example, we had long thought that our way of life depended on oil, thus control of oil was one of the greatest sources of power across the globe. The fear of reserves running out frightened us but also galvanised alternative thinking. Now we are confident that power (in the mechanical and political senses) does not have to be synonymous with oil. Incredibly, oil companies are now suggesting that we'll never have cause to drain all reserves (i.e. it will be uneconomic to do so) as we shift to a new way of working with other natural resources.

So change does happen, big change. We will all see a lot of change over our lifetimes, and while sometimes it can feel disempowering, we can feel small and helpless, there is one thing that you are absolutely in control of – your own body. It's the main thing you have, and you can take responsibility for it and treat it however you choose.

Your skincare and the care you take of your body is a great way to demonstrate your values to the world. You'll find that when you demonstrate you care about something, others around you will take interest in and start caring more too, particularly if they share the same beliefs and truths as you. Give it a go and see the love flow back when you start taking good care of you.

Ready to start taking care of yourself? It all starts with falling in love with your own skin. Be amazed, and truly grateful for the wonderful ally that's with you every day.

Beauty and seduction, I believe, is nature's tool for survival, because we all protect what we fall in love with

LOUIE SCHWARTZBERG, AMERICAN DIRECTOR, 1950-

Part 1
Vital Skin

CHAPTER 1

in praise of skin

Your skin is your largest organ. It's easy to take for granted, only noticing when there's a problem such as a blemish, an itch or dryness. It's easy to overlook the amazing role skin performs.

Skin is our container – our outer skin – the boundary that separates us from the physical world, holding all our molecules together. It is our embodiment; our complete, contained self. In this role it is definite and yet flexible: definite about its own structure and strength yet accommodating to all the movements of the body. Quite phenomenal when you stop to think about it.

But it's so much more than a simple container.

Skin protects

Our skin is like armour shielding us from the harsh elements and pollutants of the world around us. It protects us from the external onslaught of bacteria, viruses and chemicals.

The clever arrangement of cells on the surface of the skin forms a solid barrier, as the tiles of a roof shelter a home.

Left to its own devices, skin will maintain a natural pH of around 4 or 5. This slightly acidic environment is hostile to bacteria, providing us with a first line of defence. We call this protective wall our skin's 'acid mantle'. As many skincare products alter our skin's natural pH, often pushing it higher up the scale to a more alkaline level, much of our skincare regime tends to focus on correcting this pH shift to maintain the right pH levels for the acid mantle to do its work (more details on page 13).

Skin waterproofs

When you splash yourself with water, or get caught in the rain, you don't dissolve. Instead the water forms droplets that sit on the surface of your skin or slide off. This is because our skin is constantly self-lubricating with an oily, waxy substance called sebum. This is produced in the inner layers of skin and secreted through the sebaceous glands on the surface to form a waterproof layer.

Skin is a sunshield

Skin cells contain melanin that offers protection against UV. You can see the melanin responding to sunlight as you begin to tan. Of course, this doesn't provide all the protection we need from UV light, so we still need to take care, covering up exposed skin or adding additional UV protection through safe products.

Skin nourishes

One of the unique functions skin performs is to take in vitamin D, converting this from sunlight into an important nutrient for our body. Vitamin D receptors in the brain are found in the areas that are linked to depression, indicating a connection between vitamin D and happiness. Low levels

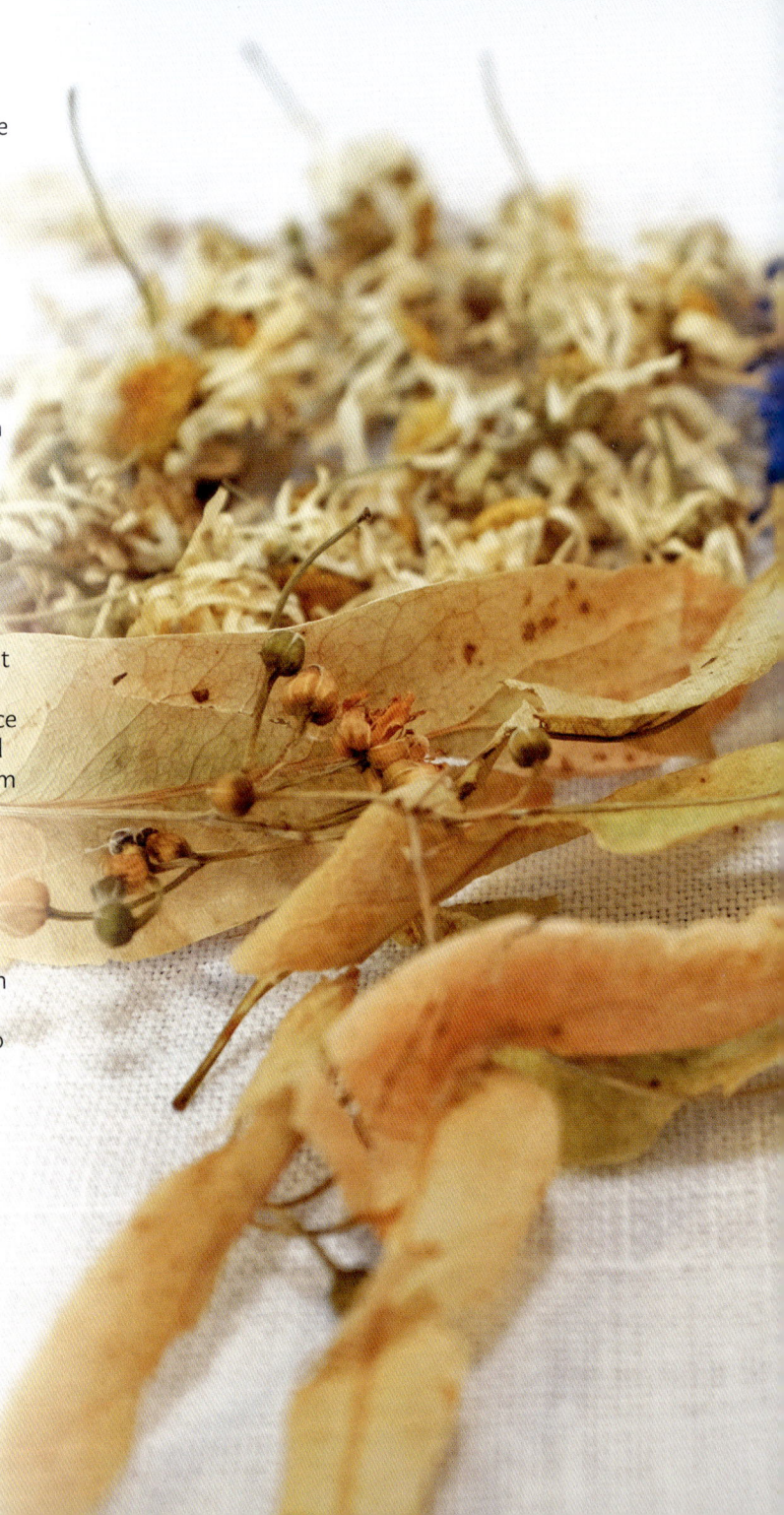

A traditional recipe for witches flying ointment, though I don't recommend trying this yourself: Caper surge sap, henbane extracts, deadly nightshade and aconite with goose grease ...

... Rub it on a broomstick and sit on it – the feeling could be akin to flying. Caper surge sap is caustic and would act as a vector for the other ingredients to pass through the skin. Henbane and deadly nightshade contain powerful hallucinogens and aconite is narcotic. The combination would have been exhilarating.

of vitamin D have often been associated with depression in clinical tests. This is one of the many reasons why going out for a walk on a sunny day can help cheer you up.

Skin absorbs many more forms of nourishment from the environment too. Substances are taken in to feed the body from the air, which is why local air quality can have such an impact on our skin: we come back from a trip outdoors with rosy cheeks or find being at the seaside gives us a radiant glow.

Substances can be absorbed from whatever comes into direct contact with the skin; creams, balms and lotions, for example. For this reason you should treat skincare like food; only put on your skin ingredients that you would be prepared to eat, drink or cook with. Knowing this can give you a new perspective when reading the ingredients listed on skincare products.

The absorbing and ingesting quality of skin is not new information; it's been known for hundreds of years. Much folk medicine makes use of poultices that bind substances to the skin knowing they will be drawn in for good effect. Superstitions of witches flying on broomsticks were probably fuelled by hallucinogenic plant substances concocted into ointments and rubbed on their broomsticks that then took effect when absorbed through permeable skin.

Skin purifies

One of the vital roles played by skin is to purify the body, emitting unwanted toxins. What we experience as perspiration is the natural process of carrying away salts and other substances in a continual cleansing process. Skin is just one of the waste-disposal systems our bodies have, and they tend to back each other up. Therefore, if something internally isn't functioning efficiently (e.g. lungs, liver, kidneys, lymphatic system or large intestine) our skin may pick up the slack. What this can actually mean for us is spots. Skin can become overwhelmed in its toxic-clearing function and so we get outbreaks of spots as more and more toxins are pushed to the surface. To stop skin suffering in this way, we should look after the internal processes to relieve the burden on our hard-working skin. Other indications of skin struggling to keep up with our body's toxins are blemishes, pasty skin colour or dark circles under the eyes.

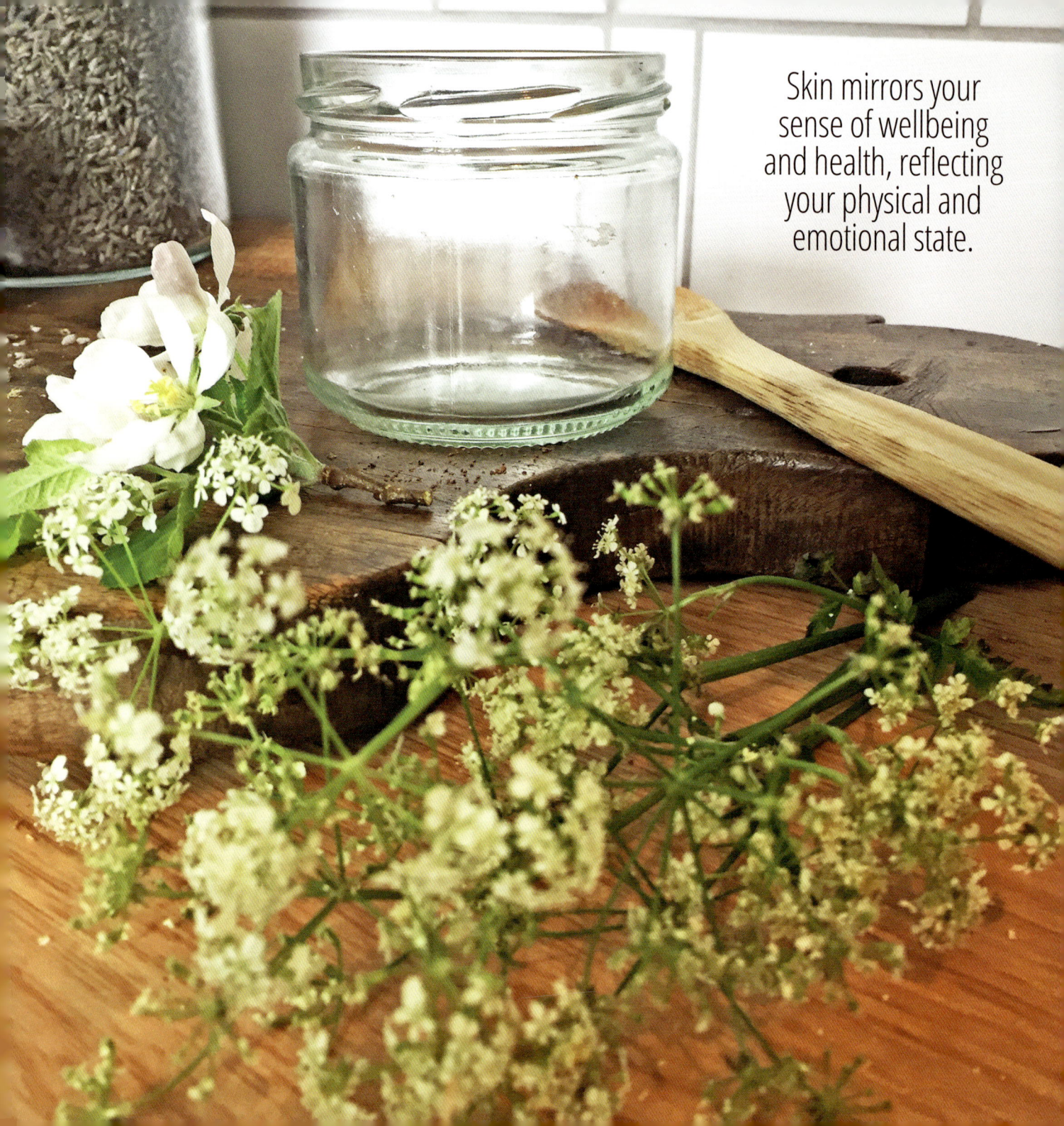

Skin mirrors your sense of wellbeing and health, reflecting your physical and emotional state.

Skin regulates temperature

As humankind has moved around the globe we have adapted to the different climatic conditions we encounter – sometimes through practical adaptations (the clothes we wear, the shelters we build) but also, long-term, through physiological adaptation – our bodies change to suit the environment we live in. In this way we are able to live in all climates from tropical to Arctic. Wherever we are, it's important for our internal organs to maintain a body temperature of 37°C. If it's cooler than this, skin will contract muscles under the hairs that cover our bodies to make them stand upright (piloerection) and thereby trap more air as insulation to keep us warm. If it's hotter than 37°C, skin will take away heat by sweating. We colloquially use the term 'cool' to imply someone who performs well under pressure, indicated by the way they don't sweat. This is factually correct – those who are 'cool' actually do have cooler skin so their need to sweat doesn't kick in as soon as those who have warmer skin.

Naturally plants have adapted to these different climatic conditions too, though, as they are not mobile like humans and animals, the adaptations are not universal; plants have evolved very specifically to suit their local environment. This gives us a vast wealth of different plants to select from in seeking nourishment for our skins and bodies. It is logical that those plants living and adapted to the same climatic conditions as ourselves should be our first and best resources as these will have greater a affinity to us through experiencing the same environment. For this reason, I always look to plants that have grown in temperate regions when creating products for my skin.

Skin is sensitive

Our skin contains touch receptors, constantly relaying information to the brain about our surroundings. It is through our skin that we get the most vivid experiences of pleasure and pain. Touch is an enormously reactive sense; we are very quick to respond to what we touch, whether that's the soft pile of rich velvet, the dry sliminess of a reptile or the ferocious heat of a hot pan. We can retain the memory of touch through a lifetime, able to imagine what places and things in our past felt like. Touch is also, of course, the key bonding mechanism between mother and child, it is an innate need. Many babies and children take comfort from having a precious item to hold or touch. This need for touch is so vital to us it has a name, skin hunger; we need the intimacy of touch to feel in connection with others.

Skin is super sensitive

Sometimes our skin responds with an almost sixth sense – we get goose bumps or shivers as we detect something in our environment, or an undertone to a story that puts us on high alert. As the point of intervention between us and the outer world, our skin provides an early-warning detection system that connects to our unconscious in ways we do not really understand, but we can feel it. It's a trigger for our conscious brain to kick in and choose how to respond – fight or flight.

Skin communicates

Our skin can act like a public-service broadcast system telling us, and the world, about our state of health – whether we like it or not. Stress or anxiety can lead to flare-ups in our skin that are difficult to hide from others, especially when on the face or hands. You may find people asking with concern 'how are you?', or suggesting you need a break or a holiday, or look 'worn out'. Conversely, we may return from a relaxing holiday and find people commenting on how radiant we look as our skin reflects an inner calm. With thoughtful skincare, radiant and relaxed can become your every day appearance.

Blushing is a form of communication too. It occurs when the blood vessels closest to the surface of the skin widen, allowing more blood to come to the surface. It is completely involuntary, triggered by the sympathetic nervous system. As something that you can't control it is a very honest response and tends to engender trust. Blushing indicates feeling and concern for others, it suggests humility and modesty. Blushing is responded to by others as a friendly gesture, a good form of conciliatory communication.

The scent of your skin is another critical form of communication, often operating subconsciously. We rarely notice the pheromones our skin emits within a milky substance from our apocrine glands under our arms, around our nipples and in our groin. For others this scent characterises you; it is your unique identifier. This can be a key component to attraction, which is why synthetic versions of the pheromones are put into perfumes.

Unfortunately, perfumed products can mask our natural scent thereby potentially reducing our attractiveness. It is better to work with our natural scent. Keeping clean ensures there are no bacteria to turn the scent sour so you should be emitting good, nice aromas. If you want to enhance these, work with the more subtle, plant-based scents from natural products that are in sync with your body.

Skin warns

Listening to our skin and looking out for how it reacts to things can provide vital early-warning to situations that are potentially harmful to our bodies. For example, it is often through a reaction on our skin that we can tell if we've eaten something that we're allergic to, used a product that doesn't suit us, encountered allergens in the atmosphere, or have been in the sun for too long.

When I was pregnant with my first daughter I developed a potentially fatal liver failure; where the only indication that anything was wrong was itchy skin. Noticing this was the prompt to act and, with intense medical attention and care, she was saved. Eighteen months later I sensed that itchy skin again. Curious, I did a pregnancy test, and learnt my second daughter was beginning her way into the world.

Skin is self-maintaining

Skin performs all these amazing functions while also looking after itself through a system of self-care and regeneration. Over a period of about 28 days (it varies with age) our skin is able to create enough new cells to totally replenish itself. These cells are produced internally and are gradually pushed to the surface in an unending cycle of renewal. Through this process skin can gradually heal and transform wounds, scars and burns. By working with our skin and its natural processes of regeneration we can enable a continually fresh and lively appearance that is a true reflection of ourselves.

Skin is amazing. It performs all these functions with us hardly noticing. So when we do feel troubled by our skin, we can think of it as communicating with us, alerting us to something we need to address and put right, either physically or emotionally. Skin is aware and it is our constant friend. We should take the time to really get to know our skin, to listen to it and look after it.

> Skin is a complex living organ that is intricately connected to other bodily systems.

I appreciate simplicity, true beauty that lasts over time, and a little wit and eclecticism that make life more fun

ELLIOTT ERWITT, FRENCH PHOTOGRAPHER, 1928–

CHAPTER 2

why it is vital to look after your skin

It is vital to look after your skin. You can do this simply by knowing the vital things your skin needs. It's an approach that blends head and heart. Use your head to understand how skin works, and to know your own skin; use your heart to guide what you prioritise in looking after yourself and the world. Then you'll focus on the vital things.

Understand your skin and you can make informed changes, which may well involve very little intervention from you. However, it will be the right support for your skin, at the right time, helping it maintain a healthy balance. Starting from a position of knowledge is the strongest way to maximise your potential for success.

Use your head:

- At a general level – know how skin functions so you can work with its natural system
- At a personal level – know how your own skin functions, and listen to it

The first step is relatively easy to achieve – we've already started thinking about the wonderful things skin does; how it does this is covered in the next chapter, so read on and within 10 minutes you will have the basis of your generic understanding.

Step two is not a 'done it, tick it off the list' kind of action. Make it a habit to think about your skin and listen to what it is telling you.

These are the basics for your unique, self-managed skincare. It has to be unique because it's your skin. Facts about how skin works are common to us all but your own skin condition is unique because it has so many different factors impacting upon it, all of which vary throughout your day, across the weeks and seasons and through your lifetime. Your skin is affected by:

- What you eat and drink
- How much sleep, rest and exercise you get
- How relaxed or anxious you are
- The environment you spend your time in: your home, your workplace, time spent in the city, countryside or coast
- The weather, and how exposed to or protected from it you find yourself
- Your choice of clothing and fabrics
- Your choice of cleaning and skincare products
- Your exposure to other products, such as washing-up products, household cleaners, paints, polishes etc.
- The activities you choose: do you garden? Does your sport impact on your skin? Are you very 'hands-on'?
- The time and attention you give to your skin and self-care

Clearly, your combination will be unique, and therefore your skin's needs are unique. Only you can tell what's best for you but changes in any of the above factors can all have an impact.

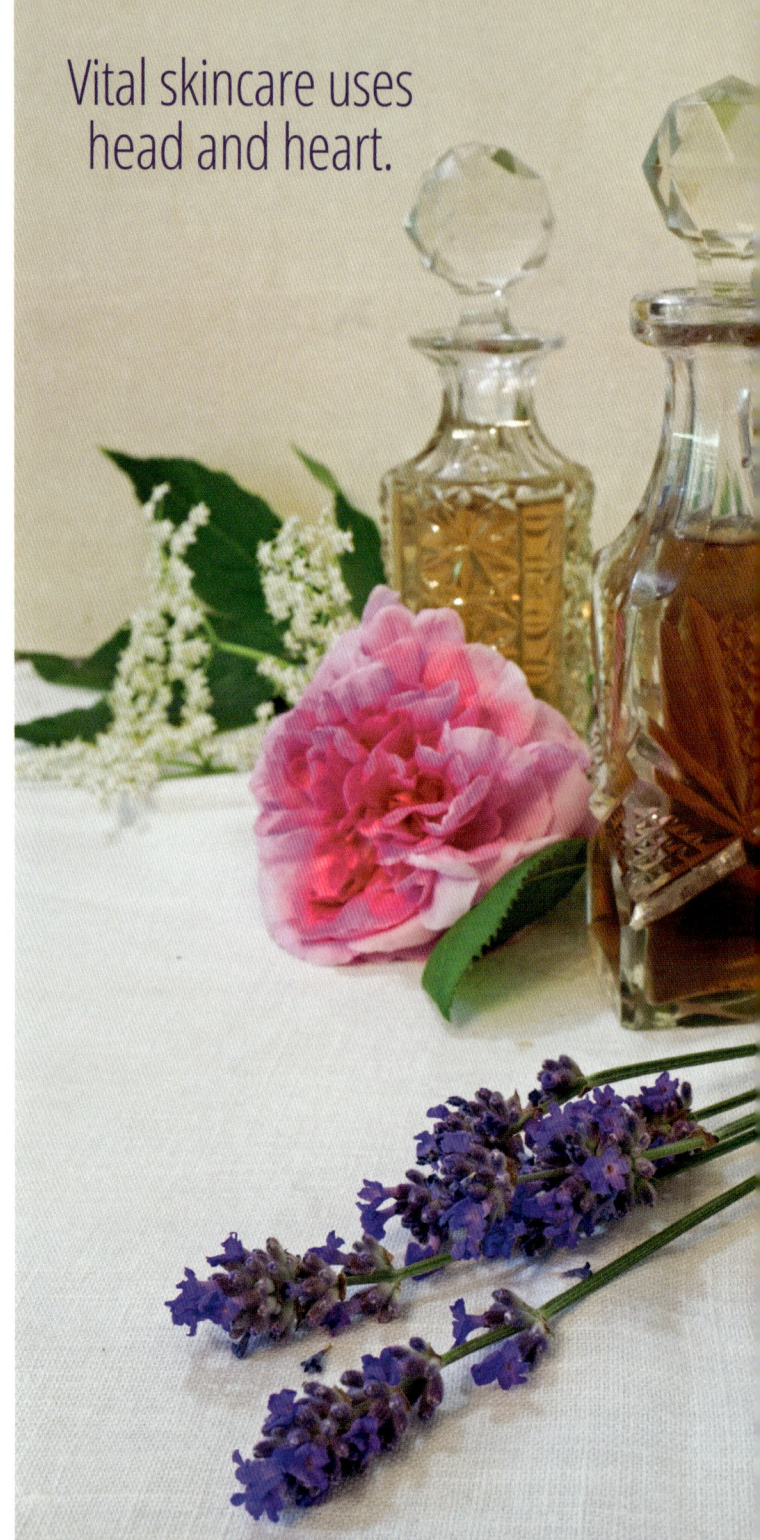

Vital skincare uses head and heart.

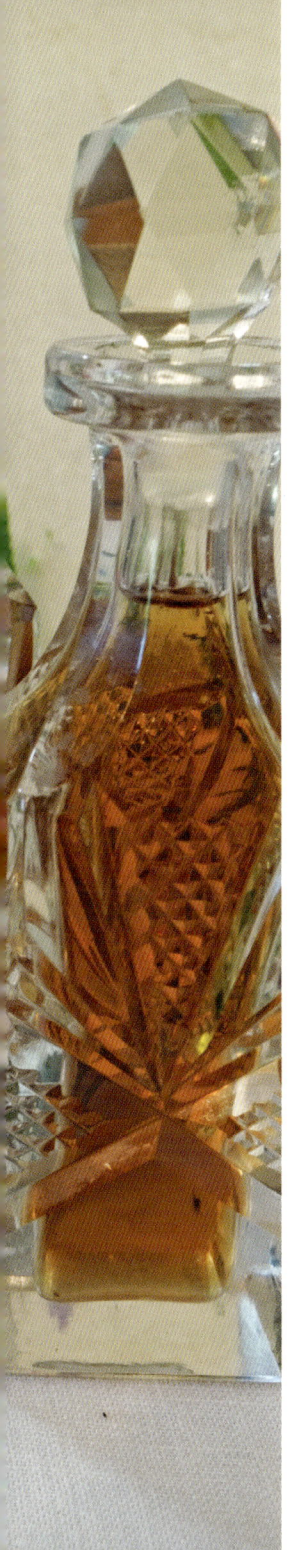

One of skin's fantastic properties is the ability it has to nourish: to absorb in elements from the atmosphere and from what we slather on our bodies. What you put on your skin – whether intentionally through skincare, beauty and cleansing products; or unintentionally through the environment you live and work in, and the things you touch – can end up in your bloodstream. There is a debate as to whether this is less impactful than the food we eat – because it is not all absorbed, or more impactful – because it is absorbed directly without enzymes to break it down. But we can be certain that it is having some impact, or we wouldn't react to skincare products at all.

A lot of things can impact us daily through our skin: the environmental pollutants from industry and transport; the chemicals leached from synthetic materials used in construction of almost everything; the solvents, cleaning products, paints and odorising compounds that filter through our airstreams on a continuous basis; the chemical fertilisers that reach us through the air and through non-organic food. Let's not panic, but there is an awful lot out there we could be worried about. The best thing we can do with our worries is put them into boxes:

- There's a box for: things I cannot influence
- A box for: things I can influence but do not have control over
- And a box for: things I can control

Be aware of what's in the first box, but do not spend your time and energy agonising over it (unless you can shift it to the second box).

Find friends who have a similar-looking second box to you and work with them to magnify your influence.

But put most of your energy and focus on the third box, the box you can control. The box potentially only you can control, the one that really needs you.

Manage this box well, and it will build you as a person, it will change how others regard you, and it will give you the strength to tackle some of the stuff in the other boxes.

So when you look at your own third box – what's in it? What can you control with regard to the potentially hazardous elements that you encounter and absorb on a daily basis?

This is where we come to the critical interface between you and the outside world: your skin. This is your first line of defence against environmental pollutants. And yet we typically bombard it with potentially hazardous products on a daily basis. Our deodorants may contain ammonium sulphide (ever noticed rashes or swollen or cracked skin?), our lipsticks may be photosensitive or have indelible dyes (familiar with cracked, dry and peeling lips?), our aftershaves and toners are primarily alcohol (which irritates and dries out skin). Skin products, hair products, baby products even, have the potential to secretly harbour carcinogens, neurotoxins and reproductive toxins – so they could mess with our health, our brains and/or our reproductive capabilities. It's worth being aware of what you're letting yourself in for.

A typical woman uses around 12 different products on her skin every day. For a man this may be less but still the average is around six. Every one of these products will have a list of ingredients, maybe a dozen, many of which you may not be able to pronounce, not all of which we know about the effects of. In many cases, the majority of these ingredients are there for the purposes of keeping the product stable, so it will look and feel just the same on the day it is made, the day you pick it from the shelf in the shop (however many months later), and the day you find it in your bathroom cupboard (even if that is a few years later).

Why would you want your skin and body to absorb ingredients that are largely focused on maintaining a product's stability? This is especially worrying when they tend to be the very ingredients that our skin reacts to; do you think our skin is trying to tell us something?

It is completely understandable that these ingredients are in the products. The alternative would be opening the pot one day and finding mould spores through your cream, which is certainly not something you'd want to use. So the preservatives and stabilisers have a purpose. But we still have several choices.

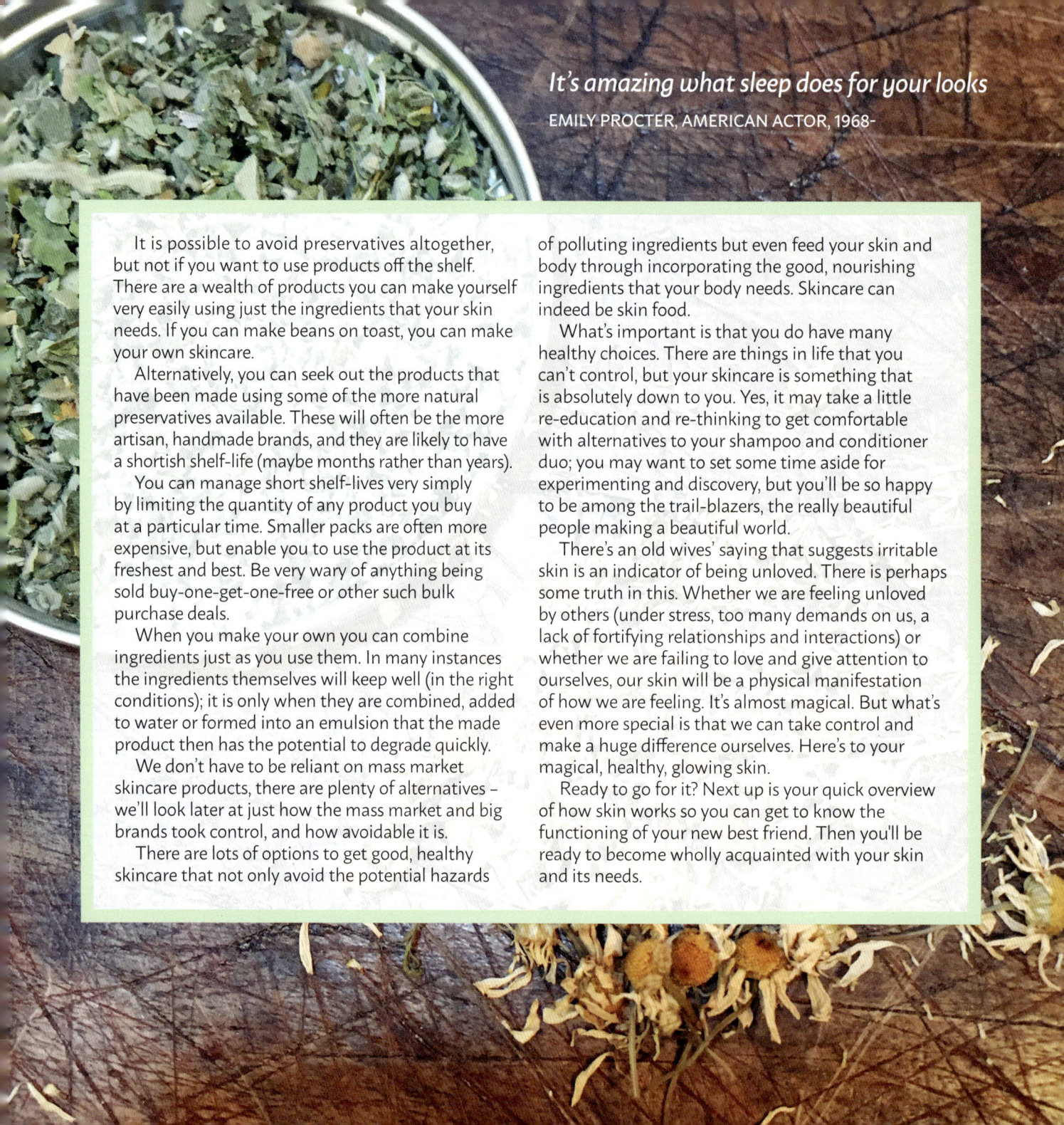

It's amazing what sleep does for your looks
EMILY PROCTER, AMERICAN ACTOR, 1968-

It is possible to avoid preservatives altogether, but not if you want to use products off the shelf. There are a wealth of products you can make yourself very easily using just the ingredients that your skin needs. If you can make beans on toast, you can make your own skincare.

Alternatively, you can seek out the products that have been made using some of the more natural preservatives available. These will often be the more artisan, handmade brands, and they are likely to have a shortish shelf-life (maybe months rather than years).

You can manage short shelf-lives very simply by limiting the quantity of any product you buy at a particular time. Smaller packs are often more expensive, but enable you to use the product at its freshest and best. Be very wary of anything being sold buy-one-get-one-free or other such bulk purchase deals.

When you make your own you can combine ingredients just as you use them. In many instances the ingredients themselves will keep well (in the right conditions); it is only when they are combined, added to water or formed into an emulsion that the made product then has the potential to degrade quickly.

We don't have to be reliant on mass market skincare products, there are plenty of alternatives – we'll look later at just how the mass market and big brands took control, and how avoidable it is.

There are lots of options to get good, healthy skincare that not only avoid the potential hazards of polluting ingredients but even feed your skin and body through incorporating the good, nourishing ingredients that your body needs. Skincare can indeed be skin food.

What's important is that you do have many healthy choices. There are things in life that you can't control, but your skincare is something that is absolutely down to you. Yes, it may take a little re-education and re-thinking to get comfortable with alternatives to your shampoo and conditioner duo; you may want to set some time aside for experimenting and discovery, but you'll be so happy to be among the trail-blazers, the really beautiful people making a beautiful world.

There's an old wives' saying that suggests irritable skin is an indicator of being unloved. There is perhaps some truth in this. Whether we are feeling unloved by others (under stress, too many demands on us, a lack of fortifying relationships and interactions) or whether we are failing to love and give attention to ourselves, our skin will be a physical manifestation of how we are feeling. It's almost magical. But what's even more special is that we can take control and make a huge difference ourselves. Here's to your magical, healthy, glowing skin.

Ready to go for it? Next up is your quick overview of how skin works so you can get to know the functioning of your new best friend. Then you'll be ready to become wholly acquainted with your skin and its needs.

CHAPTER 3

how skin works

Understanding how skin works is step one to having great skin. You want to be able to help skin do its fantastic job, so you need to know how it is structured and the processes that help it function.

The acid mantle

Our skin is sealed with a natural hydrolipidic (that's oil and water) coating, known as the acid mantle.

The oil and water are naturally produced by our skin (more on this below) but the production can vary over time, so we can support skin by providing oils and water if required. Many people are fearful to add oil to their skin, dreading the oily skin associated with spots and an unattractive sheen. This is a misplaced fear, perhaps derived from the commonplace use of synthetic oils that do not absorb into the skin. The trick is to use natural plant oils, as many of the natural, innovative and effective products on the market do today. Plant oils work in a similar way to our own oils so can support our natural systems. There are many, many other benefits of plant oils that we'll come to in later chapters. Our own natural production of oils changes with age, environment and health, so our need to support and supplement with plant oils will change over time. As we're looking for plant oils to work in sympathy with our own oils, it makes sense to use those which have grown in similar environments to us. That's why I favour seeking oils from plants that grow in a temperate climate.

The 'acid' part of the acid mantle refers to the pH value of skin. This is one of the most important things to know about in order to care properly for skin. pH (hydrogen potential) is measured on a scale from 0-14, from acid to alkali. A neutral pH is 7, anything above this is alkaline (the higher the number, the more alkaline); anything below 7 is acid (the lower the number the more acid). Skin has a slightly acidic pH of around 5.5 (it will vary a little from person to person). This acidity is critical to favour 'friendly' bacteria that will help protect our skin from invasion by other pathogenic microorganisms.

5.5

Whatever we do to our skin, we must aim to maintain this pH if we want skin to provide protection.

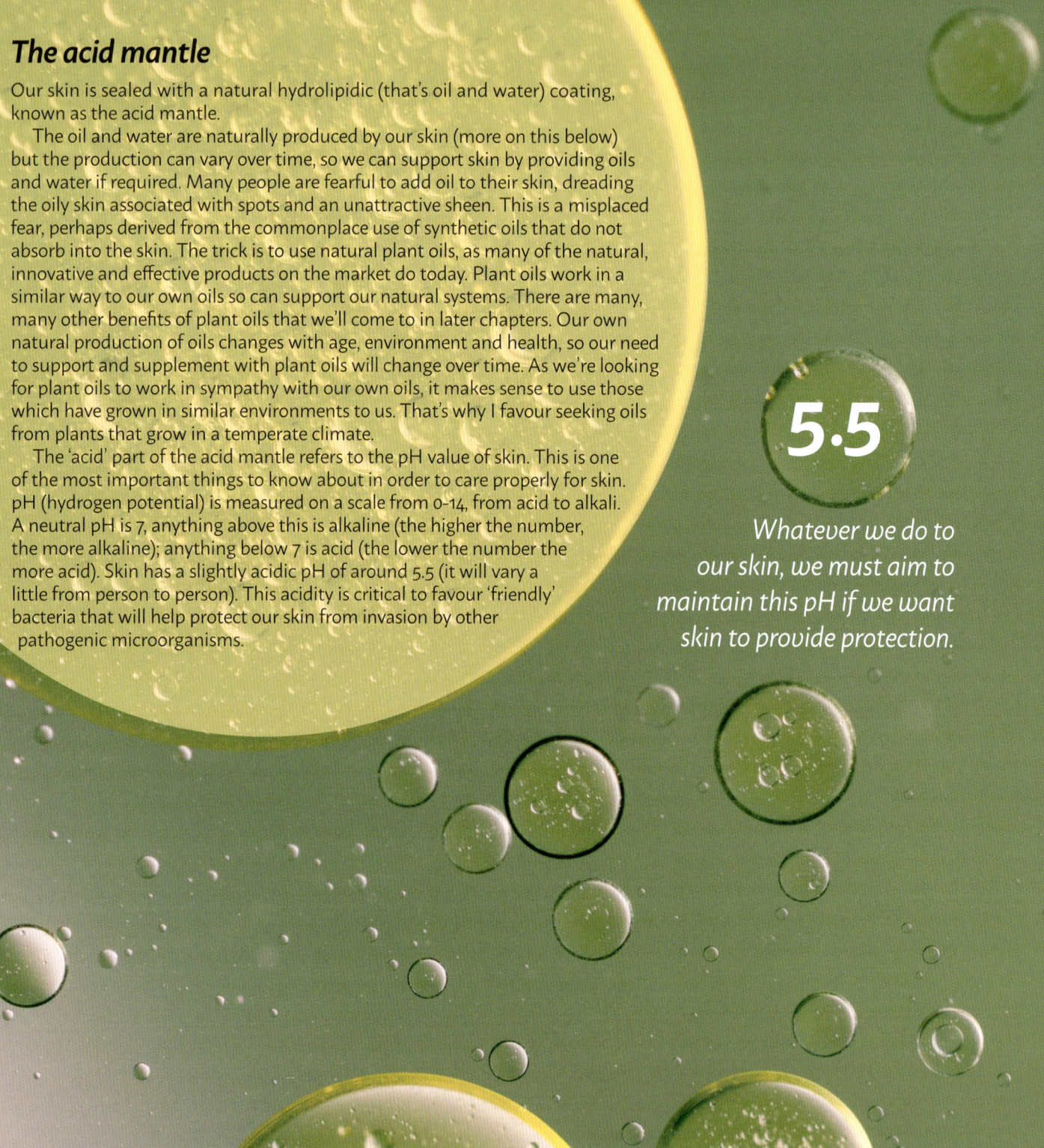

Skin's layers

Skin has two distinct layers, plus a third base layer. The effects we notice on the surface of our skin will likely have their cause deeper down.

The two main layers are the dermis and above this, the epidermis.

The epidermis

The outer part of our skin, the layer we can see, is called the epidermis. This word comes from Greek and adds 'Epi' meaning 'on, upon, above' before 'dermis'. Thus the epidermis is the layer that lies above the dermis, it is our protective covering.

The epidermis itself has four layers of cells, each performing a different function.

Right on top, the outer layer is a very thin layer of cells. This is called the *stratum corneum*, which is Latin for 'horny layer'. It's not actually horny but the cells are very tough. By the time cells are in this layer they have travelled up through the skin and lost most of their moisture. They are therefore flat and scale-like and are held together with the waxy substance, sebum, to form our waterproof and germ-resistant covering. At this stage the cells are called 'squamous cells'. The thickness of this layer varies on different parts of our body. The soles of our feet may have a thick layer, and feel quite hard; our eyelids have perhaps the thinnest layer and the skin there is very delicate.

Strong detergents, alkaline soaps, buffing and the wind are constant challenges for this outer layer, potentially inflicting damage on the structure of well-organised cells and impacting their protective properties. We notice the resulting rough skin or soreness. Ideally we should intervene before this time to prevent such damage by choosing more caring products, using barrier creams and lubricating oils, wearing gloves and warm or protective clothing – all the things our mothers said we should do while we happily laughed and shrugged off their fussiness!

Thankfully these effects are not permanent. We are continuously losing cells from the *stratum corneum*, they are dead and simply flake off. A component of household dust is our dead skin cells. Some people say about 70% of dust is skin – it's not that high, as there are lots of other things in dust. Looking after your skin and helping it shed and renew in the shower or bath can mean you reduce dust around the house, but the real bonus of course is beautiful smooth skin.

If we're constantly losing skin cells, we need to be replacing them. This is the wonderful self-renewing property of skin. At the base of the epidermis is a layer called the *stratum basale*. Here we find stem cells that are constantly dividing to make new ones; it's a skin cell factory. These plump, round new cells are called 'basal cells'. The new cells rise up through the epidermis, like bubbles in a champagne glass, and form a new outer layer. During this process the cells are forming keratin, a tough protein. This process takes about 28-35 days (the older you are, the longer it will take. For teenagers it can be just two to three weeks) which means our outer skin is completely refreshed each month or so. Therefore, whatever action you take, you can expect to see a significant difference within a month. Complete skin renewal takes about seven years so you may find your skin behaving quite differently in phases of your life, partly due to it being a whole new set of cells to get to know.

We can help the epidermis in its shedding and replenishing by practicing exfoliation. This loosens the dead skin cells and removes them, exposing the fresher new cells beneath. The more evenly these cells lie, the smoother the surface will be, which enables light to bounce off and gives skin a glowing, luminous appearance.

In between the *stratum basale* and the *stratum corneum* are two additional layers. The lower of these is the *stratum spinosum* which houses spiny keratinocytes that help bond other cells together. Above this, the *stratum granulosum* has cells that produce a waxy material that aids in waterproofing the skin.

On those thickest parts of our skin mentioned earlier – the soles of our feet and palms of our hands – there is an additional layer. This is the *stratum lucidum*, a translucent layer that gives extra thickness.

The dermis

Our true skin is a thick layer of living tissue below the epidermis. This contains connective tissue, blood and lymph vessels, nerve endings, sweat glands and hair follicles. Sometimes you may hear it referred to as the 'corium', but it's more commonly known as the 'dermis'. It is fed by very thin blood capillaries that bring oxygen and take away carbon dioxide and other waste.

The dermis acts as a cushion for the epidermis. How plump and soft our skin feels will be a result of the quality of the dermis and its combination of both collagen and elastin. These two substances are made in the dermis in special cells called fibroblasts. They work in alliance, collagen being tough and resilient, elastin being supple and stretchy. Each of us will have our own balance of these two. This will have a significant influence on what our skin feels like. Generally, the older we get, the stiffer these become; we see this on the surface of our skin as wrinkles.

Three noticeable substances are created in the dermis and emitted out of our bodies through the pores in our skin. These are sweat, sebum and scent.

❊ Sweat

This is a watery fluid and is incredibly important for regulating body temperature and carrying toxins from the body. Eccrine glands are responsible for secreting sweat. They are found all over our bodies but are particularly concentrated in the soles of our feet and the palms of our hands. Antiperspirants are designed to stop sweating (perplexingly some people even suggest you should put antiperspirant on at night so they have time to activate and therefore keep you sweat-free in the morning; some are even designed to stop sweat for 48 hours). When you understand how important sweat is to the body, it seems illogical to intervene to prevent it, as the toxins will only have to find another way out (which may mean spots and other eruptions on the skin). Sweat has got a bad press because it is associated with unpleasant body odour. The bad smells only come when the sweat is ingested by bacteria. So to control the odour, control the bacteria (through washing) and leave sweat to do its good work.

❊ Sebum

This is an oily substance that moisturises our skin. It is secreted through the sebaceous glands that are also all over our bodies but tend to be larger on the face, scalp and shoulders. It is the protective and lubricating nature of oily sebum blended with watery sweat that many manufactured moisturisers are looking to mimic, which is why they are typically based on an emulsion, the critical combination of oil and water. When our natural oil and water production is functioning well, we consider ourselves to have well-balanced skin. Skin naturally corrects its emitting of these two in response to temperature and environment (all the nerve endings in the dermis make skin highly sensitive to changes). This explains why our skin can behave erratically when we spend time in and out between hot and cold places, or when we go on holiday to a different climate. Sebum production really kicks in during puberty, and lessens from middle age onwards, so we tend to have drier skin as we get older. Very few of us have 'well behaved' sebaceous glands, as they are very sensitive to hormones.

❊ Scent

Besides the avoidable sweat-related body odour, our bodies produce their own real odours. These are secreted from the apocrine glands which tend to be in the hairy parts of our body (especially groin and armpits). These only start functioning in puberty as we start to form our own distinctive characters.

Subcutaneous fatty layer

Just as every building needs a good sub-structure, our skin has good solid foundations in the layer of fatty tissue that lies below the dermis. It's from this tissue that we get our smooth, sensuous contours, as well as good insulation for our bodies.

This layer is the starting point for much of the functions of the dermis. All the nerves that manage the hair follicles, glands and receptors in the dermis have come through the fatty layer. Arteries and veins in the fatty layer are the roots of the capillaries in the dermis.

The cleansing function of skin begins in this layer as the fatty tissue is bathed in clear lymph fluid that gathers up debris and waste such as old cells, toxins and bacteria. When this is functioning well, we look clear and refreshed; when it slows down we can start to look puffy and in need of rest. It's then that we should take notice and work on our lymph system to get things moving again.

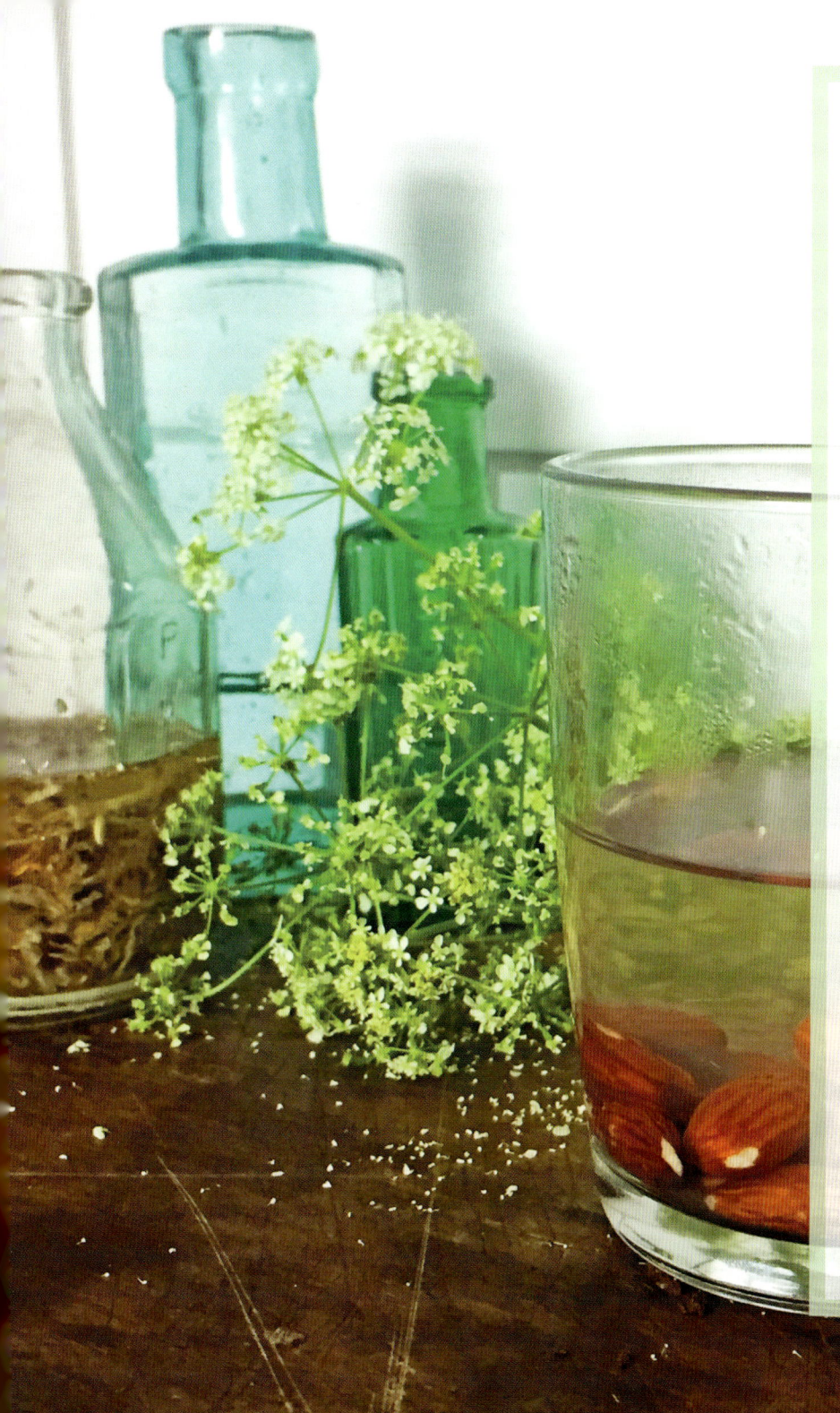

The lymph system

Our lymph system is similar to our blood system in that it is a means for fluid to travel around our bodies gathering waste and distributing materials to where they are needed. It's remarkably efficient design when you think about it, like the everlasting lazy river.

To function these systems depend upon continual flow, a constant momentum. The blood system has the heart to regulate and maintain this flow, constantly pumping to keep blood on the move. The lymph system has no such pump or engine, it's reliant on muscle contractions and good breathing to keep going. It's therefore much easier for the lymph system to get sluggish or clogged. This is where we need to intervene and help, as a well-functioning lymph system is critical for vibrant, healthy skin.

A poorly functioning lymph leads to a build up of toxins below the skin's surface, which we see as redness, puffiness, irritableness or spots. Long-term it can create cellulite, the lumpy bumpy skin texture that's so difficult to correct. Act now to work with your lymph system and keep it flowing. Prevention is better than cure.

There are lots of ways to get our lymph system going, one of the simplest is body brushing which is why this is raved about by those wanting lovely looking skin. There are good approaches to diet to help lymph too, and a focused spring clean is especially recommended. Handily, nature provides lots of fresh herbs at that time of the year that you can use in teas to detox and cleanse and bring your body out of its winter cocoon.

Essential fatty acids

The membrane of each skin cell contains essential fatty acids (EFAs) and cholesterol. Maintaining levels of these two substances is essential to healthy skin and bodies.

While we can manufacture our own cholesterol, our bodies do not produce the EFAs, so we have to provide them through food and skincare. Unfortunately, we can also damage EFAs through UV exposure, toxic chemicals in cigarette smoke and environmental pollutants. However, we can also protect EFAs by introducing antioxidants, such as vitamins A, C and E.

Without EFAs, skin loses water at an alarming rate and soon becomes dry, flaky and itchy. Eczema often flares up when these nutrients are in short supply.

Omega 6 and 3 fatty acids work together to keep the skin soft, velvety and resistant to the dehydrating effects of the elements. While Omega 6 fatty acids work well when applied to the skin, such as in moisturisers, Omega 3 fatty acids work best from within, so we should look to foods with Omega 3.

There are two basic EFAs: linoleic acid (an Omega 6 fatty acid) and alpha-linoleic acid (an Omega 3 fatty acid). All others can be made from these two. Linoleic acid may be converted into gamma-linolenic acid (GLA), and is found in large quantities in evening primrose and borage oil. Alpha-linoleic acid may be converted into eicosapentaenoic acid (EPA) and docosahexaenoic acid (DHA), which is found in oily, cold water fish. Prostaglandins (hormone-like substances) are also made from EFAs. They support the immune system, enhance energy production, influence fluid balance and control inflammation.

As their name implies, essential fatty acids are vital to the functioning of our body. To maintain a good supply of EFAs:

- Introduce them to our bodies through diet and skincare (good sources are sunflower and pumpkin seeds, linseeds (flax), hemp oil, nuts (especially walnuts), soya beans, leafy vegetables and oily fish)
- Protect them through managing our environmental exposure
- Protect them through adding antioxidants to our diet and skincare

Oxygen

We can often overlook the simple effects of a good supply of oxygen to our skin. We know oxygen is vital to our body functioning: when oxygen levels in our blood drop we feel breathless, dizzy, lethargic, nauseous and faint on exertion. There's a similar effect on skin: without enough oxygen skin becomes pale and lifeless; with energising oxygen skin exudes radiance and vitality.

Our supplies of oxygen are affected by our environment (air pollution – indoor and out) and our behaviour (shallow breathing and inner tensions). For remedies, we need to change our environment (visit places with clean, fresh air; use simple, natural cleaning products, reduce artificial scents) and behaviour (exercise and meditative breathing practices). Oxygen helps our skin come alive with a healthy blush. We can also give ourselves a boost with circulation-enhancing herbs and essential oils to restore a natural glow.

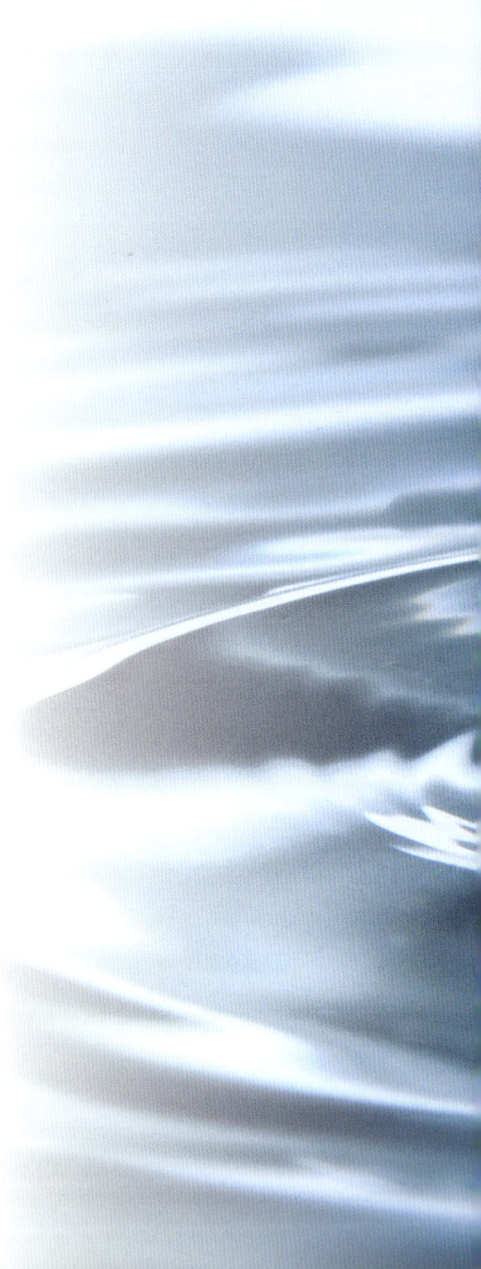

Water

Our bodies are about 70% water. Our skin helps manage that water by keeping it contained, and managing its loss. We lose water in the process of flushing toxins out of our bodies so we also need to continually replenish. Our skin cells start off plump and full of fluid at the base of the epidermis but are hard, flat and dry by the time they reach the outer surface – a result of water lost. All resources go to service vital organs first, skin last. Which means, if we skimp on water, the first place to suffer is our skin.

So now you know the basics of how your skin operates, what it needs and the functions that you can support.

We'll look later at how to provide this support and the techniques, ingredients and approaches that can get the best results for your skin.

When we do this you'll need to make some choices about what suits you best, so before we move on to the practical advice, I'd like to give you some context for your decision-making. It's so easy for us to just follow the crowd and act unquestioningly. We can gain perspective by stopping for a moment to think about how our current skincare products came about and why.

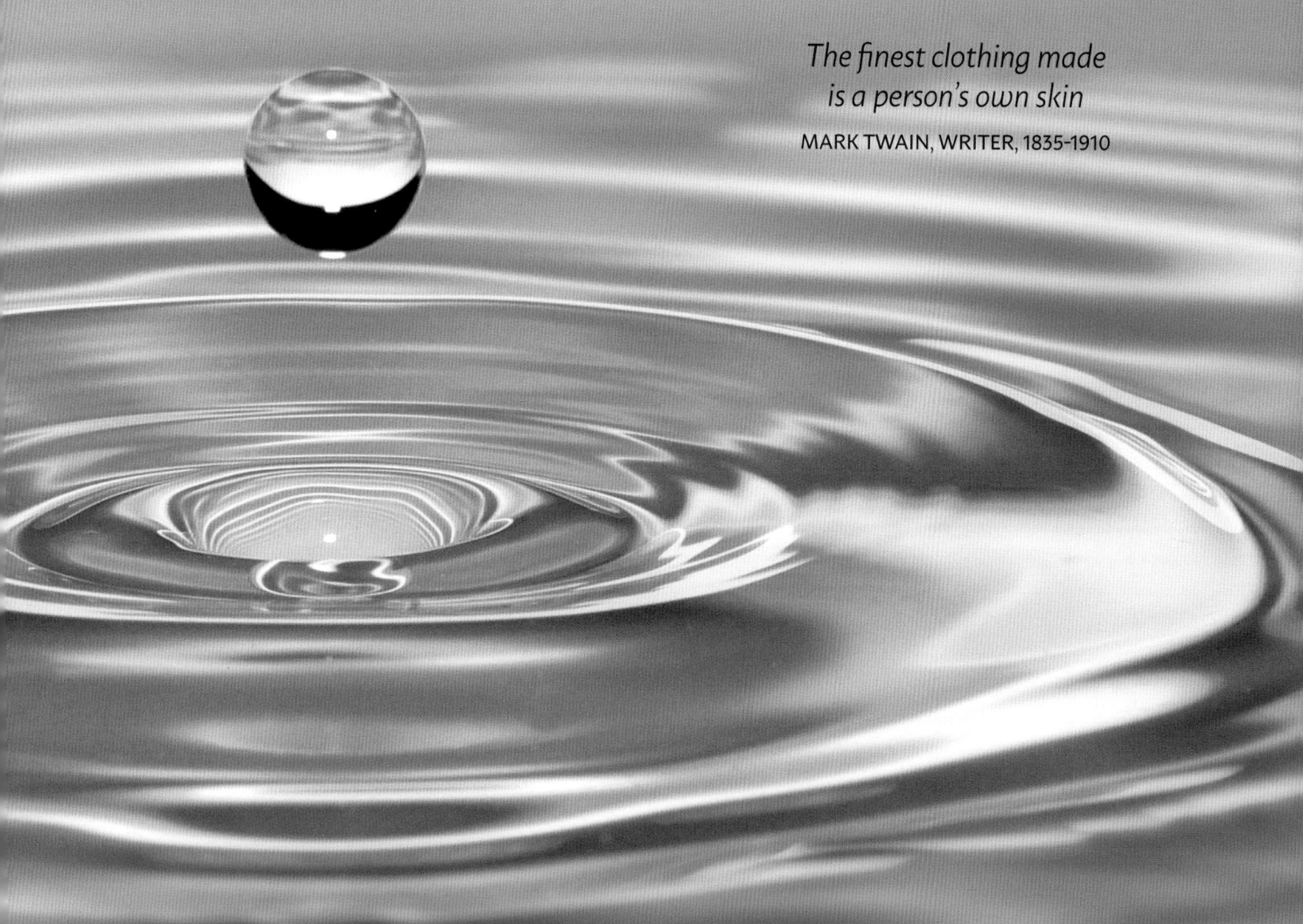

The finest clothing made is a person's own skin

MARK TWAIN, WRITER, 1835-1910

Part 2
Vital Products

CHAPTER 4

from handmade to off the shelf and back again

Just a couple of generations ago, making your own skincare was the preferred, or perhaps only option for most people. Today almost all skincare is bought off the shelf. How this shift came about deserves consideration, as does what it means for the ingredients in our skincare. Another trend across this period of time is the increase in reported skin sensitivities (one in three people now claim to have reacted to a skincare product). Can the two phenomena be related?

The dominance of off-the-shelf skincare is a massive cultural change, akin to how mobile phones swept through our psyche. Over less than two decades they went from being obscure novelties for the few, to the accepted means of communication. Most children leave primary school these days already equipped with their mobile phone. Along the way, letter writing has subsided; we rarely put pen to paper to make an enquiry or thank a friend, believing a text will do. We're losing the art of letter writing, the necessary tools are not to hand around the house, we forget the 'correct' forms to use in addressing people and signing off – the formula of letter writing. So it is with skincare. A quicker, more covetable approach has swept through society and we've switched en masse without pausing to think about what we're losing, or whether the new approach really has the quality and personal benefit of the former way. There is something grounding and fulfilling about deliberately investing time and thought into creating a good thing – like a letter, or a pot of face cream.

In the past, most people lived in small communities, villages, maybe with just 20 or 30 families together. You would be born, grow up, live and die among the same group of people: they'd know you, and you'd know them, all your life. Which meant that anything you did or said would be remembered (for better or worse) and your persona would be formed from all the incidents along the way. People often ended up with names, or nicknames, based upon their inherent characteristics. This is how we get surnames like Armstrong, Whitehead, Leader, and so on. Your reputation was built upon deeds and stayed with you forever.

Here's an extract of contemporary writing from *Cotswold Tales* by Alan Sutton:

"In country districts where every man's identity is known to all the parish, every action of every individual is commented upon by the neighbours, with a degree of eagerness amazing to, but not experienced by, those who dwell in populous towns."

Information was passed from generation to generation. Living among the same fields, hedgerows and woods they could instinctively share their gleaned knowledge about what grows where, when it's ready to harvest, how to use and how to look after it: essentially how to use the natural larder and provisions store.

I was reminded of this on a walk with a friend. We'd made a steep climb up through beech trees and emerged at the top of the hill into a meadow that rolled down into the valley below. A little stream meandered through the valley, curling

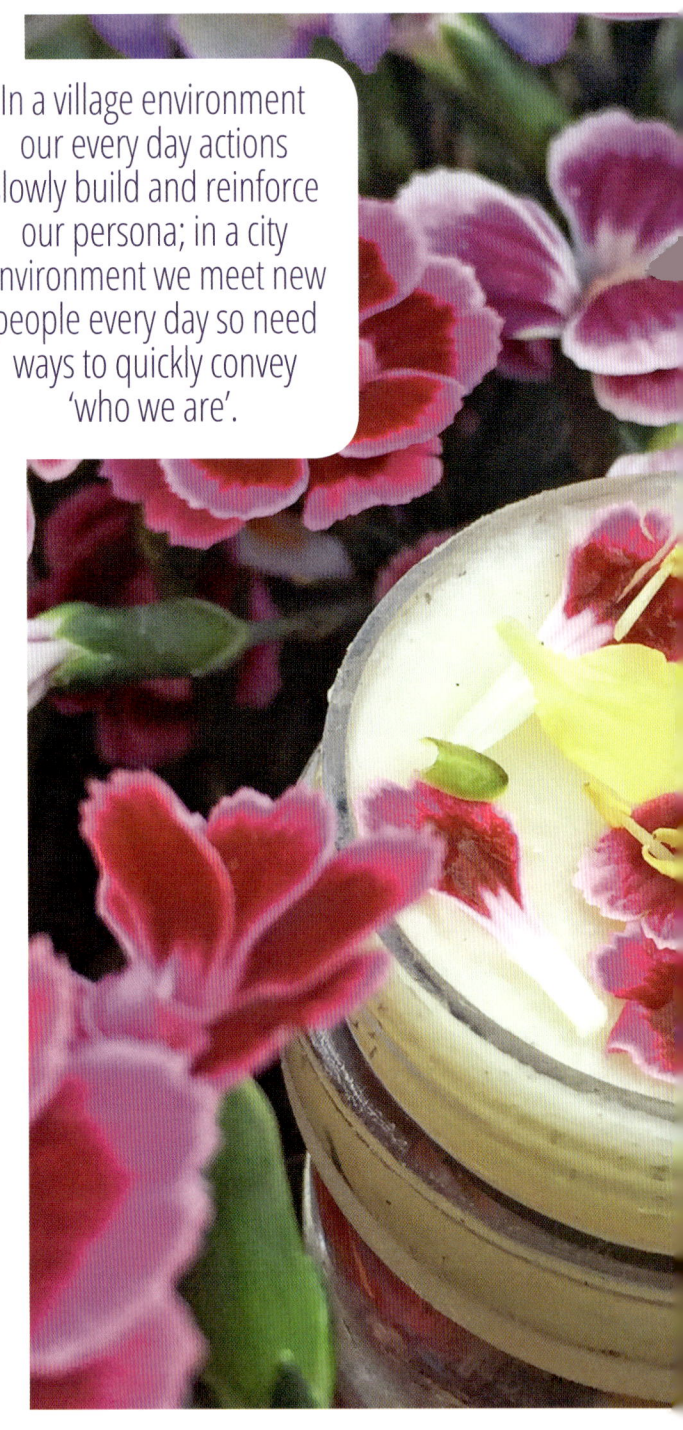

In a village environment our every day actions slowly build and reinforce our persona; in a city environment we meet new people every day so need ways to quickly convey 'who we are'.

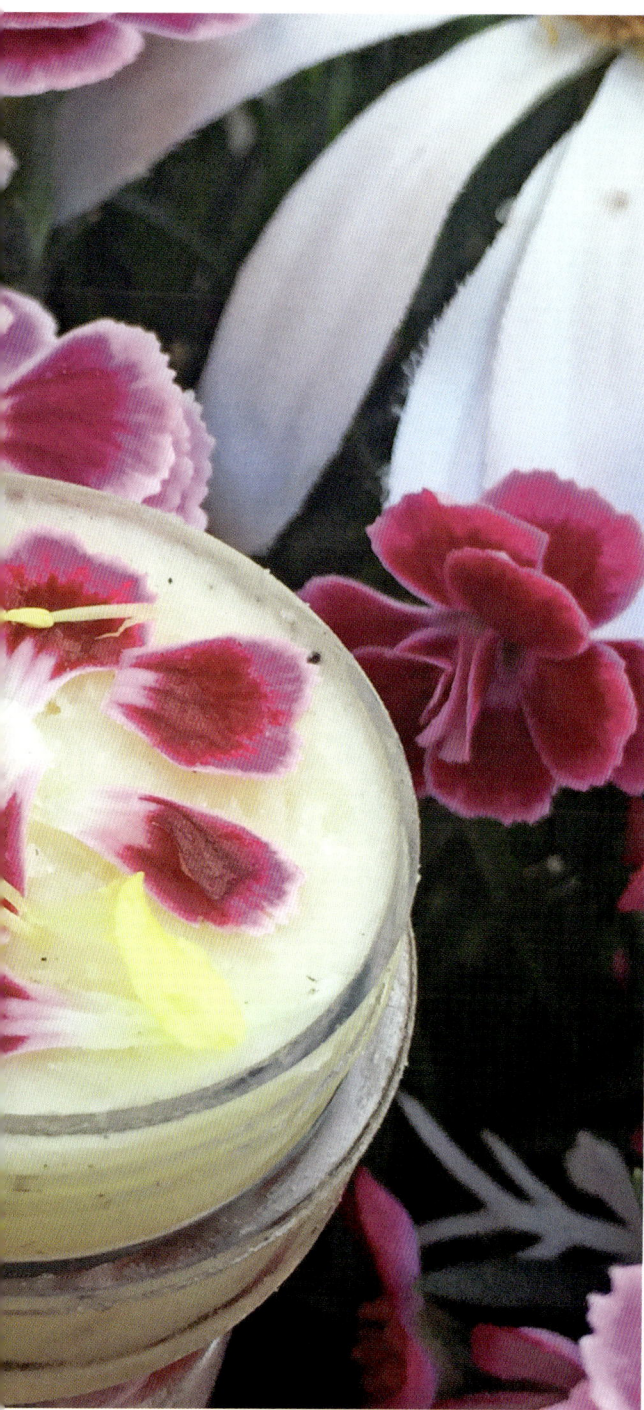

back and forth past farms and a favourite pub. My friend told me how Audrey, the lady who used to live down the road from her, knew that watercress grows wild in that stream. It's natural that it would, as it has just the right conditions, but it takes local knowledge and exploring to find it at the right time. This information is shared with caution; those relying on their precious natural resources will take care of them, ensuring their sustainability. A more short-term economic model, concerned with global supply and profit, is too demanding for the fragile seasonal ecosystem. We have abandoned ways that don't work on a mass scale; however, they're still perfectly good on a personal scale.

The changing economy created larger towns and cities. With industrialisation, people moved out of their villages, away from those they'd known all their lives, into places full of strangers. There they needed to get work and form social bonds as quickly as they could. There was no time to prove your worth over years of good humour or hard work; you were hired or fired, liked or disliked, based on what you did right now. This brought a new emphasis on appearance.

It was a fundamental shift from being judged on **what we do** to being judged on **how we look**. The importance of a 'good first impression' started to become an obsession. Publications would be full of hints and tips of how to make yourself look good, things to be aware of, although much of the advice may now seem quaint or simplistic, it started a formula of information sharing which we continue to follow through magazines, websites and social media. We're constantly looking for advice on how to look good.

How did we meet these needs, away from the grandmother, mother, aunt or sister who would typically have made creams and balms to treat and protect skin and all sorts of conditions in their country kitchens? Knowledge of how to make these things, and importantly access to the necessary ingredients, did not transfer to the cities. Stepping away from the countryside environment leaves the stories and our connections to them behind. The shared experience is lost, the knowledge is lost. Separated from our hedgerow store cupboards and family expertise, we were forced to purchase from shops, do without or find alternatives. Many of the natural, foraged ingredients just can't be bought over the counter, so gradually our needs have been met by pre-prepared solutions in jars and bottles.

It is the same story with the food we eat. Without home cooking, convenience foods began to appear in greater quantities: gravy granules, sliced bread, and packet soup were all handy substitutes for the good homemade stuff.

The space was there for entrepreneurial businesses to provide and promote solutions, some of them with more promise than foundation. Advertising began to grow as its own commercial industry using billboards, adverts in magazines and newspapers and promotions on packaging – techniques very familiar to us now. As a fledgling industry, there was little regulation then. A business could make spectacular claims about the benefits of its product, often with hand drawn imagery designed to be eye-catching and persuasive, not accurate. A willing, gullible public, full of individuals with their own private worries, fears and neurosis would lap this up. Maybe they were sceptical, but they wanted to believe. They wanted the miracle cures and the brilliant impacts. So, to give them every chance in a harsh and difficult new world, they convinced themselves, and bought.

Some of the classic examples of this kind of persuasive advertising have been studied by sociologists in the U.S. They highlight, for example, a 1917 advert for Woodbury Facial Soap which encourages women to 'Get A Skin You Love to Touch … and that dashing men will love to kiss'. This is cited as the first time 'sex' was used to sell a product.

Again, in 1922, Woodbury's were advertising with the line: 'all around you people are judging you silently'. They were joined by other brands, such as Williams Shaving Cream company telling its audience: 'critical eyes are sizing you up right now' and 'let your face reflect confidence, not worry! It's the 'look' of you by which you are judged most often'.

The cult of personality and our obsession with movie stars and glamour dates to this time too when there was the growing belief that 'people who pass us on the street can't know that we're clever and charming unless we look it'. Instead of the guidance on inner virtues that pervaded the 19th century (when positive characteristics included charity, order and chasteness) the new 20th century virtues were charisma, attractiveness and charm.

A host of products were created to help us achieve that all-important good first impression. In 1922, Palmolive was showing us on adverts, 'The girl women envy and men admire'. Ever-practical Ponds told us in 1924, 'They learned to have the prettiest skins. Girls in business are as fresh and lovely at 5 as at 9'. A year later, Lifebuoy Soap proclaimed 'Popular Men and Women. They are the ones who take care of themselves – healthy, attractive people. They are constantly moving upwards, making new friendships, holding old ones. Everybody seems to like them. And nothing is so attractive as personal cleanliness'. Pepsodent Company toothpaste traded on 'How Pretty Teeth affect the smile' and

> Societies in Europe were making a big shift from village to city living in the decades either side of 1900. By the early 20th century this was bringing about big changes in our personalities and ways of relating to each other.

in 1927 Listerine frankly said 'Dandruff is inexcusable … And now it is avoidable'. The ultimate slick product, Brylcreem, was created in 1928. By the time its first TV ads were created they had the jingle 'Brylcreem — A Little Dab'll Do Ya! Brylcreem — You'll look so debonair. Brylcreem — The gals'll all pursue ya; they'll love to run their fingers through your hair!'

And so the mass conversion took place. New people arrived in towns and cities; they needed work and friends, they needed to make a good first impression, they needed advice and support. Preying on this, businesses stepped in with advice, knowing a need is always an opportunity for profit. They employed and professionalised the art of persuasive language and techniques; their claims, messaging and imagery become more sophisticated. As a result, more people were convinced by their claims and bought their products. Product use then became the norm, and expectations grew as people sought to prove themselves and improve their lives. Encouraged by their popularity, businesses innovated new products and promoted their features, creating their distinctive niche and generating loyalty. Products soon became associated with personality.

Of course, these products needed to be readily available in an easy-to-use form, so new packaging was devised and formulas adjusted to ensure a reasonable shelf life. In some cases, products may have been bulked out to give a perception of better value, or ingredients substituted to simplify production or reduce costs.

Today the majority of people live in large communities, cities and towns, with thousands of families. Critically, this is a very fluid population, people come and go all the time: it is rare to be born and live in the same place all your life. Our characteristics are assessed in the moment, so our appearance is critical.

It's easy to see how dependent we've become on our beauty brands. They helped us establish ourselves into city living, they're a crutch to us, helping us confront a harsh world. However we have a habit of believing the great messaging, wanting the promises to be true and convincing ourselves. It's time to think a bit more about this.

We're a lot more sophisticated than we were in the early days of the 20th century. In fact, we've moved on from impressions being made simply based on the person stood in front of us at that moment. We have social media now. All of our online messaging and sharing enables us to build the village-like connections and display a lifetime of interests and activities to anyone we encounter and choose to share with. Beauty is no longer skin-deep as we have the means to reflect our lifestyle, choices and ethics in our online collection of events and images. We're not judged now on a single moment but on thousands of them.

This changes our relationship with the world and gives us space to really be ourselves. We need a sustainable, consistent approach, a way to show our character without the exhausting, confusing relentlessness of constant reinvention and presentation. We need to be comfortable in our whole selves, confident in the choices we make, content that we post and like, and share and comment on what is collectively building our persona to the world. It's a way of living in which thinking about what we do, rather than blindly following and believing, is the foundation of our character.

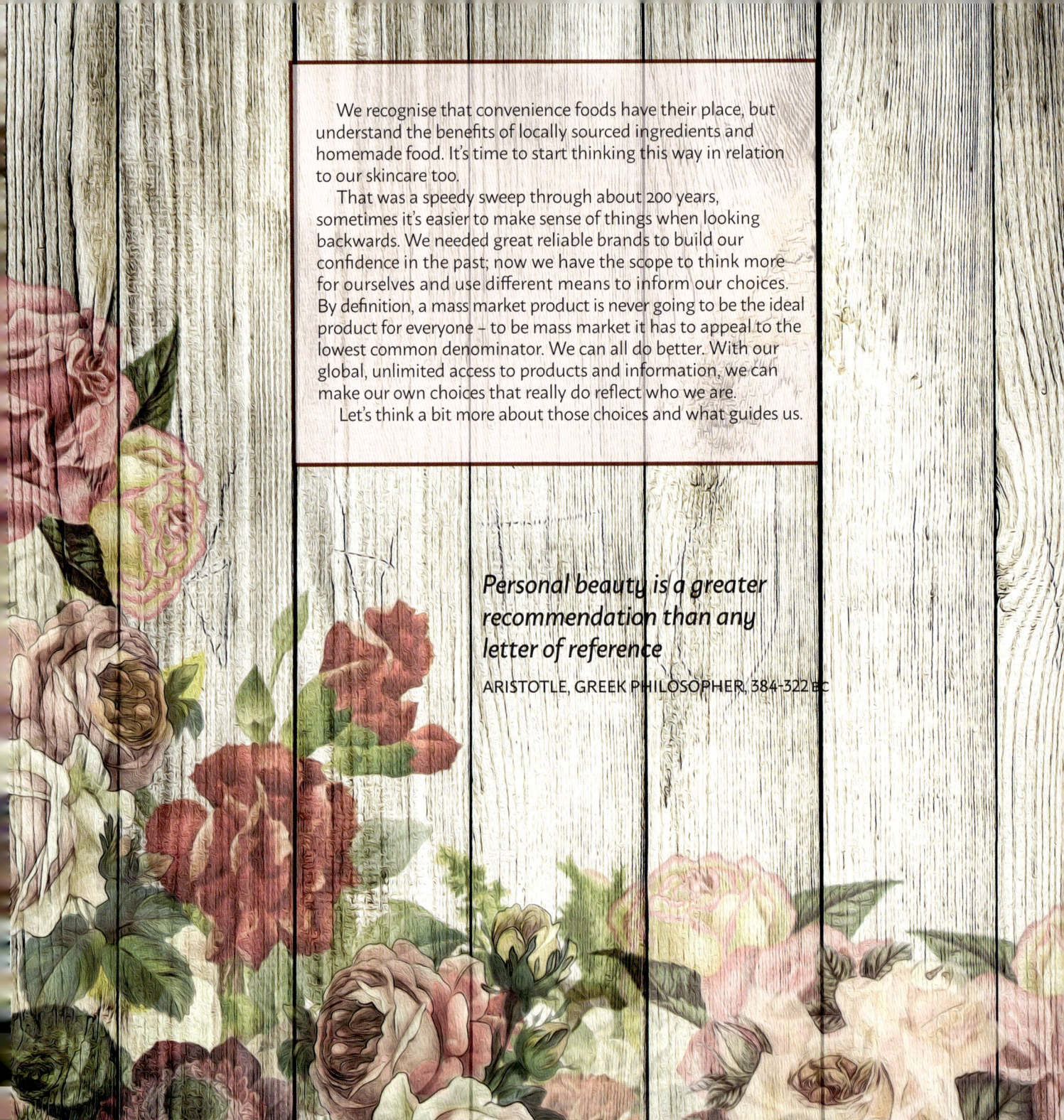

We recognise that convenience foods have their place, but understand the benefits of locally sourced ingredients and homemade food. It's time to start thinking this way in relation to our skincare too.

That was a speedy sweep through about 200 years, sometimes it's easier to make sense of things when looking backwards. We needed great reliable brands to build our confidence in the past; now we have the scope to think more for ourselves and use different means to inform our choices. By definition, a mass market product is never going to be the ideal product for everyone – to be mass market it has to appeal to the lowest common denominator. We can all do better. With our global, unlimited access to products and information, we can make our own choices that really do reflect who we are.

Let's think a bit more about those choices and what guides us.

Personal beauty is a greater recommendation than any letter of reference

ARISTOTLE, GREEK PHILOSOPHER, 384-322 BC

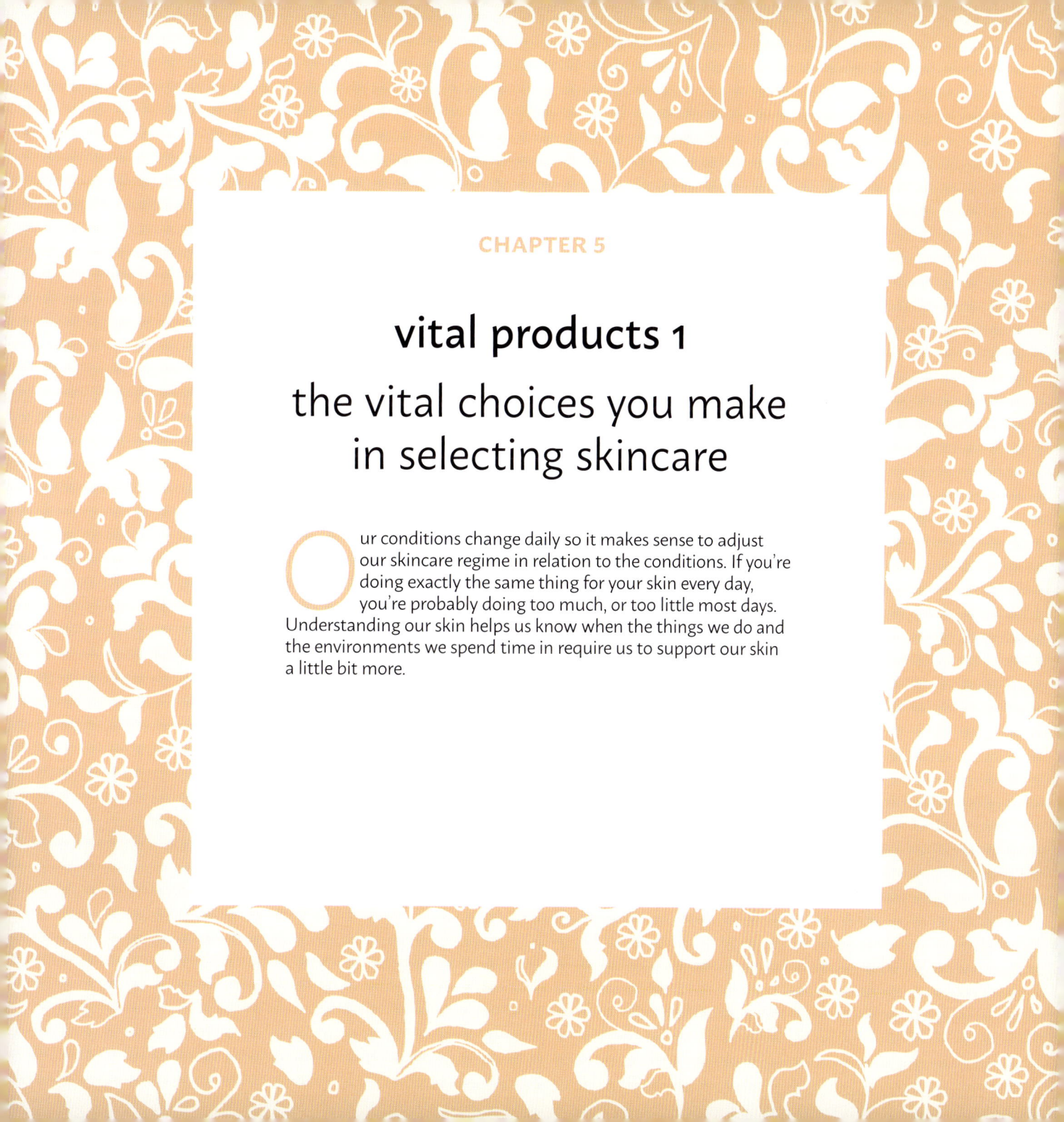

CHAPTER 5

vital products 1
the vital choices you make in selecting skincare

Our conditions change daily so it makes sense to adjust our skincare regime in relation to the conditions. If you're doing exactly the same thing for your skin every day, you're probably doing too much, or too little most days. Understanding our skin helps us know when the things we do and the environments we spend time in require us to support our skin a little bit more.

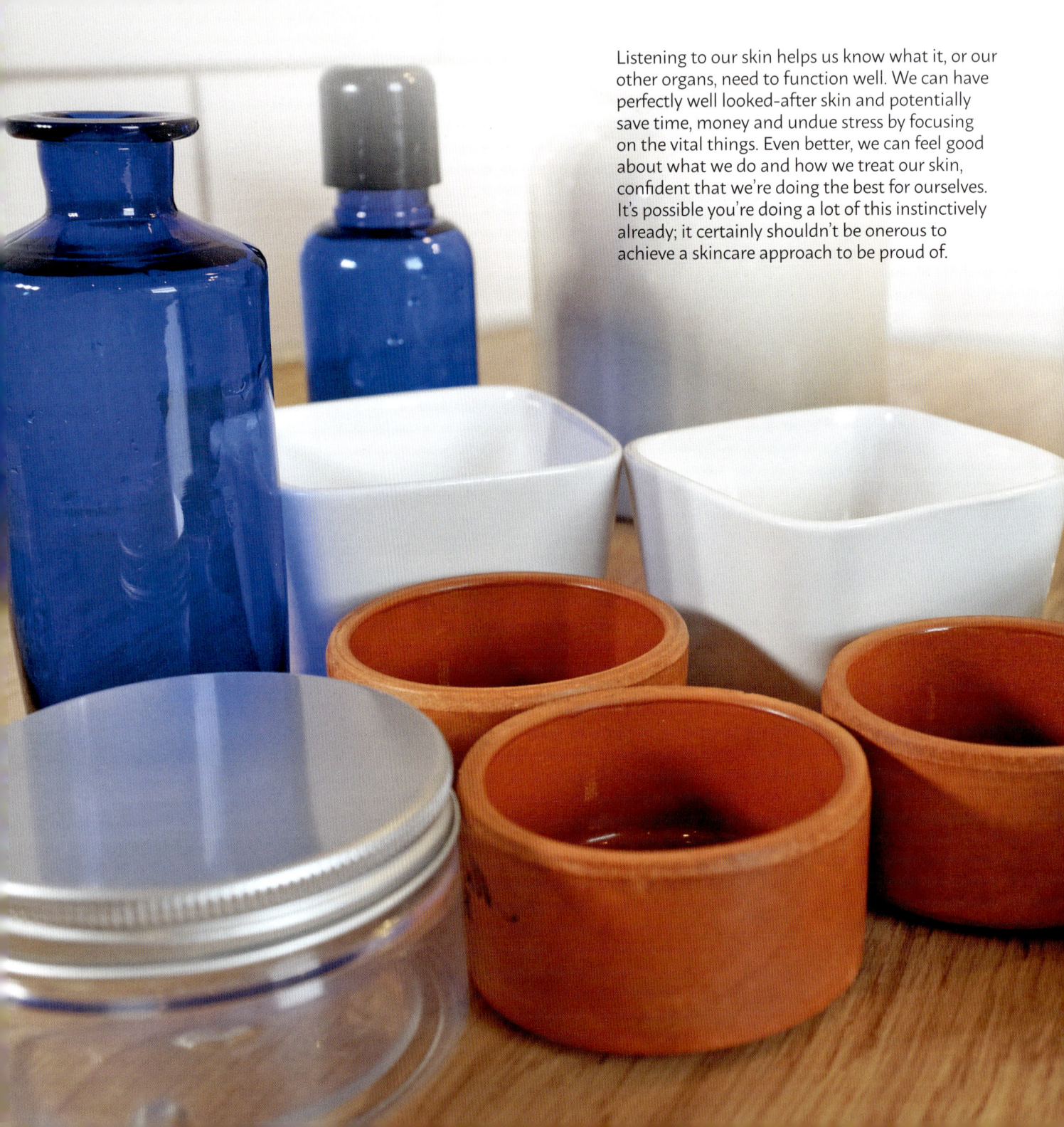

Listening to our skin helps us know what it, or our other organs, need to function well. We can have perfectly well looked-after skin and potentially save time, money and undue stress by focusing on the vital things. Even better, we can feel good about what we do and how we treat our skin, confident that we're doing the best for ourselves. It's possible you're doing a lot of this instinctively already; it certainly shouldn't be onerous to achieve a skincare approach to be proud of.

Considering how much is covered in magazines and online, skincare is a remarkably private affair. From whatever age we learn to use the lock on the bathroom door, we're on our own finding out for ourselves.

I like to ask people 'who or what has been most influential to you in creating your skincare routine?'. The surprise is that I hear as much about people they don't want to follow as I do about positive role models. At least half of those with positive role models tell me about their grandmothers, and those from a generation who were less commercially led, and more inclined to make their own.

It seems that despite magazines and the Internet bursting with beauty tips, detailed instructions and advice on what and how to do everything – from taming our eyebrows to filing our nails – these media outlets are not core influencers. These are just noise. We want to learn from people, and this includes the thought leaders in skincare like sadly missed Anita Roddick (founder of The Body Shop) and Liz Earle (founder of Liz Earle Beauty Co and Liz Earle Wellbeing), and the vloggers, but it is mostly our mothers, grandmothers and friends. We look to these people as much to learn what not to do as to learn what to do. Ultimately, if we're doing our own thing, it has to be right for us.

For many of us, developing an approach to skincare happens by default. Skincare just isn't something we talk that much about, so we're left to our own devices to figure out what to do. Our practice evolves from an accumulation of ad hoc tips, advice and product trials.

There are parallels with sex education. In my traditional schooling there was very little advice or instruction about relationships and sex; we were left to work it out for ourselves. It's amazing how much we could read between the lines of a *Jackie* magazine! Thankfully, a generation on, I find my daughters being given much more guidance and access to information. The result is confident people, able to converse and make their own choices from a position of knowledge; wary (in a good way) and more comfortable to do what suits them.

That's the change we can make in skincare. To shift the balance so our information is not all derived from adverts and promotions. To open the conversation so we can inform ourselves and understand how our bodies work and what they need. To change our slapdash approach to trying any product we come across and instead think about what we want and why. To create the confidence to make our own informed choices, connect with the things we value and take pride in (rather than fear) our own uniqueness.

Are you one of the many of people who takes your amazing skin functioning for granted, never really giving it a second thought? Or maybe you are obsessive in your skincare regime and maintenance, constantly aware of potential polluting hazards, their impact and how to avoid them. Typically our attention to skin waxes and wanes – maybe you've a special event you want to look your best for which encourages you to put more time and attention into your skin; possibly you're upset by physical manifestations of spots, soreness, dryness or itchiness and experiment with all manner of things to correct and heal; maybe you're living with scars or wounds which need your patient care and acceptance.

When I start talking skincare with people I find myself being asked questions as fundamental as 'how should I clean my face?' –We're confused even on the basics. There is too much information to be able to decipher what's best, and we forget to listen to our own skin. It's also difficult to differentiate between product claims and easy to be convinced by promise and flash-words like 'natural' and 'laboratory tested'. It's normal to think that, because it's a name we recognise, it must be good.

A friend asked me what she should do for eczema and proceeded to run through the list of prescribed and over-the-counter remedies she'd tried from steroids to creams and lotions. She said there was only one thing that had made a difference. Not surprising. Everything mentioned up until that point had been petrochemical-based or laced with ingredients known to cause reactions. The one product that had been effective and not caused more irritation was the one based on natural plant materials. She hadn't realised the difference between the products listed because they all had recognised names, so she'd thought she was using the 'right' stuff.

When seeking a remedy or a new beauty product, don't look at the name on the front, look at the ingredients on the back and make your decision based on that. It's important for your health, comfort and budget.

A peep inside the cupboard

I am so grateful to all those I've interviewed for sharing their personal routines and preferences with me, allowing me to rummage through their jars and bottles and makeup bags – surprising me on a number of occasions. It's intimate stuff. All the more so because everyone is so different. We all have our accumulated collection of things tried, things gifted, things abandoned and things relied upon. The stories of why we choose one thing or another, what we do or don't like. It's an internal, unspoken narrative that we live with subliminally everyday: each time we use a care product, take a shower, wash our hands, read an article, seek a new product. Most people did say they spoke to friends and family about skincare, but ultimately their practices were their own. Every choice a personal one.

This to me is so encouraging. It may feel like there is mass indoctrination about what you should or shouldn't do with regard to skincare, but in reality, we're doing things our own way. The choice and the freedom is ours.

Choosing your own skincare

When you look at the amount of competition in the skincare market (just pause for a moment and think about how many different brands you can name) it's clear there are so many options for us. It's wonderful to have individuality, but this wealth of options and choices can be bewildering. With so many promises to listen to and a plethora of ingredients to recognise and understand, it becomes a complex environment to navigate.

Those who are most confident in their skincare routines, most clear about what they do and don't need, what's right for them, are those who have a sound belief system guiding their choices. Often these are hard-won life stances, arrived at after much trial and consideration. Confident users appear to be wedded not to a specific brand, but to certain principles.

There are some who conclude that less is best – they want their skin to 'breathe' and will only use the minimum; some who are guided by previous difficulties, even skin cancer, and so now prioritise care and protection over look and feel; some who are environmentally led to seek natural products in sympathy with their skin, and kind to the world around them. Their confidence comes from knowing why they are making the choices they do; it's a compass enabling them to navigate the diverse skincare landscape.

We can be constantly picking up tips. So we need our own framework of understanding to file the ideas and to distinguish those that will or won't work for us.

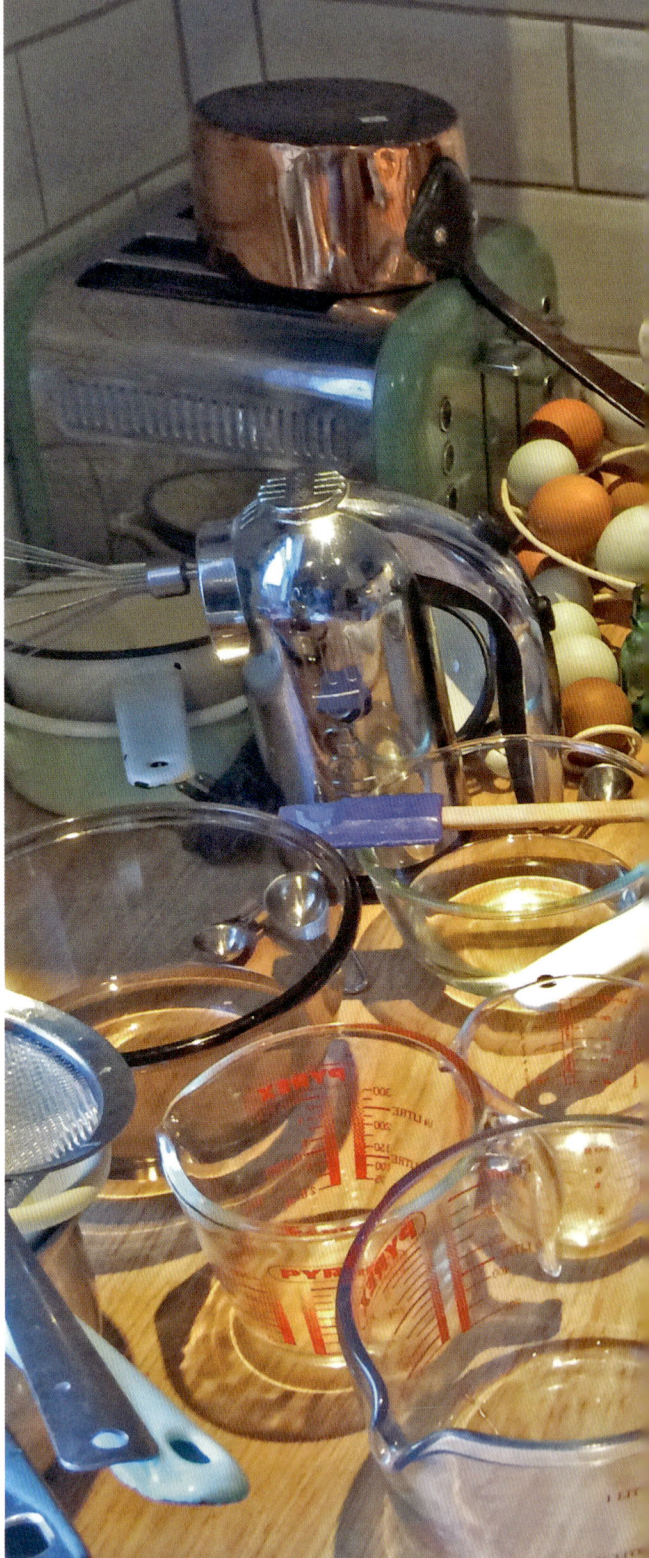

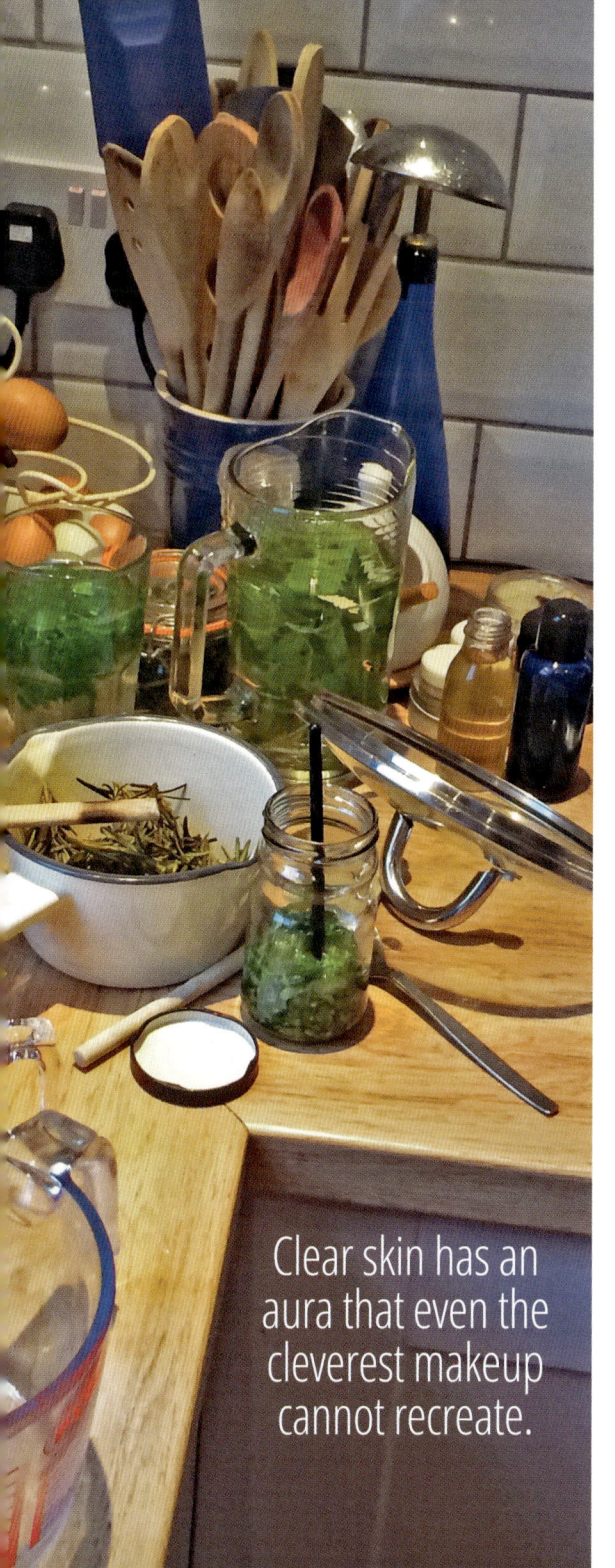

Clear skin has an aura that even the cleverest makeup cannot recreate.

Find your own way

Each one of us has unique skin, so we have to find what's good for us, look to our own needs, and not compare with others. Our skincare should reflect our individuality.

This is the reason many people have given me for not sharing skincare tips and advice or taking product recommendations from others; what suits one person doesn't necessarily suit another. We can share advice on the options available and the considerations that guide our decisions, but ultimately, we each need to make our own choices, in the full and intimate knowledge of our own skin.

We do this by listening to our skin and recognising its needs. When you have the confidence to know you're making the right choices each day for your skin it shows. You can do this by knowing the ingredients, and by understanding how to integrate skincare as a beneficial part of self-care: knowing all the needs good skincare is fulfilling for you in nurturing body, mind and spirit. There's more about this in the next chapter.

All in moderation

With more holistic thought we can be a lot more effective and efficient in our skincare. But is it possible to be fully responsive to every need and situation? How much attention should we be paying?

In the world of personal technology – a microchip to solve any problem – the trend is beginning for digital feedback systems. We're now going beyond fitness tracking of heartbeats, footsteps and sleep patterns to monitoring skin conditions. Clearly it's true that your skin is changing and responding to the environment all the time, so to manage it at an optimum level, you need to be aware of those changes constantly. Some gadgets will even refer to weather predictions to provide you with recommendations about the right products to use for your day's skincare needs.

Do we really need digital interceptors (beyond our own digits, of course) to tell us how our skin is? Do you find the weather forecast more reliable than looking out of the window? We come with our own sensors built in, our skin has specialist cells in the dermis: touch corpuscles, touch receptors, heat receptors, cold receptors, pressure corpuscles and nerve endings to sense pain. What's more, these are naturally programmed into our brain so we constantly listen and learn from them and adapt our behaviour accordingly. It's pretty much automatic, we just need to tune into it and trust it.

With the multitude of products and ingredients bursting with promises about what they can do for our skins, the most important thing is to make your choices with knowledge and understanding. Time taken to really know and understand your skin can save you years of fruitless and potentially uncomfortable, embarrassing or maybe even dangerous product trialling.

The natural beauty revolution

When you think of skincare like food – both nourishing your body and affecting your health and wellbeing – you can apply similar choices to both. We love food that is freshly prepared and made from local ingredients. This is how the best skincare is too.

You won't find that message coming from the big brands because of course they can't produce freshly prepared skincare from local ingredients and give it a shelf life around the world.

But they've recognised the change in consumer mood to wanting healthier skincare products, and ones that are better for the environment too.

Natural and organic skincare is such a massive growth area now, which is why they work to meet what consumers want. Natural ingredients are frequently referenced in promotions, along with a lot of investment into researching their benefits (much of which is confirming traditional beliefs). All these off the shelf products will still have preservatives and ingredients that are included for the benefit of the product, rather than for the benefit of your skin. Making your own, fresh at home, avoids that and gives you the choice as to whether you want ingredients to be local, organic, fresh, or all three.

The natural beauty revolution is happening anyway; the question is whether you want to be part of it. It's your choice, naturally.

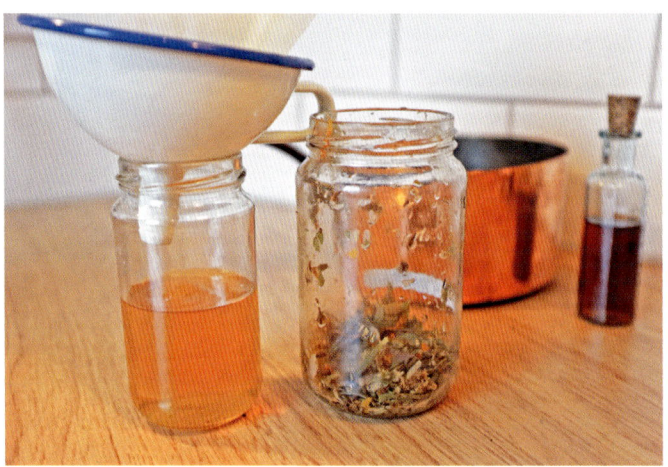

Progress is man's ability to complicate simplicity

THOR HEYERDAHL, NORWEGIAN ADVENTURER, 1914-2002

CHAPTER 6

blending your own

Maybe you've been curious about making your own skincare for a while, or perhaps you've had a go already. Or maybe the thought has never crossed your mind, because you never realised you could.

I believe it's great to have the ability to blend your own skincare and to make it part of your repertoire. If you're on the verge of trying but need more convincing, or if you want to convince others, here are some thoughts that might persuade you.

What will blending your own do for you?

Confidence, control and choice

You need to know what you're putting on your skin (and into your body). If you blend it yourself you can see, touch, smell and feel the real ingredients. You know where they came from and how much of each is in the product. You can be confident that you're using ingredients that will feed and nourish your body.

Blending your own gives you back control. You can make your own version of pretty much anything you could buy and you'll know exactly what's in it because you'll have chosen the ingredients you want to use.

Freshness

Just as we like freshly prepared food and recognise the benefits of good fresh ingredients, our skinfood has more vitality for being freshly made. When you create something yourself you can use it the moment it's made. Your product does not need a 'shelf life' to cover the time it spends travelling from factory to shop to you, it just needs to last for the time you'll be using it.

Less preservative

You have the choice of making a product with no preservative (if you're going to use it all in a few days) or with minimal preservative, just to maintain it in good condition over the few weeks or months of your use.

Simple

The bigger things get, the more complicated they become. Products get more complex as they are refined for multiple, mass markets and less precise as they seek to suit all. Products are standardised and less able to respond to personal needs. Skincare is one of those examples in life where bigger does not mean better. Small batches produced for a specific need will always be far better for you than a mass produced product.

Specific to you

You can tailor your product to be exactly how you like it, and contain more of the ingredients you love; none of the ones you react to. You can choose the scents you prefer, add the boosts your skin needs and create your product to the consistency you like to use, which you may choose to vary through the year.

Cheap

On a simple cost basis, skincare that you blend yourself is going to be cheaper than what you can buy, and much, much cheaper than what you can buy of a similar quality. There are also hidden benefit savings because you make just what you need. You also make what you know will be good for you (rather than trying something and having to abandon it when it doesn't suit) and you can minimise packaging costs.

Fun

Let's not forget the joy you can have in blending your own, the sense of creation, the thrill of finding the right ingredients and experimenting. The excitement of sharing with others and using something that you have created yourself.

Good for the environment

When you're choosing ingredients that are beneficial for your body, they're likely to be good for the environment too, or at least not harmful to it, as plastic microbeads, phytoestrogens and other chemicals have been proven to be. What's more, there will be little waste if you're just making what you need and you haven't incurred the environmental costs of transport and packaging. As an additional bonus, sourcing ingredients from your local environment naturally increases your awareness and desire to take care of it.

Full of love

When you know care and attention has gone into making something there is a greater sense of care in using it. You can sense the love encapsulated within it, essential in a self-care routine that is all about showing love for yourself. Even if you haven't always the time to blend it yourself from scratch, using products that you know have been made with love by others can have a similar effect, if you appreciate the care and attention that has been taken.

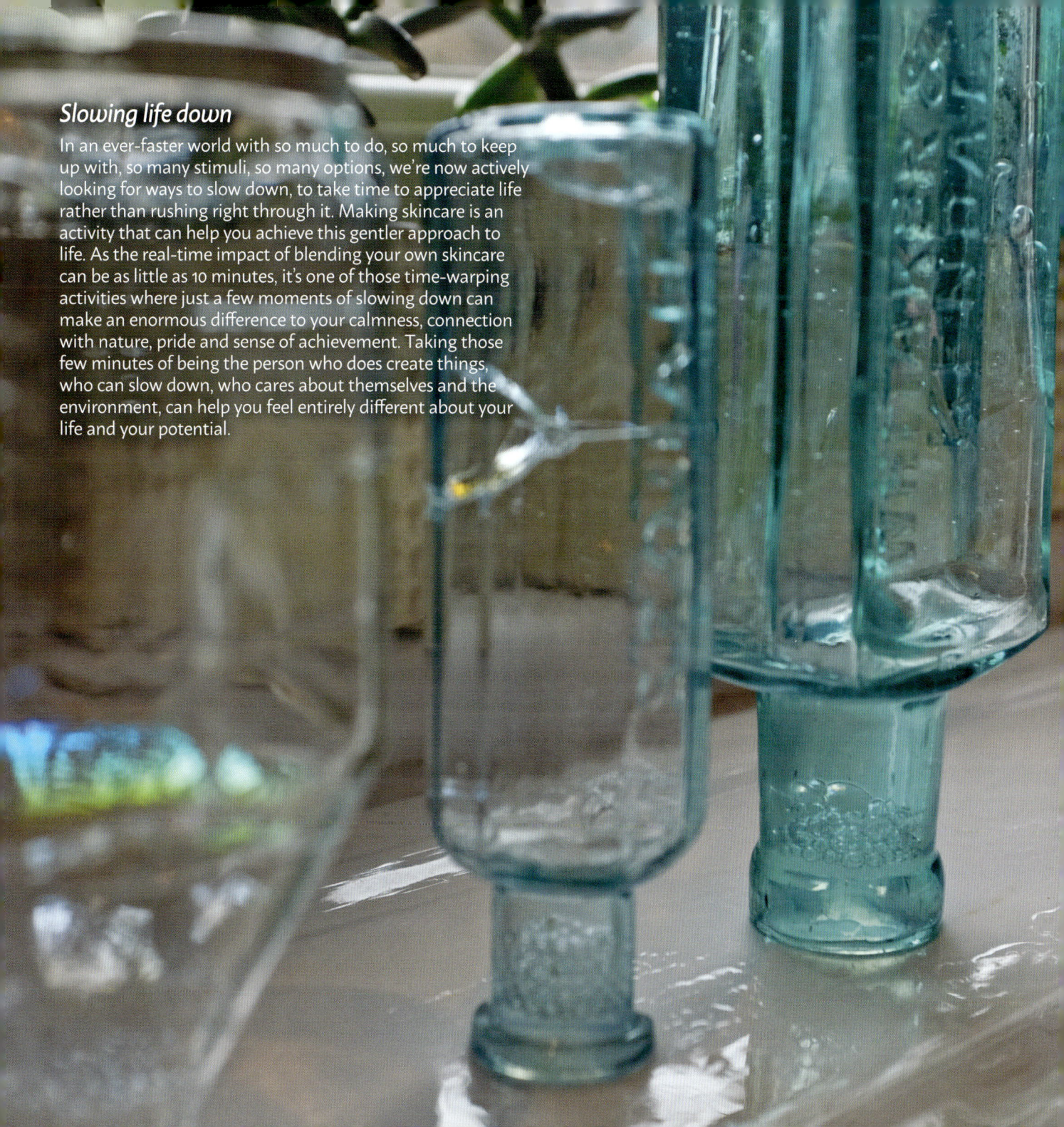

Slowing life down

In an ever-faster world with so much to do, so much to keep up with, so many stimuli, so many options, we're now actively looking for ways to slow down, to take time to appreciate life rather than rushing right through it. Making skincare is an activity that can help you achieve this gentler approach to life. As the real-time impact of blending your own skincare can be as little as 10 minutes, it's one of those time-warping activities where just a few moments of slowing down can make an enormous difference to your calmness, connection with nature, pride and sense of achievement. Taking those few minutes of being the person who does create things, who can slow down, who cares about themselves and the environment, can help you feel entirely different about your life and your potential.

Those are some of the direct benefits of blending your own skincare, however there are wider ways in which blending your own skincare can build confidence, connection and happiness.

Here are some of the most basic human needs and desires that blending your own skincare can impact upon:

✳ *Self improvement*

In the physical sense of having better skin, and a healthier body; and by way of learning new skills and useful knowledge to help yourself and others.

✳ *Identity*

The choices you make in the skincare you use every day demonstrate your values and positively reinforce them as you're reminded of your good choices in your regular routines and daily practice.

✳ *Honesty*

Have you ever sat down to enjoy delicious home-cooked food and have someone around the table ask 'what's in this?' to which the chef is able to respond with a list of ingredients and perhaps a quick resumé of how it all came together? Natural skincare made by you is just like that, it makes a virtue of every ingredient included and you can be happy to tell people what's in it and how simply you made it.

✳ *Transparency*

When you start with an empty pot and decide yourself what goes into it. When you know what each of the ingredients is doing for the product and for you and what the difference would be with or without it. That's transparency, that's knowing what you're putting on your skin.

✳ *Freedom*

You have absolute freedom when blending your own to tailor exactly to your needs including what suits you, making the quantity you need and using it as you like.

✳ *Simplicity*

You can keep the ingredients list and the techniques for combining them really simple; and the product you create free of confusing complexity, making it much easier for your body to assimilate and benefit from.

✳ *Entertainment*

Blending your own skincare is a great way to spend a morning or afternoon, by yourself or with friends. It can be calming working with natural ingredients, fun seeing it all quickly come together and of course, lovely then to use.

✳ *Excitement*

For those that 'get the bug' there can be a real 'kid in sweet shop' excitement that suddenly it is possible to make whatever you choose, as there's such a variety of different things to try and experiment with. If you've felt that sense of 'closing doors' that comes when you realise that so much of what you can buy off the shelf may be harmful to you, this is suddenly reversed when the world of healthy opportunity opens up in the knowledge that you can blend your own really great products.

✳ *Creativity*

We all have a basic instinct to create, and can get a real boost from knowing we've made something ourselves. From the product ideas to the ingredient combinations, the scents you add and the way you present your products, there is limitless potential for creativity; have fun with it.

✳ *Connection*

The greatest connection I get from blending my own skincare is connecting with my environment.

By using the herbs, flowers and plants that grow in the same conditions as me – things I can gather from local fields and hedgerows – I am bringing nature into my daily life, harnessing the goodness in it and making it part of me as my body absorbs the creams and lotions I apply.

I've also found natural skincare a great point of connection with others, the kindred spirits who too have become worried about the chemicals going onto their skin and are happy for mutual support in seeking good alternatives – share the knowledge, they'll love you for it!

Social interaction

Making stuff is fun and can bring people together, either in the making process or in the sharing of what is made. Just as you'll discuss meal ideas with friends and share recipes, blending it yourself benefits from that social interaction. Talking to others about skincare and products (a sharing most often confined to family members or very close friends) is part of quite an intimate bond. The conversation increases and widens when you share your experiences of making.

Social status and recognition

As you improve your own skin's appearance, your newfound confidence will not go unnoticed. One of the most wonderful boosts you can get is when someone genuinely comments on how lovely your skin seems or how healthy and happy you look. You're also gaining expertise which will change the way people think about you as you become a go-to person for advice.

Security

Firstly there's the security of knowing what's going into your products. Secondly, there's a security of supply. We're in pretty turbulent times at present; who knows where the world is going next, or what resources will become in short supply or inaccessible to us. There is a security in the ability to build self-reliance. Knowing how to use the resources growing around you to provide for your basic needs is a treasured skill and potential source of comfort.

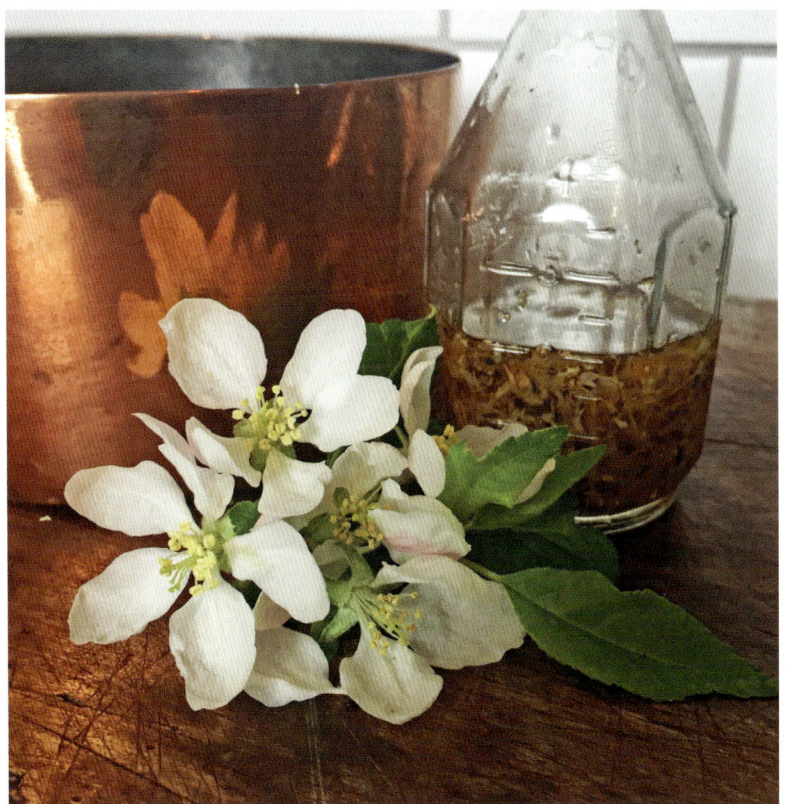

Fairness

Many of us have grown our awareness about how products are sourced, made and traded. We've begun to ask questions about who created this? Under what conditions? How was the environment affected? Is this right? We heatedly get concerned about who gets access to what – why is there surplus in some areas and famine or deprivation in others? Blending your own skincare is not going to solve this, but it is a small statement about wanting to be thoughtful about what you use, not simply going along with the consumerism that has contributed to injustice in the world.

Making your own skincare isn't just another activity on the to-do list, it helps sustain a good, fulfilled life. It can be a defining part of who you are and how you connect with the world.

So why aren't we all doing it?

I spend a lot of time doing demos of skincare making, helping people understand it by seeing and doing, trying and testing. It's wonderful to witness people move from a position of unawareness to excitement and conviction in the space of less than an hour. However, amid the less convinced, there are three common worries that emerge:

- What if it goes wrong?
- I haven't got the right kit
- I haven't got the time

"But I can't ….", "… it might go wrong"

Many recipes are so simple, there are very few things that can go wrong. But if they do, why is that a problem? Stuff does! Not everything you cook is perfect. You learn from your mistakes and it is very rarely unusable. You're making for yourself, so you can forgive yourself. Even if it doesn't look perfect, it can still work fine.

You can also take steps to help you be more confident it won't go wrong:

- Keep it simple – the process may at first be unfamiliar to you, but really it can be as easy as making a cup of tea
- Follow a recipe
- Understand the ingredients
- Use a kit where everything has been prepared and measured for you so the process becomes a lot simpler and foolproof

"I haven't got the right equipment"

Most of what you need to make skincare will be in your kitchen already. A few exceptions may be:

- A double boiler (which is easy to improvise using a heatproof bowl over a saucepan)
- Micro scales to weigh small quantities of ingredients (often you can use tablespoon and teaspoon measurements instead, or use a pre-measured kit to eliminate the need to weigh altogether)
- Pots to put the finished product in – there's lots you can experiment, improvise and have fun with. If it can be sterilised, you can probably use it. There are plenty of suppliers online where you can find specialist containers, so don't be held back

"I haven't got the time"

Time is such an interesting thing. We never seem to have time for anything, and yet we all have a full 24 hours every day. Time is the one thing that is allocated absolutely fairly to us all; it's how we use our time that differentiates us from each other.

I became so fed up with our general obsession with 'time' that a few years ago I decided to simply take the word out of my vocabulary! It made sense: time is an illusion after all. As Einstein taught us, "a minute in the company of a beautiful lady is entirely different to a minute on a hot stove". You've probably had occasions when you've rattled through a number of tasks in just a few minutes; and other occasions when somehow, despite starting with a clear day, you didn't seem to get done what you wanted, you couldn't settle into your activity. It's not about the time available, but about the mood you're in, the energy you have or the attitude you adopt at that moment.

Time is just something we invented to help us make sense of the sun and the moon; we've now forgotten to refer to the sun and the moon, which is a foolish omission, as they govern our energy. Maintaining a connection with them is what keeps our key resources (time and energy) abundant.

The rhythms of the moon take us through our daily and monthly cycles, it's the basis for our months. The moon controls the tides and movement of water across the planet, which is bound to impact upon us as we are 70% water.

The sun gives us our seasons as the intensity of its energy changes throughout the cycle of the year. Plants and many animals and insects respond to this innately. Where we sit on the globe will affect how much of the sun's intensity we encounter, which is why we have an affinity with the things that live and grow at similar latitudes to ourselves. We have cocooned ourselves from much of the changes through our insulated buildings and electric light sources, but we can still feel a change in pace and lifestyle contrasting summer to winter, autumn to spring.

Connecting to nature and the lunar and solar cycles can provide a different perspective on the resources we have available to us. Time is not a finite thing, but a constant presence. Our energy can naturally ebb and flow, as all things in nature do, and we can respond and reflect that as we go about our tasks.

It may feel like it will take a lot of time to master the art of blending your own skincare. This need not be so, you can get going very quickly – after that, it's a question of how much time you want to put into experimenting and adapting recipes to suit yourself.

If you are trying to remedy a particular skin problem, you will find a solution quicker by learning a bit about the natural ingredients that can help and putting them to use, than you will by trying out a series of commercial products, hoping to hit on one that suits.

When you buy off the shelf it's 'hope and wish'. Try something, it doesn't work, try something else. Or worse: try something, it produces a negative effect, try something else to counter the effect, and so on … a constant cycle. It takes time to work out which ingredients affect you, or do you good. Even when you work that out, you may then have difficulty finding the right product with the right combination of ingredients for you. It's time consuming, frustrating and there's no guarantee of success.

When you blend for yourself, it's thoughtful. You know what you're making and why, and you know what you want it to do and what ingredients in it are going to help that. It works, or it doesn't. You could do better, so you make adjustments to your formula and you make it better. It's a constant improvement.

Time invested in selecting good products or gathering ingredients and blending your own is positive time, it can energise and fuel the rest of your life, keeping you going. Your self-care time is absolutely essential for your health and wellbeing. When you feel good you can move mountains in no time.

Time to go natural

Don't be content to grab a pot of something from a shelf and make do. You can do a lot better for yourself; take care of your skin and it will take care of you.

There is beauty when something works and it works intuitively

JONATHAN IVE, ENGLISH DESIGNER, 1967–

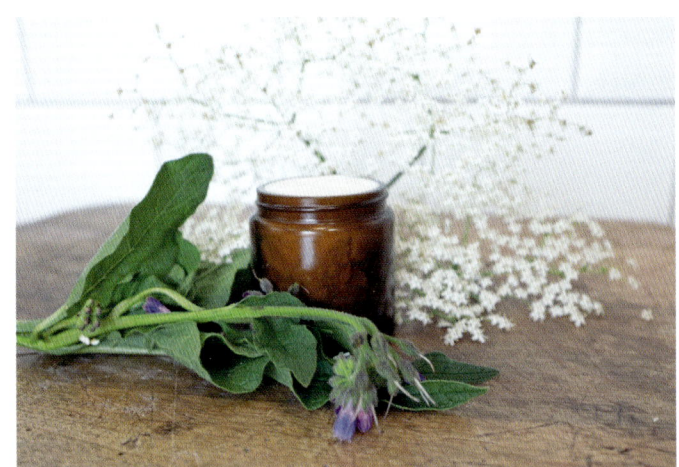

CHAPTER 7

vital products 2
which products are vital to you?

What you put on your skin and into your body is a reflection of your perception of self-worth. Taking care over the products you select demonstrates taking care of yourself. This isn't a showy thing. It's not about having the right bottles on the shelf to impress others. The person you demonstrate your self-worth to is yourself. You're the person who needs to believe it.

The vast majority of people I've spoken to, across all ages and genders, did not think of themselves as having a skincare regime. They had a set practice perhaps, some things they did every day, or most days. They had some special interventions that they might do on occasions. Very few felt confident that they had the best solution; there was a general hunger to find more products they were comfortable with and could be proud of. It's a subtle, unconscious thing but the accumulated difference of each day using a product you doubt or have little regard for, compared to each day using a product you have confidence in and love has a real multiplier effect over time for your wellbeing and positivity.

Through conversation, I've discovered some have a favourite product, used for a number of years, but their loyalty does not extend across the whole product range. There's a lot lurking in cabinets and wash bags that we have no loyalty to at all. Products would be tried and abandoned, used or forgotten at will. Where loyalty existed, it was based on ethics such as non-testing on animals or good ingredients. People used the brand as a shortcut for trusting that their values were being upheld. Loyalty based on the product effectiveness did not extend far. For example, the trusted mascara didn't lead to a love of all the makeup in that range.

Your skincare personality

Our behaviour in selecting skincare, as with many things in life, is by no means entirely rational. In an interview situation when asked to consider which products you'd be most likely to try from a new skincare brand, typically people were happier to cite hand cream as an easy thing to change but were most nervous about making changes to face creams. It was surprising, therefore, when launching my new skincare brand, including day and night face creams, body cream, hand cream and foot cream, that the day and night creams, intended for use on the face, were always my sell-out items. Maybe their names 'Face the Day Cream' and 'Marshmallow Dream Cream' along with the story of their beneficial ingredients is enough to overcome those nervous to try new products for the face. Maybe there are other trust factors – I sell more of the face creams when selling direct (through stalls and skincare parties), more of the hand cream when selling through anonymous online channels. This shows we can't necessarily accept the first, most rational answer, but need to look deeper into what is really motivating our actions.

Do you buy with your head or your heart? While you've probably got an immediate answer to this, reality is likely to be a complex blend.

Here are some techniques to help you uncover your skincare personality. They involve sorting and categorising all your skincare items, so you'll need to gather them all into one place. That's soaps, hair care products, deodorants, shaving creams, moisturisers, hand creams, lip balms, spritzers, perfumes, aftershaves …

There are printable sorting aids available online (www.fieldfreshskincare.co.uk). Download your copies of these as you gather all your items together.

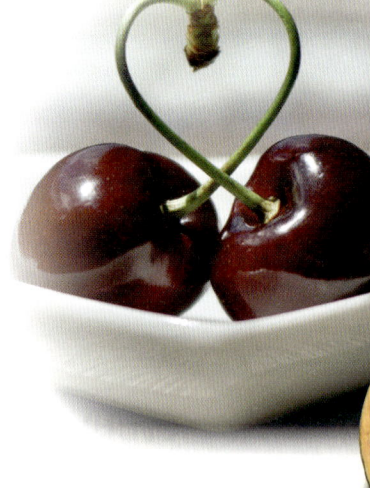

Exercise 1: Head and heart

Sort your products into two groups:

1. **Head**: bought for a rational reason.
   e.g. Most easily available, best value, on special offer, packaging and size that suited your purpose.

2. **Heart**: bought because you loved it.
   A magical enticement – the scent, the feel, the packaging, the promise, the brand or product story, the ingredients you seek or trust.

   ▹ If the product was given to you by someone else, consider how you think about it

   ▹ If you can't remember your motivation for purchasing, check the sell-by date. Chances are it is not at its best and should be replaced with something fresher

   ▹ If both head and heart played a part, create a middle category and ask yourself both the head and the heart questions below

Now pick two different coloured pens, one for positive thoughts and the other for negative thoughts. Use these to jot down your responses to the following questions:

For each 'head' product, consider:

▹ What filtering influenced your selection?
e.g. Were the options available to you limited by: the place you bought from, the budget you set, promotions, or other factors?

▹ What were the main influences on your purchase decision?
e.g. Your previous experience, what others have said, or what you believe they think, what you've read or seen in advertising or in use

For each 'heart' product, check with yourself:

▹ Do you feel wonderful when using these, do they bring magic to your day?

▹ Have they lived up to their promise?

▹ How will you feel when your current supply runs out?

And remember, there's probably a bundle of products that you've liked in the shop but not been enticed enough to buy. Why was that? What reasons stopped you then?

❈ Conclusions to Exercise 1 – Are you head or heart?

Which category has more products: head or heart? Do you have more negative or positive comments? Find the box that most relates to you:

		MAJORITY OF PRODUCTS	
		HEAD	**HEART**
MAJORITY OF COMMENTS	**POSITIVE**	**Least Worst** You're a practical person, know what you need and look for products that simply meet those needs. *In the next exercise, find out which products you can use with healthy confidence.*	**Heart's Desire** You love your products and like to be charmed by them. *In the next exercise, find out which products offer health and happiness.*
	NEGATIVE	**Quest for Best** Have you been holding back? Give yourself permission to indulge a bit in the products you love. *The next exercise can help you find products to boost your wellbeing.*	**Unfulfilled Dreams** You have an optimistic tendency to be enticed by promises. *Use the next exercise to know what products can keep you smiling.*

VITAL PRODUCTS 2: WHICH PRODUCTS ARE VITAL TO YOU?

Exercise 2: Ingredients check

The packaging may look good and say wonderful things, but you'll only know if the product is really great for you by looking at the ingredients.

Ingredient lists might look dense at first, but with practice you'll get used to recognising some names and deciphering what you need to know. Legally, all ingredient lists have to use the 'International Nomenclature of Cosmetic Ingredients' (INCI). Just like plant naming, this often uses Latin to ensure commonality of naming wherever the country of origin. Encouragingly, sometimes you'll find a 'common' name is included alongside the INCI name to help you recognise ingredients e.g., Butyrospermum parkii (shea) butter.

It is also a legal requirement to list ingredients in quantity order, largest first. You'll often find Aqua (water) quite high up on the ingredients list, while some of the active ingredients highlighted on the front may be low down, and therefore included in relatively small quantities. A long list of ingredients needn't be off-putting in itself. What's important is how many of the ingredients are there for the benefit of your skin, compared to those there for the benefit of the product, either as bulking agents or preservatives.

In evaluating your product, consider the proportion of natural to synthetic ingredients, the type and level of preservative used, whether there are any specific ingredients you either love or take exception to, and whether you have any qualms about the sourcing or method of production for particular ingredients. For example, palm oils have come under scrutiny for destructive and exploitative practices, glitters have been criticised for their impact on the environment, and those adhering to vegan principles will choose to avoid animal products in their skincare.

To complete this exercise, look at your products by application and use the table to help note the ingredients' function and your judgement on whether you are happy to see the ingredient or wary of it. By creating a table for each product you want to understand, you'll be able to see at a glance how your different products stack up, which will help in rating your priorities.

Seek out the components you know will be in the product. There are likely to be:

- A preservative
- Ingredients to help the product's function
    e.g. surfactants (foaming agents)
    emollients (for moisture and sheen)
    occlusives (for protection)
- Ingredients to provide scent and character to the product

	Preservatives	Surfactants	Emollients, humectants & occlusives	Scent, colour, character	Botanical ingredients	Other
Especially check in:	All products Soaps Toothpaste	Shampoos Cleansers	Creams Lotions Balms Shampoos	Shampoos Makeup Creams		
Wary						
Happy						

Here are some of the ingredients that go into my 'wary' boxes:

Preservatives: Parabens and diazolidinyl urea (which may cause skin irritation), DMDM hydantoin and methenamine (known allergens) triclosan and triclocarban (hormone disrupters) and borax (now banned and a likely carcinogen).

Surfactants: Sulphates – the three main ones being sodium laureth sulphate (SLES), sodium lauryl sulphate (SLS) and ammonium lauryl sulphate (ALS) (which can cause irritation and are synthesised from petrolatum), Cocamide DEA/cocamide diethanolamine (a carcinogen) and triethanolamine (TEA) (an allergen).

Emollients, humectants and occlusives: PEG compounds (designed to penetrate the skin, so able to take other ingredients deeper with them too); petroleum-based products e.g. petroleum jelly, paraffin oil, waxes or liquid, mineral oil, microcrystalline waxes (because they lack vitality, being essentially dead, and because our use of petroleum-based products is unsustainable) and propylene glycol (which may be associated with respiratory difficulties).

Scent, colour, character: Any mention of 'fragrance' or 'parfum', plasticisers such as dimethicone, phthalates and the lightening agent hydroquinone.

- Don't look at what it says on the front of the label (e.g. terms like 'natural' or 'lab-tested' or calling out specific ingredients), look at what it says on the back in the real ingredients list.
- A short ingredients list can be a good sign, but always look at the detail.
- It will be difficult to find any products without some ingredients that you may question (unless you're making fresh yourself). You'll need to evaluate and compromise. The lower down on the list they appear, the smaller proportion of the product is made up of that ingredient (but some things can cause sensitivity even in small quantities).
- Some ingredients sound OK, but may cause sensitivity e.g. 'limonene' (a constituent of essential oil but a known allergen).
- Some ingredients have unusual names but are fine to use e.g. sodium cocoyl isethionate (a surfactant based on coconut oil, which is considered one of the less irritating surfactants, especially if used at low percentages).

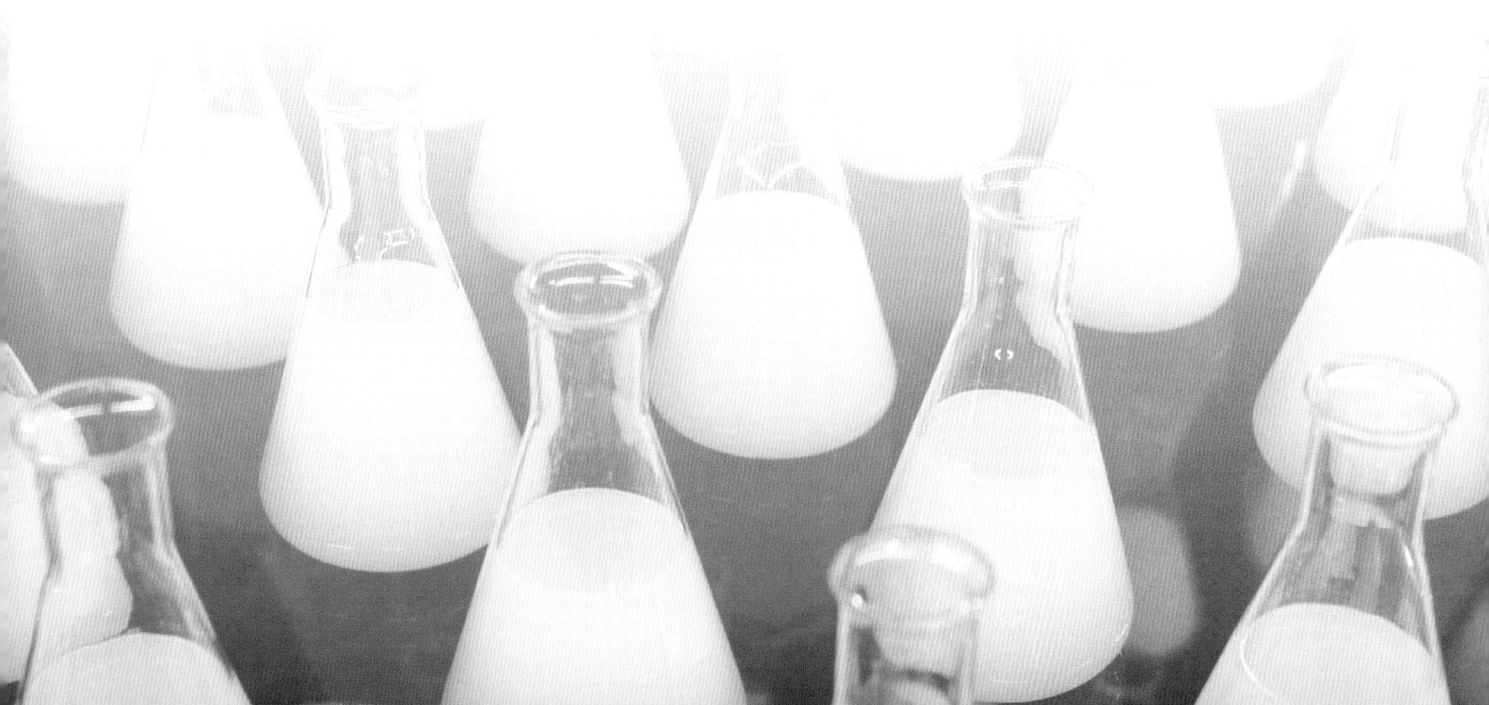

Evaluate each product and note your comments and give them a grade. As you're the person who needs to be happy with your product selection, the 'grading' of each product is entirely up to you. Here's an example of how to grade from 'be happy' to 'be wary':

5 You're entirely happy with the product, the ingredients in it and the claims made for it.

4 You are content to use this product, recognising that the ingredient choices are a reasonable compromise between good ingredients and performance quality.

3 You have some concerns about ingredients in this product and will reduce your use of it over time, so long as you can find a better alternative.

2 You have significant concerns about some ingredients in this product and will minimise your use of it while seeking an alternative.

1 There are certain ingredients in this product that mean you do not want to use it at all.

Application	Product Name	Contentment with ingredients	
		Score	Comments
Cleansers	A		
	B		
	C		
Moisturisers	A		
	B		
	C		
Hair products	A		
	B		
	C		
Bath products	A		
	B		
	C		
Balms	A		
	B		
	C		
Other	A		
	B		
	C		

How many individual items do you have listed? Can you reduce it to just 20? Twelve is the average number of items a woman will use in a day so for most people reducing their whole skincare repertoire to 12 items will be a squeeze. If you're smiling because you're below 12 already, check if you've covered all bases in terms of what your skin is likely to need. You should probably have an example of most of the product types on this 'use frequently' list and at least something from the 'use occasionally' list.

✳ *Use frequently*

- SPF protection
- A facial cleanser
- An exfoliator
- A body cleanser
- Shaving kit
- Toner or aftershave
- Moisturiser
- Deodorant
- Shampoo
- Conditioner
- Toothpaste
- Bath products: oils, salts, bath bomb, etc.
- Perfume or cologne

✳ *Use occasionally*

- Hand cream
- Lip balm
- Foot balm
- Masks: face, hair, hands, feet
- Healing creams and ointments
- Nail polishes
- Nail polish remover
- Hair dyes
- Massage oils

How are you doing? What does your top 20 look like? Put a star next to your favourite 12 items. Are there any gaps where you don't have a favourite product, or would like to find better?

Take these thoughts into Exercise 3.

Exercise 3: Bin / Ban / Plan

Having considered what you love and don't love about your products, what you want more of and what you want less of, you can make your informed choices about what to Bin, what to Ban and what to Plan to use more.

Go through your products for a final time and decide:

BIN – for anything out of date, or that you simply don't use or don't want to use. If it's a perfectly good product but just not right for you, give it to a friend who'd appreciate it.

BAN – if you identified ingredients, brands or product types that don't suit you, resolve not to buy them again. Now you know what you're looking for you can be particularly vigilant while still keeping your mind open to new possibilities.

PLAN – the changes you want to make. Looking at the patterns emerging in your chart should help direct your next steps. Where have you got real gaps without a product satisfying your needs? Where would you like to find new alternatives to try? Would you like to make the changes through finding new products to buy or by making products yourself?

A clear-minded approach to your own needs will help sift through the many beautiful packages and persuasive marketing to find your perfect product.

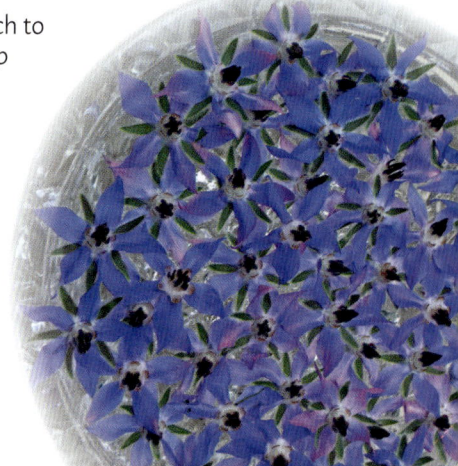

Borage flowers

Transitioning

Integrating new products into your regime often requires a transition period to get your body, your skin and yourself used to a new approach.

It's tempting to make wholesale change, and to eradicate all troublesome chemicals from our lives. But this is often too daunting, too huge or too difficult to achieve. Instead, think of the one or two products that you can really make a difference with. These may be something you use every day, or something where you are particularly concerned about the non-natural version and the effect it is having. Make this simple change your goal.

Making the change

We use our skincare products daily. They become part of our trusted routines, and even part of how we define ourselves. It's a crutch that we can be reluctant to let go of. Do it for the right reasons – your own reasons – to transition successfully. Know what's vital in your skincare.

It won't always be simple. You're not guaranteed to hit on the right product straight away, and you may have to change your routines a little to accommodate them. For example, layering natural oils can provide wonderful hydration and protection for dry skin, but you'll need to allow a few minutes between application and getting dressed to let them sink in. Which may mean changing the order of routine morning tasks to make the best use of that time.

The first thing to do with any product is a patch test. There are more details on how to do this overleaf. Once you're happy there are no immediate sensitivities, start bringing the product into normal use. Make a conscious effort to use the product and think about it with each application. It takes 66 days to establish a new habit, over time you'll create a new normal that you're happy with, that's 'your way'.

At best you'll love the product and make it a staple go-to. Or perhaps you will choose to build it into a repertoire of balancing, complementary products to use in a cycle. Even if you decide you don't get on with it, because you've chosen the product thoughtfully and used it consciously, you will know exactly why it's not your thing and can bring that information to your next, refined product choice.

Where you can, share your experiences – with friends and family and in online communities – so you get support and advice through your transitioning and can provide the help, encouragement and guidance that others need too. We need to make our own decisions about what's right for ourselves, but we don't need to fathom it alone. Documenting it can be fun too. It may be small steps but over time you'll be able to look back on big, positive change.

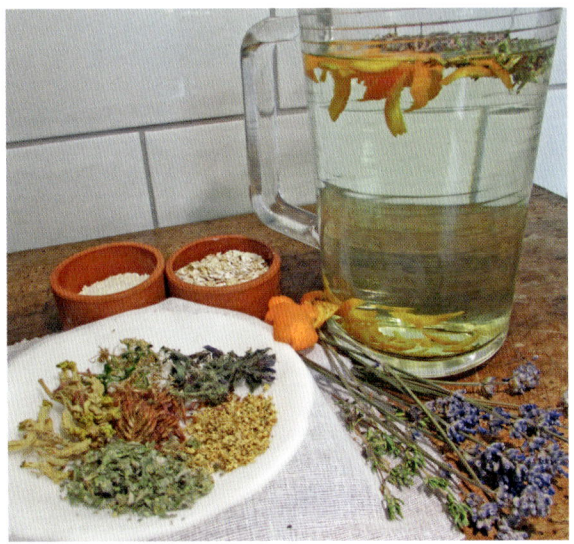

Ingredients for Duchess and Dairymaid Skin Softening Bath, see page 173.

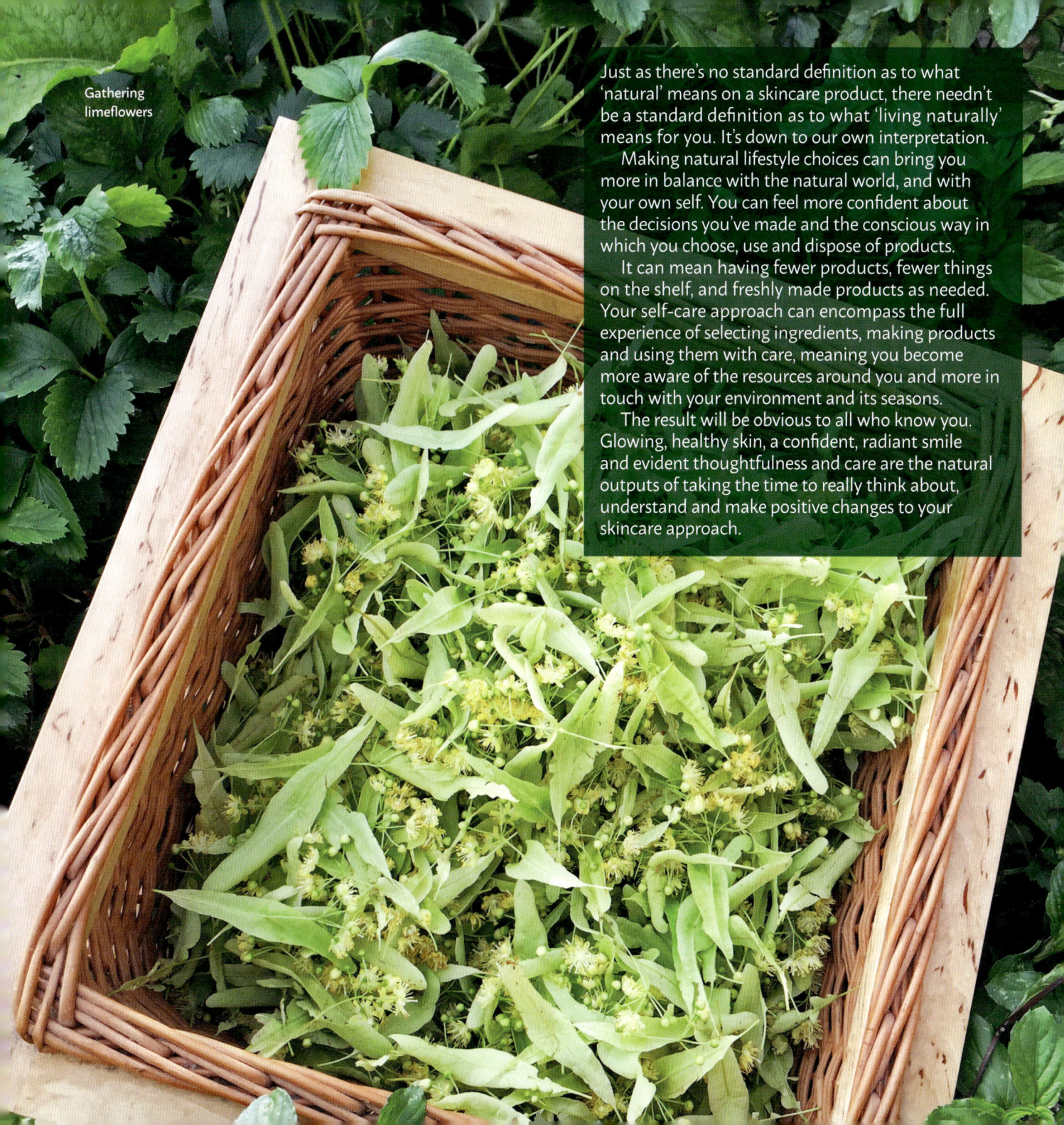

Gathering limeflowers

Just as there's no standard definition as to what 'natural' means on a skincare product, there needn't be a standard definition as to what 'living naturally' means for you. It's down to our own interpretation.

Making natural lifestyle choices can bring you more in balance with the natural world, and with your own self. You can feel more confident about the decisions you've made and the conscious way in which you choose, use and dispose of products.

It can mean having fewer products, fewer things on the shelf, and freshly made products as needed. Your self-care approach can encompass the full experience of selecting ingredients, making products and using them with care, meaning you become more aware of the resources around you and more in touch with your environment and its seasons.

The result will be obvious to all who know you. Glowing, healthy skin, a confident, radiant smile and evident thoughtfulness and care are the natural outputs of taking the time to really think about, understand and make positive changes to your skincare approach.

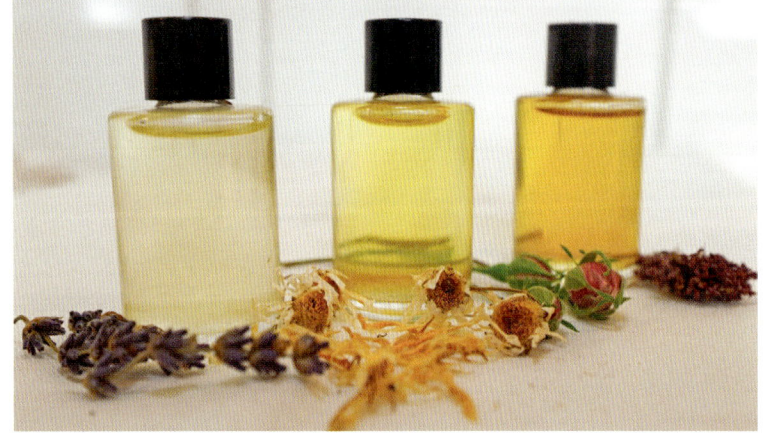

> *Beauty is only skin deep.
> I think what's really important is finding a balance of mind, body and spirit*
>
> JENNIFER LOPEZ,
> AMERICAN SINGER, 1969–

Patch testing

Everyone has his or her own unique skin so it's impossible to say how an individual will react to a particular ingredient. While many of the ingredients with known, more universal, sensitivities are avoided in natural skincare (the artificial fragrances in particular, as well as many preservatives and additives) it is still possible that you may react to a natural ingredient.

Plants and herbs are potent; it's why they're included as active ingredients in our skincare. Generally, their effect is positive, but we should also cautiously find out if we have reactions to any particular ingredients.

What is a patch test?

A patch test is a means to understand whether you are sensitive to any particular products or ingredients. It simply involves applying a small amount of the product, or ingredient, to a small area of skin and observing if there is any reaction.

It should be performed whenever you use a new product or ingredient. A patch test gives personal information about how you respond, and may be different to the response of others. Don't rely on results from others, find out for yourself.

In a patch test you apply a small amount of the product to a relatively hidden area of skin. Then you wait to see how your skin responds. Any reaction will be obvious within 24 hours.

The patch test results tell you whether it is advisable, or not, to use the product tested and what kind of reaction, if any, you can expect.

It will not tell you why you react that way, but further research can help decipher that and help you make an informed decision about which ingredients to use or to avoid.

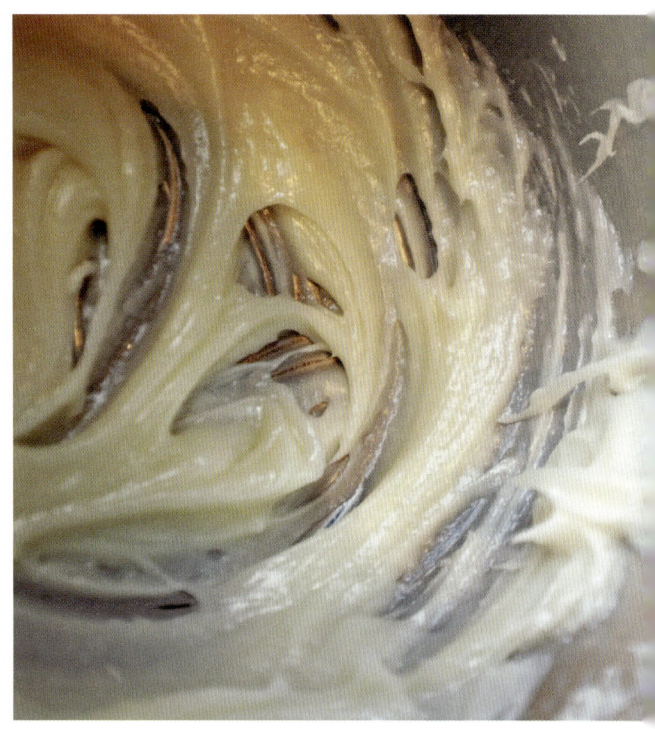

How to do a patch test

A patch test should be performed in conditions as close as possible to the way in which you intend to use the product. For example, when testing a face product, test on an area that is like the face, but more discrete, such as the side of the neck. This area will still have the thinner, typically more reactive skin of the face but is not so visible, in case a reaction does occur (while still being visible for you in a mirror to inspect the results).

Other good 'hidden' and yet sensitive areas for testing are the inner wrist, inner elbow and the back of your knees. You could choose to test in two separate areas for comparison.

If you know you are sensitive in a particular area, this is where to test a product for irritation, again looking for the most discrete position possible. Similarly, if you want to test to see if a product will affect a particular condition, such as acne or clogged pores, test in the area where you are most likely to experience this.

Keep the area of your patch test quite small, about two to four centimetres squared. This is large enough for you to spot any reaction but small enough for you to be able to deal with it quickly if necessary, and not too obvious to those not looking for it.

1. To begin your test, first clean the area.
2. Use a cotton bud, brush or cloth to dab a small amount of product onto your test area and then cover with a waterproof plaster

The reaction may happen immediately, or it may take 24 hours or longer to respond. If it's an ingredient you're particularly concerned about, wait at least a day between performing the patch test and deciding whether to use the product.

If you feel at all uncomfortable during the test period, remove the plaster and cleanse the area. Otherwise wait 24 hours and then remove the plaster. If there is no visible irritation you are OK to go ahead and use the product.

As you become aware of which ingredients are best for you, you will be able to proceed with confidence. The simpler the ingredients, the easier this is.

How to respond to a positive patch test

A positive patch test is one in which you do see a reaction to the ingredient tested. This may, for example, be redness, itching, swelling, hives or irritation.

If this occurs, **firstly**, wash the area thoroughly with plain water and don't use the product. Apply a soothing oil if necessary, such as sweet almond oil or olive oil.

Secondly, note the specific ingredients in the product so you can gradually test each one, eliminating ingredients that are fine. This will help you identify the ingredient that does not agree with you. Use this as guidance for what to avoid in the future. Read the ingredients list on every product and identify the name(s) of your problem ingredient.

Thirdly, for deeper understanding, do a little research to understand the family that your sensitive ingredient comes from, find out if plants related to it have a similar effect for you. You may even be able to isolate the constituent part of the plant that you react to and find out if that is present in any other ingredients.

Finally, when it's appropriate to – and if you feel you'd like to – return to the ingredient you're nervous of to check if your reactions have changed. Sensitivities can come and go through life. Sometimes sensitivities are brought on through hormonal changes (especially in puberty, pregnancy and menopause) and may abate later; or they may impact seasonally or in combination with other ingredients or in specific applications. So it's possible that a permanent, blanket ban is not necessary. But only do what you are comfortable with.

The more you know about yourself and your responses to ingredients, the more you can progress with confidence in creating and using the skincare that is absolutely right for you.

Enjoy learning about your skin, its needs and the herbs and oils that can help it, and do keep performing patch tests to build your confidence.

Part 3
Vital Skincare

CHAPTER 8

vital skincare – simple as 1, 2, 3

Vital skincare is simple. Know the three determinants that make your skin what it is; and know the three simple practices that are vital to keeping it naturally healthy.

Three determinants that make your skin what it is

1. Genetic factors: the skin you're given
2. Lifestyle: the impact on your skin of what you do each day
3. Care: how you have looked after your skin

Our skin is continually responding. This dynamic context gives each of us unique requirements, and necessitates a personal and adaptable approach to our skincare. It's never fixed, there's constant change as we move through the days, seasons and years. But nature is always looking for equilibrium, so working with nature is the swiftest and most secure way to maintain your perfectly balanced skin.

The three determinants each change at a different pace. Your skin cells gradually evolve through your lifetime; your activities and environment are constantly changing; and the way you look after your skin may fluctuate based on your time, energy and interest on any day of the week.

Determinant 1: The skin you're given

We often hear of 'skin types'. For example, aestheticians will refer to oily, dry, sensitive and combination skin. There are many terms and grades. Each of these are an attempt to create a simple view of the huge variety in human skin and the variety of needs that we collectively possess.

Why is this done? Primarily it is to enable a single entity (whether that's a beauty expert giving advice or a company with a product to sell), to understand, and communicate a message to many people. To do that effectively, it's necessary to have classifications and groups to simplify messaging. Product ranges would be vast, and advice endless, if every actual skin type was catered for. So highly generic groups are created. This keeps product lines simple and developmental and manufacturing costs lower, but it is also what makes finding the perfect product for you harder.

You'll find the way this classification works will vary from one supplier to another, each aesthetician will have their own way to consider skin types. The truth is, any classification is going to be arbitrary, more useful to the giver of advice and products than the receiver. We don't fit into neat boxes.

Thankfully, you only have to deal with one skin type – yours. And you know that there are times when it feels oilier and times when it feels drier, areas that are more problematic or sensitive and perhaps ingredients that you are wary of through experience. Your skin will have a natural predisposition based on your genetics. The way your skin functions will evolve with you, and respond to how you treat it. Your skin may change over the years, typically getting drier as you age and naturally produce fewer oils and have slower cell regeneration. So your needs will change through the decades.

In reality, our skin is much more complex than a skin-type label allows us to recognise, and varies across our body (we all know our own problem patches). Focus on your needs and seek products for particular skin situations, rather than a generic skin type.

As your skin finds its own natural balance, problems such as excess oiliness, dryness and sensitivity should start to disappear. You'll need fewer corrective products then.

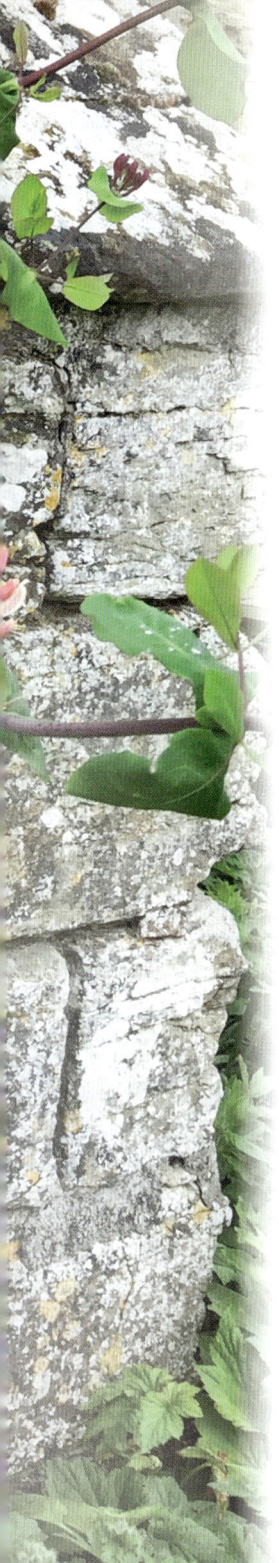

Determinant 2: Lifestyle: what you do each day

Each day's individual combination of factors from your rest, diet, environment and clothes impact on your skin. We looked in Chapter 2 at all the things that can make a difference. Now we can look in more detail at some of the factors.

❋ What you eat and drink

Our diet provides water, Essential Fatty Acids (EFAs), vitamins and antioxidants, which are all vital to skin health and minimise the effects of ageing. The more of these we can incorporate, through our food and our skincare, the better.

Borage seed oil is one of the best sources of gamma-linolenic acid (GLA), an Omega 6 fatty acid. It also contains a variety of A, B D and E vitamins.

❋ Sleep and rest

Is there a better feeling than waking up from a contented sleep feeling fully refreshed, energised and ready to face the day? There's no doubting the rejuvenating impact of sleep and the positive impact it has on our mood and energy levels. It also shines through in our skin.

The familiar tell-tale signs of an accumulation of poor sleep are dark circles under the eyes, puffiness, and a greater propensity to spots and blemishes. Some of this is a response to the psychological impact and stress created through not sleeping. Some may be associated with the non-skin-friendly activities that are keeping us from our beds (working late in front of a screen, racing around in lots of different environments and drinking alcohol). While some are simply due to skin not getting its restorative down-time. Well-rested skin is more even and less prone to flare-ups.

At night our skin's pH drops a little which is an indicator for the skin cell renewal process to begin. In peaceful sleep, skin is able to focus on restorative work in a relatively stable environment, different to its defensive daytime work. It's good therefore to use skin-nourishing treatments just before bed to assist with the cell regeneration that takes place as you sleep. Good additions to nighttime skincare include vitamin A (retinol) to work against the wrinkles of sun-damaged skin, vitamin C (an antioxidant) to minimise free radicals and so reduce oxidation, skin-conditioning vitamin E and moisture-enhancing hyaluronic acid.

> Elderflower has traditionally been used as a treatment for eyes. In laboratory tests, elder was found to be a good treatment for dark circles and puffy eyes due to its rutin content (a flavonoid) and antioxidating and anti-inflammatory acids. An extract is now being created to bring these benefits to eye treatments.
>
> *Personal Care Magazine* May 2017, Emmanual Coste, Jean-Francois Nicolay – Exsymol, Monaco: Dark circle and puffy eyes treated with elderberry.

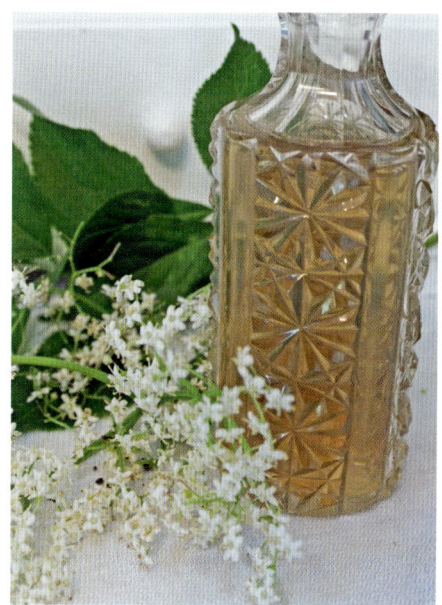

Elderflower water, see page 89

❋ Stress and relaxation

These are two sides of the coin with equally negative and positive effects on our skin.

STRESS

- Stress makes our adrenaline kick in and causes the body to pump our muscles with blood, this means less blood available for the skin that becomes pale. We see this in a sudden way after shock or in a more gradual way when stress and strain is relentless.
- If we're angry or irritated, anxious or excited, our sebaceous glands can be triggered to produce more oil. Often the cause of blackheads or pimples forming just before an important occasion.
- In extreme cases our muscles will stiffen as a result of stress, inhibiting oxygen and nutrient flow to the skin as well as removal of waste. Our skin looks sluggish, and lacks vitality, which is true, as our systems have slowed down. Cell regeneration also slows down, meaning as old cells reach the surface they're even drier and duller.
- Constant stress lowers our immune system over time and we become more sensitive to irritants in our products, for example, reacting to perfumes.
- Stress takes its toll on our skin over time as 'worry lines' become etched in, muscles become used to the frown and less elastic skin settles into its regular form.

RELAXATION

- Taking a lighter view on life can help us look more youthful just by the way emotions flit over the skin instead of lingering. The pace of fleeting emotions caught in social media snapshots is part of what gives them a youthful edge. Detaching ourselves from stress in this way can be rejuvenating, but we require more than a relaxing evening or holiday to achieve a lasting impact.
- When we are content it visibly shows in our skin.
- There's a beautiful added bonus in using natural products on our skin as, when we think about what these mean to us, it can connect us to nature and a well of inner calm.
- Being relaxed helps to clear our mind and think about what we need. Our intuition is sharper, we can tune into our instinct and choose for ourselves, unpressured by external influences.
- When we relax, life flows better and so do our internal systems. We function more efficiently.
- Calmness shows on the outside and serenity is beautifully attractive.

❋ Environment

Very few of us are lucky enough to spend our time in a clean environment. We all build up grime on our skin during the day that will need to be rinsed off at night before the toxins can be absorbed into our bodies.

Indoors, central heating creates a warm, dry environment that is also very dehydrating.

Outdoors, our skin can 'breathe' but generally needs some protection from the elements.

❋ Weather

For those of us living in a temperate climate, skin tends to feel best in spring and autumn. At these times of the year breezes are more often warm than icy and frequent rain showers keep the ambient moisture high.

Bitter winter winds deplete moisture levels. Once the general temperatures are below 20°C (68°F), as is typical for winter, each further drop of 7-8°C (or 45-46°F) will halve the water in the air. We notice this dryness in our skins – particularly our hands and faces, the exposed parts. Skin can become cracked and bleed, or be dry and flaky. We can respond with extra moisturiser, ideally including more essential fatty acids and vitamin A (beta-Carotene) to keep skin nourished and supple.

In winter our complexion can lose tone and colour so needs greater attention. Facial masks can be great for this. In summer there may be drier conditions but it is UV that presents the greatest threat to skin as the sun is at its strongest. We need to protect well and take in extra antioxidant nutrients: vitamins A, C, E and selenium.

❋ Clothing and fabrics

Particular clothing can irritate some skin. Often it is the chemicals used in treating fabrics, rather than the fabrics themselves that cause a reaction. So be careful even when selecting natural fibres to wear (such as cotton, silk, hemp, linen and wool) that they have not been treated with something you may react to.

Common culprits can be formaldehyde, used to make wrinkle-resistant fabric, or chemicals used in dyes and flame-retardants. Also be wary of the nickel used in rivets and fastenings that can cause reactions.

Wear loose, comfortable clothing made from untreated, natural fibres, selecting colours to suit your skin tone and styles to suit your mood.

❋ Household cleaning products

Your skin will respond to whatever it comes into contact with, so look for products with ingredients that are as familiar to your own body as possible. Natural oils and plants grown in the environment that you live in will be some of the closest matches you can find.

Simple ingredients such as vinegar, lemon juice, essential oils and bicarbonate of soda can perform a multitude of household tasks as well as or better than, bottled offerings from the household products aisles of supermarkets. There's a common myth that natural is less effective. Beware, in some instances it can be highly effective. And there are plenty of non-natural products that still aren't effective.

The more aware you are of your skin, the more sensitive you will become to ingredients in all products, detecting them by smell, feel or inhaling. Seek to minimise your exposure to substances that are alien to your skin.

Steps to move to less harmful products include:

- Using less
- Adjusting our sensibilities to and preconceptions of scent: focus more on what the product does than what it smells like, don't be fooled into thinking that just because you can smell cleaning products in the room, the place must be clean. It's much easier to squirt it around than to ensure it's doing a good job. Over time your response to scent will change as you seek out more natural fragrances.
- Look for more natural ingredients
- Make your own, ideally making fresh as needed

❋ Activities that impact on your skin

Do you garden? Does your sport impact on your skin? Are you very 'hands-on'?

You don't wear your gardening clothes to go shopping, or turn up at a smart restaurant wearing climbing gear, so your skin shouldn't betray these activities either.

Build pro-active steps into your routines to take care of your skin. Wear gloves, put protective barrier creams on before the task, use scrubs and cleansers designed specifically for the purpose and moisturise. Make these a necessary part of the activity.

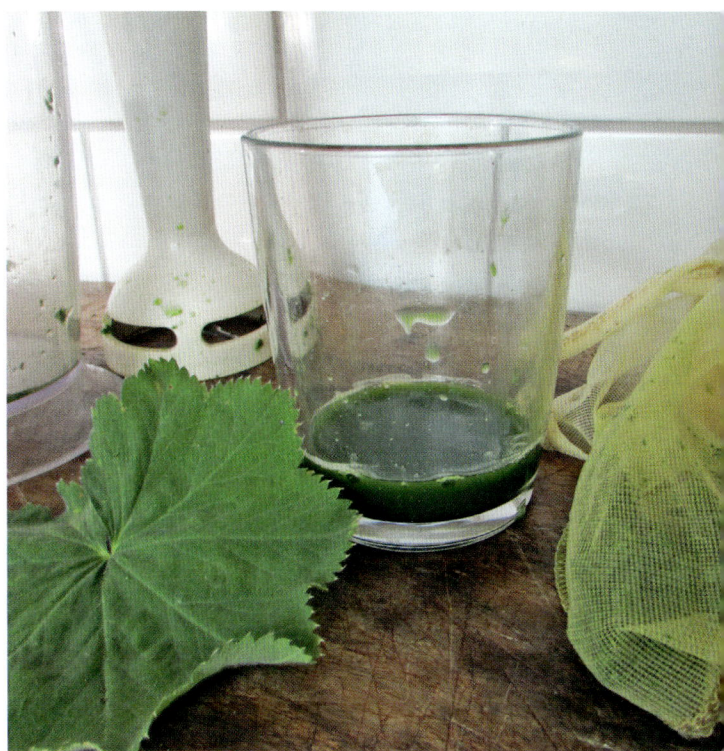

Extracting lady's mantle juice, to treat acne. See page 160.

Determinant 3: Your skincare approach

The third determinant to your skin condition is the approach you take in your skincare. The time, effort and thought you choose to put into your skincare is a combination of attitude and lifestyle. In looking for the best skincare approach, it's not the quantity of time you dedicate, but the quality of thought that counts. Doing the right things for your skin can be very simple indeed.

Your skincare approach may have changed intermittently as you take more or less interest in your skin (often prompted by a particular event in life or skin problem) and the space you have to dedicate time to self-care. Often it fluctuates between weekday and weekend, or between everyday life and holiday time.

It's never too late to make a change. Three simple practices are vital to healthy skincare.

Three simple practices

Skin is designed to function on its own in a regenerating system of self-care and maintenance. Our basic practices simply need to support skin's own system.

The three simple ways to support skin are:

1. Keep it clean
2. Keep it fresh
3. Keep it moist

Practice 1: Keep skin clean

Cleansing is how we support our skin by removing the dirt from the surface that would otherwise build up and block pores. Pores need to be clean and unclogged. Your skin has to have a free flow through its surface pores to successfully manage emitting toxins and to maintain the right levels of oil and water to keep skin supple. You know when this is compromised because spots will occur if there is an accumulation of toxins under the skin, and skin will become dry and cracked if its normal moisturising activities are impeded. Whoever we are, and whatever our skin type, cleanliness is critical.

The natural detoxifying and lubricating processes of our skin mean oils, salts and waste are continually excreted onto the surface. There, they are joined by external pollution and dirt. The moisture in our skin attracts specks of dust and particles. The grime may be from things we've added, such as makeup or sun creams, or from what we've picked up from our environment. Pollution is omnipresent so we need to be constantly vigilant to cleansing. The cleansing that we do for our skin in our daily washing, or deeper steam and clay treatments, can be supplemented by an internal cleansing of a detoxifying diet and mental or spiritual cleansing through meditation.

Cleansing is not just a functional issue. How we cleanse is steeped in cultural practice and impacted by the climate and environment we live in. So if you've ever been told 'this is what you should do', think of it as 'this is what you could do' and find the way that works best for you. That enables you to feel clean and smell fresh and that is in tune with your way of living.

Cleansing can be over-done if it works against our body's natural processes. We actually need many of the bacteria on our skin as they break down waste for us. If we try to eradicate them (with antiseptics, antibiotics and antibacterial products) nature will keep retaliating and strengthening the bacteria (good and bad). Our battle becomes harder if we work against nature.

Cleansing is good for the soul: the calmness of a relaxing, warm bath or the invigoration of a cool shower are universally understood and appreciated, our response to them is innate.

In the next chapter (see page 59) there are lots of suggestions for how to use good natural ingredients for cleansing your skin.

Practice 2: Keep skin fresh

Skin is naturally kept fresh by the constant cycling and renewing of individual skin cells. The official term for this natural process is desquamation. It's a process that can slow down with age as the web-like matrix within which cells sit becomes thicker, making it harder to shed entrapped cells. By being vigilant of this process, and using small interventions, we can keep our skin at its freshest and best. We do this simply by helping skin rid the dead cells on the surface.

New skin cells are formed in the base layers of our skin and rise up to the surface. By the time they emerge at the top, they are flat, dry and lifeless. Their rough texture reflects light unevenly, giving us a dull complexion. However, rising up just below these are new, plumper skin cells. Natural flaking sheds the top dead cells and reveals the fresh, smoother new ones beneath. When these are visible our skin looks more young and radiant, simply because it is: we're seeing younger, more vibrant cells.

In the normal course of things this is happening all the time in its own ad hoc way, so we don't really notice it. The majority of surface cells will be dead and dry, so our complexion can be consequentially dull. By stepping in and taking more control of the process – ensuring it happens evenly and at a time when we will most benefit from looking fresh - we support our skin and turn its natural processes to our advantage. So it's in our interest to keep the cycle of cell renewal working as efficiently as possible. But it has to be done with care in the right way. Too much and you'll reveal cells that aren't yet ready to do the hard work of surface cells.

These will then react becoming red, blotchy and sore. Be gentle and listen to your skin.

Actively managing the removal of dead skin cells also helps support skin's cleansing process as they're all part of the surface debris we need to remove to prevent blocked pores.

The term for our active sloughing of surface skin cells is 'exfoliation' (which reminds me of a tree shedding its leaves in autumn, a necessary stage in the cycle to forming new leaf buds and fresh green). There are two primary ways to exfoliate: physical and chemical, but many different techniques and products that can help. We'll look at these and the great natural approaches you can take for exfoliation in Chapter 10, page 83.

Practice 3: Keeping skin moist

Our skin is incredibly thirsty for oil. For thousands of years people have used oil on their skins as the only form of anti-wrinkle treatment.

We know that skin has the remarkable ability to produce oils and direct them to the skin's surface to keep it supple and waterproofed. However, some parts of our bodies are less well endowed with oil producing glands (for instance, they are absent on our lips) and our oil-producing systems can deteriorate with age or get confused by stress, which we notice as resulting in less or more oil to our skin's surface.

We are able to support our skin's own moisture and oil levels using both internal and external methods. To know when to moisturise, listen to your skin. If it feels dry, add moisture; if it feels soft, it's fine.

Your needs will change over time. Natural moisture levels are affected by travel to different places with different climates, moving through the seasons and elements, changing from indoor to outdoor conditions and stress. You can help your skin by having rich and light preparations ready to use accordingly.

Of course, there are many wonderful natural ingredients that can help you with this, and many products you can make yourself. It's worth getting to know them and experimenting with different oils, serums, lotions, balms, butters, creams and waxes so you know which to use for best effect. All these are explained in Chapter 11, page 99.

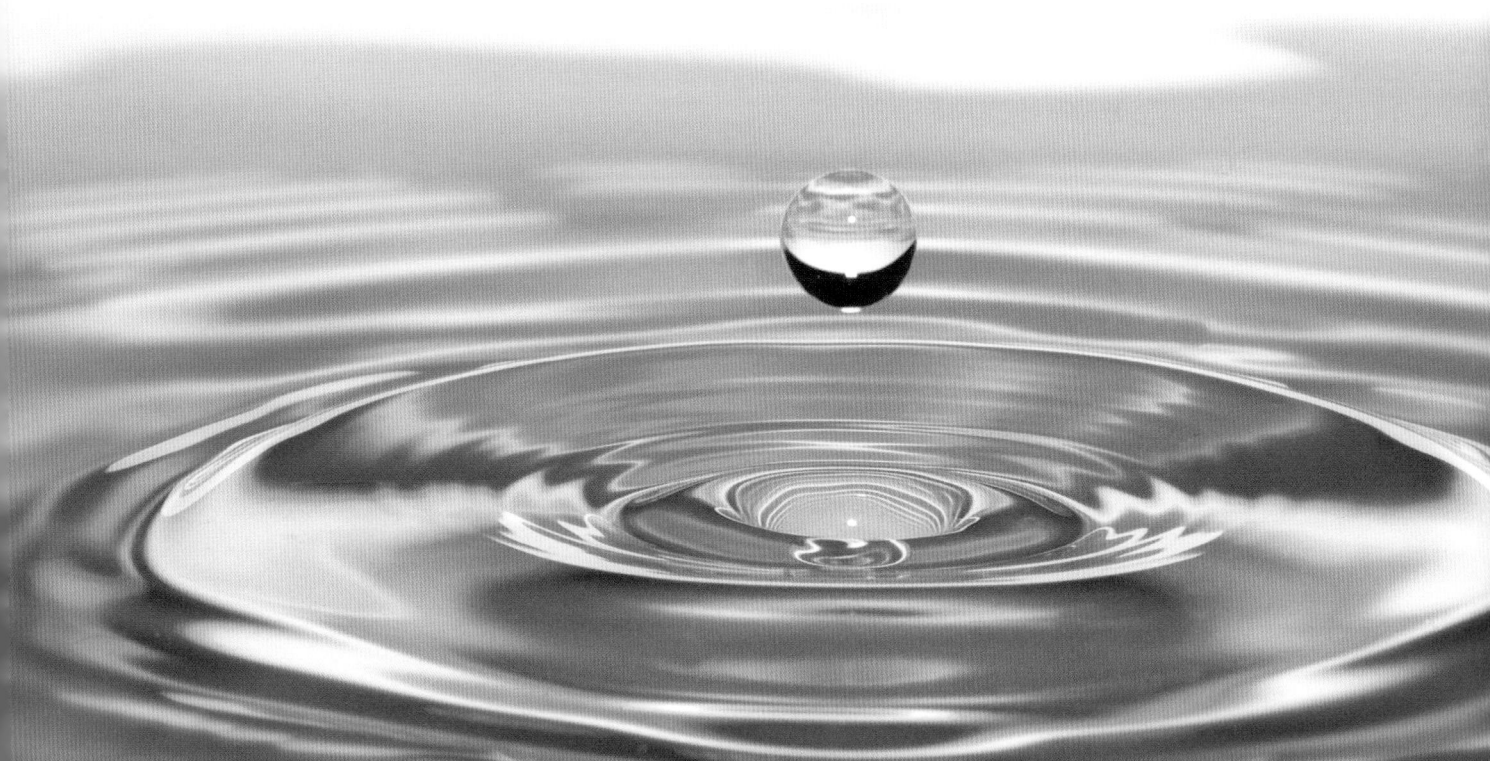

Time for action

There are so many different ways to cleanse, exfoliate and moisturise using natural ingredients, whether you need to act quickly or want to spend some time enjoying the process. The following chapters contain a selection of guidance and recipes. Experiment and find out what works with your skin.

You'll be able to get going right away with the options here, but to add endless potential and variety to your routines, you can use these basic formulas as a starting point and then substitute your own choice of herbs, plant seed oils and essential oils to suit your skin, your preference, or the ingredients available to you locally. Learn more about these in the chapters on vitality.

When changing recipes, remember to use softer, milder ingredients in products for your face, where skin can be more delicate than on your body. Also think about the scale of the area you'll be covering with the product. Faces, being smaller, need more precision treatment. It's good to use oils that don't stretch too far and are therefore more controllable. For body products it's great to use really long oils that can stretch along limbs. Our faces have a tiny amount of skin compared to our bodies so we can treat ourselves to more intense, expensive ingredients that would feel really costly to lavish all over our bodies.

Whenever you're trying something new, do it gradually, test a little area first and be patient. Look at the guidance on how to do a patch test (page 48), and also consider the thoughts at the end of Chapter 7 on transitioning to natural products.

The starter batch of recipes provided in the next chapters include ones you can whip up in an instant and use right away; as well as ones that take a little longer to prepare or use, or require some forethought. As you advance and want to learn and do more, use the guidance in Chapter 12 to know what you will need to do to blend and preserve your own natural products.

With all natural, homemade recipes, consider them as food for your skin and treat them as you would the food you make from fresh ingredients i.e. use them as you make them and store any leftovers in the fridge to use as soon as possible. Enjoy them while they're fresh. Make in small batches so you just have the quantity you need, that way you can try more recipes and sample them all at their best.

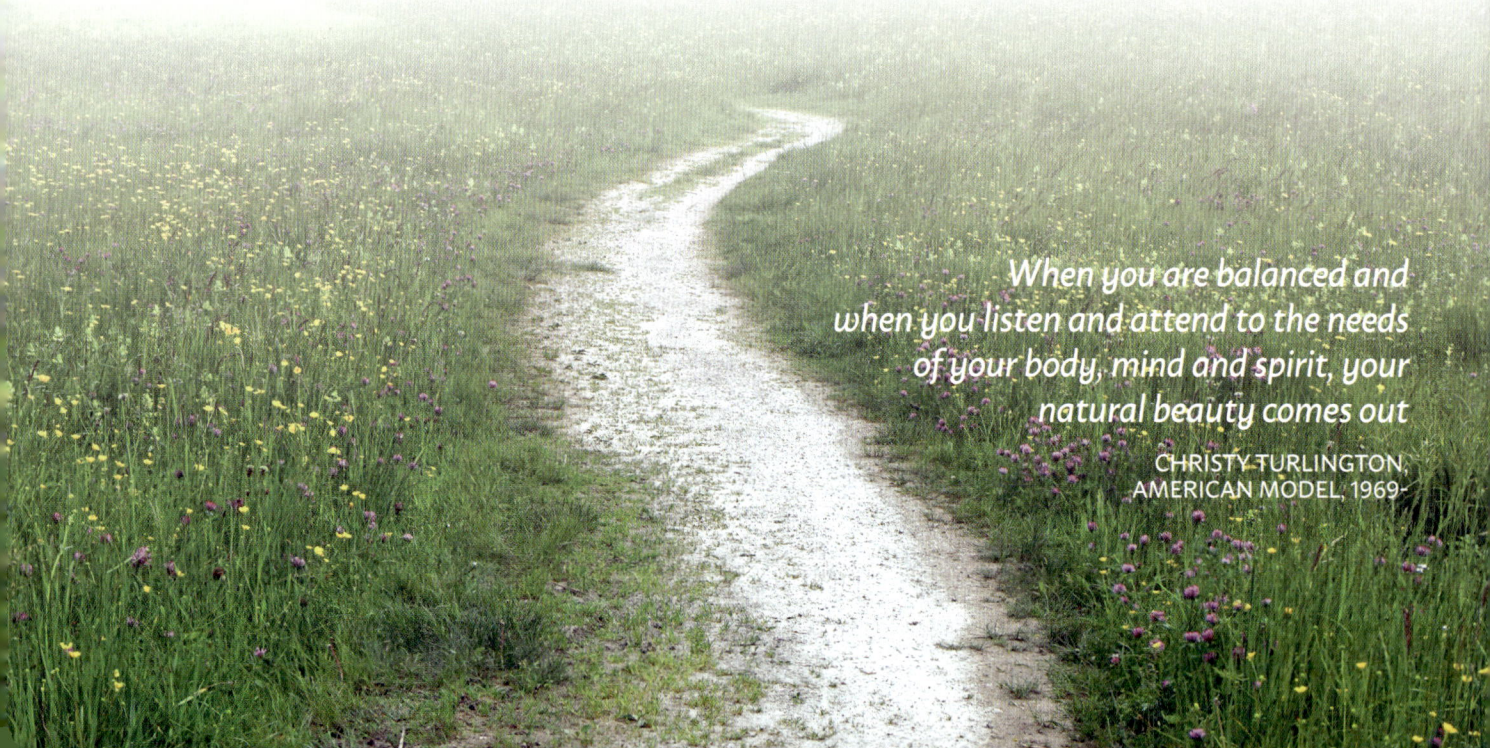

When you are balanced and when you listen and attend to the needs of your body, mind and spirit, your natural beauty comes out

CHRISTY TURLINGTON,
AMERICAN MODEL, 1969–

CHAPTER 9

cleansing

Cleansing needs to remove the daily build-up of dirt, grime and old cells from our skin. The best cleansers work alongside natural processes to do this, and enable our skin to perform at its best. It's a complex job with chemical and physical processes working together. A cleanser needs to be active enough to loosen dirt from pores; but still gentle enough to be used frequently without upsetting the delicate balance of our skin.

Why we need to cleanse

During the day, we emit sweat (with all its salts) and sebum. This coats our skin and can block our pores. It's also like a magnet to all the dirt particles in the air that will cling to our skin. This debris builds up, along with the products we add ourselves: from creams and deodorants to sprays and make up. The more we put on our skin, the more effort we should take to remove it. And the more polluted the environment we live in, the more attention we should pay to cleansing, even double-cleansing.

The better you cleanse your skin, the healthier it can be and the more effective whatever you put on top (your moisturisers, sun protection or makeup) can be. Your cleanser is therefore the most important thing in your skincare repertoire. It may only be on your skin for a short while, but its impact is great. With a little thought, the effort you put into cleansing can also provide nourishment, protection and support to your skin. It's something you do every day so it's worth taking a bit of time to understand what's involved and to make sure you're doing it right.

Factors to consider in choosing your cleansing products are:

- It's got to do a good cleansing job – sounds obvious, but worth stating, and by no means guaranteed with all commercial cleansers
- It should have minimal impact on your skin pH – quite a difficult thing to achieve as good cleansers are often alkaline, while our skin is acidic
- Ingredients should be present not just for minimal harm, but for maximum benefit
- It needs to be mild enough for daily use

Good cleansing requires both oil and water, so typically cleansers contain both.

Oil is critical as it combines with grease on the skin to dissolve it; water can't mix with oil in this way. Water is needed to dissolve dust and salts and wash away the loosened dirt and oil.

It is possible to clean with just oil – wiping it on and off again, taking the surface oils and dirt with it. However it's not possible to clean effectively with just water as it will not combine with the oils and lift them.

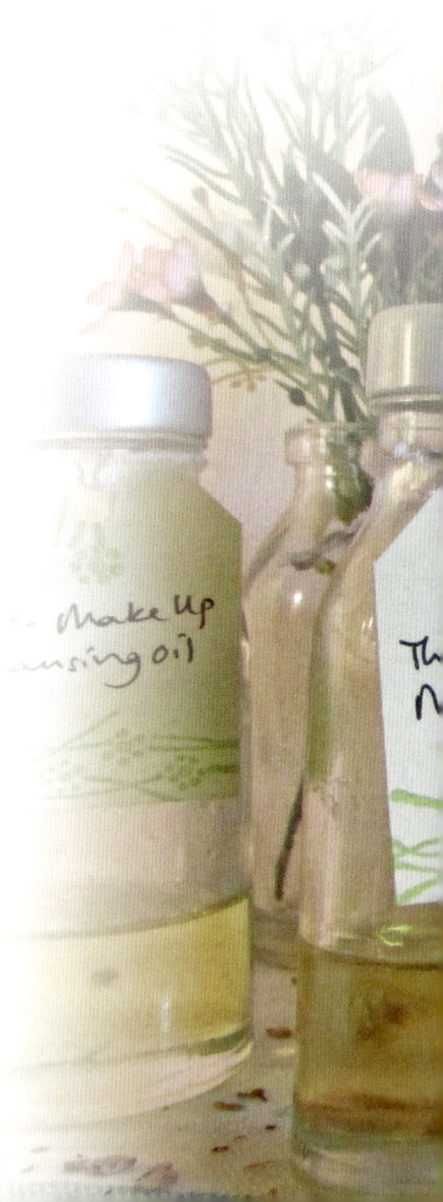

1. Oil cleansing

In a 'keep it simple' approach to skincare, oil cleansing can be one of the easiest approaches, especially if you want to make your own products. As this is now a 'trend' in skincare, a plethora of advice and techniques for it can be found online, but really it can be very straightforward.

Breakouts are often blamed on oily skin, making people nervous to use oil in cleansing. In reality, oil-free cleansers are potentially doing harm by stripping skin of its natural oils (which only encourages it to produce more). Using good, natural, plant-based oils in our cleansers can nourish skin and help it stay balanced. They can add antioxidants (to help combat signs of ageing) and vitamins; plus create even tone and smooth skin.

Oil cleansing is great for dry skin, but also perfectly good for oily skin (just use 'drier', less fatty oils).

Taking some care over your oil selection (maybe by blending your own combination of oils) can create a simple cleanser ideally suited to your skin. Look for things like their linoleic acid and oleic acid levels. Higher levels of the first are good for acne-prone skin, the latter for dry skin. You can also respond to the seasonal fluctuations in your skin by adjusting your blend accordingly.

Here are some examples of good oils to use. For more about plant seed oils, see Chapter 13.

For **Linoleic acid**: evening primrose oil (80%), thistle oil (75%), sunflower oil (70%), poppy seed oil (69%), walnut oil (60%).

For **Oleic acid**: sunflower oil (83%), carrot seed oil (80%), thistle oil (77%), hazelnut oil (75%), rapeseed oil (74%).

Soap makers have to be very conscious of the acid content of different oils so an online soap calculator website will often be a good place to find out about an oil you're interested in.

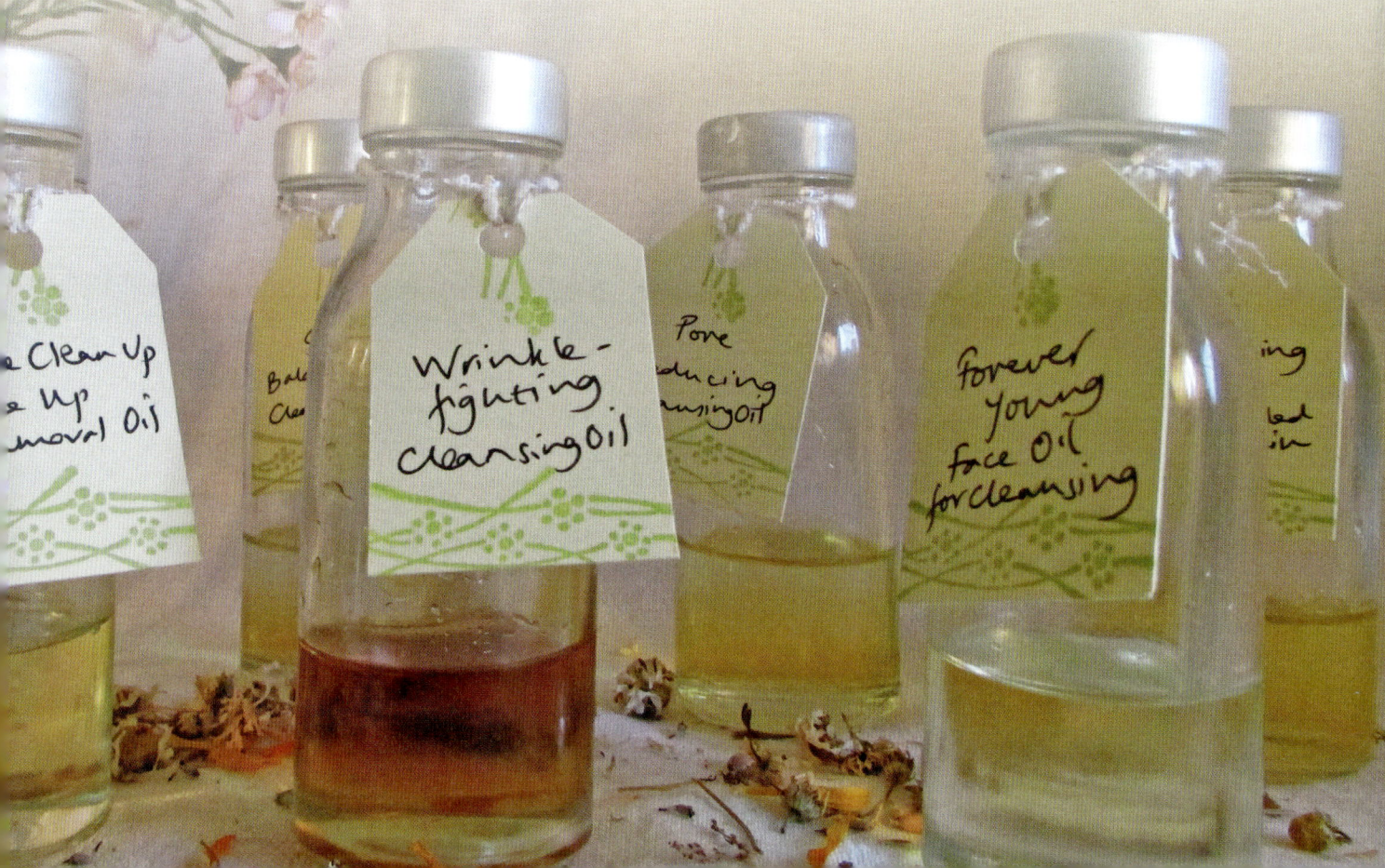

To make your own cleansing oil, start by selecting a base oil that you're happy with for your skin. Then experiment by adding supporting oils selected for their specific qualities. Making in very small quantities means you can adjust your blend to suit your skin on a regular basis.

Start with: 1 tbsp (15g) of **base** oil
and add: 1 tsp (5g) of your **supporting** oil

If there's a blend you use frequently, make it up in larger batches and store in a dark glass bottle.

Any of the oils can be macerated with further herbs to bring in their cleansing, reviving, toning, emollient, or other qualities. See Chapter 14 for how to do this.

You can also add a drop or two of your favourite essential oil to your facial cleansing oil blend for its therapeutic qualities and scent.

❋ Selecting your oils

Coconut oil, sweet almond oil and jojoba oil are 'go-to' oils for cleansing; sesame oil is seen in the Ayurvedic tradition as 'the' vegetable oil cleanser. Castor oil also has a reputation for drawing dirt to itself, making it a good inclusion in cleansers. All of these however, come from warmer climes. There are oils derived from plants that grow in temperate zones which can be just as kind and effective and, I believe, have better affinity with the skins of people living in a temperate climate.

On the opposite page is a collection of blends for facial oil cleansing based on temperate oils and herbs. Try using these, or create your own combinations.

❋ How to do oil cleansing

You can do basic oil cleansing by sweeping a single oil (for example, olive oil) over your face with one cloth or cotton pad, and then wiping away with a clean cloth. This was the way my mother cleaned her face daily, having been recommended to do so by a dermatologist following reactions to many substances. Her skin was fresh, soft, even and radiant.

If you've taken time to select and create a particular oil blend, it's worth making your application of it a calming mini-ritual:

- Pour a little oil into your palm and use your natural warmth to heat it
- Massage it gently into your skin
- Then put a hot flannel over your face letting the steam from this help draw out the dirt from the pores
- Wait until it has cooled then flip it over and wipe your face clean

If you prefer a creamier cleanser, this can be achieved by adding butters or waxes to the oil. Gently heat them to melt and combine together, then pour into a jar and leave them to cool and firm for a creamy consistency.

Massaging a nourishing oil into your skin and then wiping or washing it off removes dirt and leaves your skin helpfully moisturised. As oil has no pH level this cleansing method does not affect the pH of your skin. Do refer to the notes on toning (page 77), as you'll want to follow your oil cleansing with something hydrating.

'MAKE EVERY DAY SPECIAL' FACE OIL

Good for all skin types to use on a daily basis

BASE **Thistle oil**

High in vitamin F and linoleic acid, which makes it easy to absorb. Thistle oil is good for circulation, nourishing and helps reduce pore size.

SUPPORTING **Rosehip oil**

A treat that can be used on even the most delicate skin, it's absorbed quickly and will help reduce fine lines.

SKIN BALANCING FACE OIL

Good to bring oily skin back to normal

BASE **Thistle oil**

High in vitamin F and linoleic acid, which makes it easy to absorb. Thistle oil is good for circulation, nourishing and helps reduce pore size.

SUPPORTING **Hemp seed oil**

Great for balance and tone, softens by penetrating deeply, which helps sufferers of eczema, psoriasis and acne.

PORE REDUCING FACE OIL

Tightens pores to even skin tone and minimise infections

BASE **Sunflower oil**

Light and dry, this is easily absorbed and uplifting.

SUPPORTING **Hemp seed oil**

Great for balance and tone, softens by penetrating deeply, which helps sufferers of eczema, psoriasis and acne.

FACE OIL FOR TROUBLED SKIN

A kind, softening oil to encourage skin's natural restorative processes

BASE **Hazelnut oil**

Quickly absorbed without greasiness and instantly softening, this is toning, firming and encourages cell regeneration.

SUPPORTING **Hemp seed oil**

Great for balance and tone, softens by penetrating deeply, which helps sufferers of eczema, psoriasis and acne.

FOREVER YOUNG FACE OIL

Nourishing for mature and dry skins

BASE **Borage oil**

Moisturising, soothing, regenerating and revitalising.

SUPPORTING **Mullein oil**

Packed with vitamins, minerals, tannins and elastin to help defend against wrinkles and the elements.

WRINKLE-FIGHTING FACE OIL

Use regularly to combat signs of ageing

BASE **Camelina oil**

Hydrating and moisturising this is good for wrinkles and promoting skin elasticity.

SUPPORTING **Walnut oil**

Helps with skin regeneration, leaving skin soft and supple.

PRE MAKEUP FACE OIL

Prepare your face well to look your best

BASE **Camelina oil**

Hydrating and moisturising.

SUPPORTING **Broccoli seed oil**

Reduces greasiness while giving luminescence and glow.

'THISTLE CLEAN UP' MAKEUP REMOVAL OIL

Clean with ease and help your skin rest and revive

BASE **Thistle oil**

Meet like-with-like, thistle oil is burnt in the making of khol so great to deploy in makeup removal.

SUPPORTING **Comfrey oil**

Rejuvenating, healing and soothing to restore skin to normal at the end of the day.

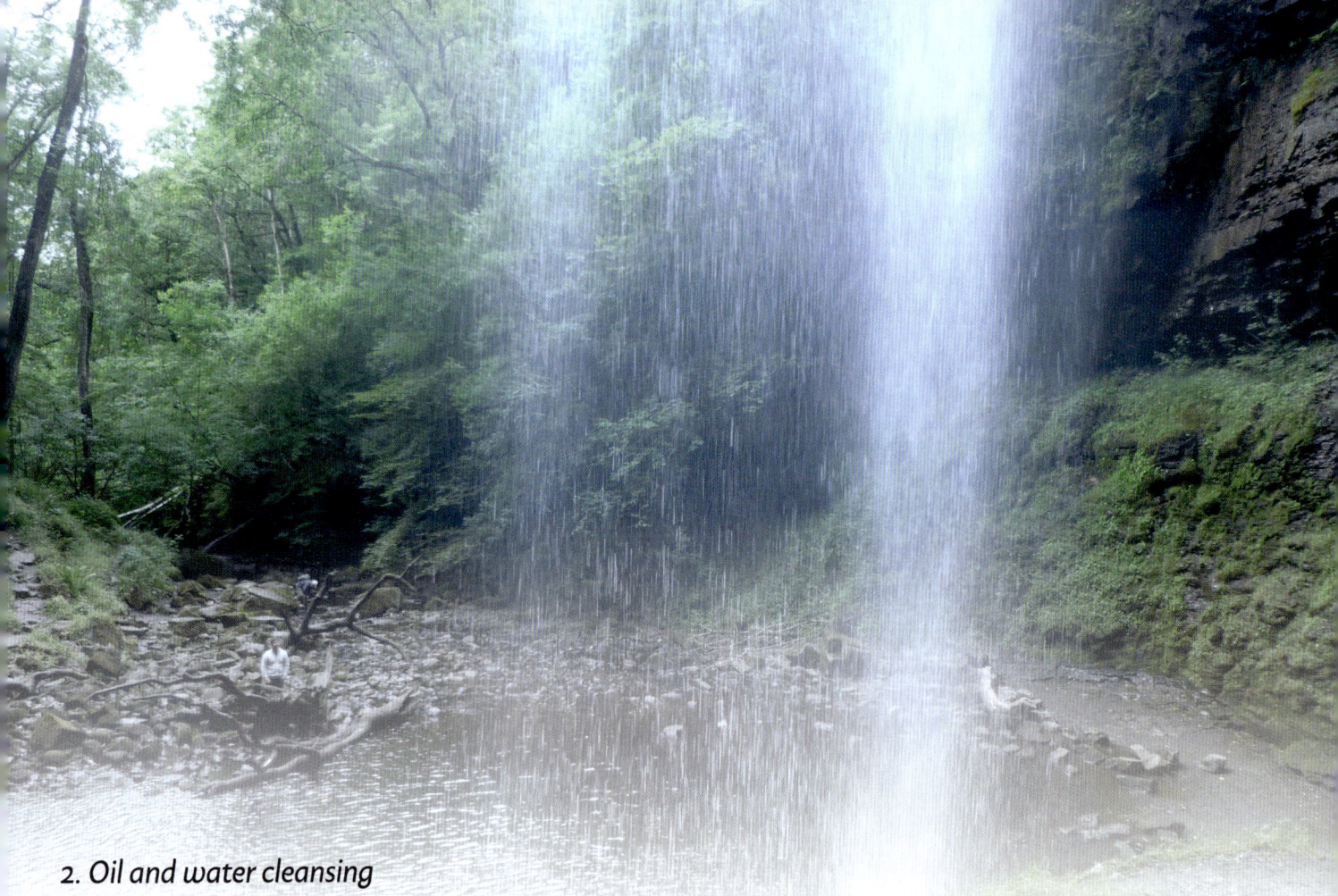

2. Oil and water cleansing

There is a psychological benefit to the fresh feeling we get from splashing water on our skin. We hold deep associations between water and cleansing: washing away. To be able to swoosh our dirt down the plug hole, we need to bring water into our cleansing products.

Oil and water cleansers will typically take the form of either a lotion (more water than oil) or a cream (more oil than water). A lotion is quicker to apply and splash off and can feel very refreshing; a cream takes more care and attention, especially to remove but it can clean deeper and also provide nourishment to the skin more effectively than a lotion. My preference is to use a quick fix, wake-up lotion in the morning and a gentle, calming cream in the evening.

Bringing water into our cleanser blends throws up two very important requirements:

1. Mastering the art of creating a stable emulsion, i.e. getting the oil and water to mix together.

A cleanser based on an emulsion has the benefit of both oil and water, a powerful duo. The closer a cleanser is to your own hydro-lipo (water-oil) balance, the more effective it is likely to be for you, which is one of the reasons cleansing is such a personal thing.

2. Protecting your product from mould and bacteria, which will form in just a few days in any product containing water.

There is advice on how to achieve each of these in Chapter 12 where we look at the chemistry of making skincare products, but here are a few simple approaches for freshly made cleansers combining oil and water.

Nero's wife bathed in asses' milk, as did Cleopatra.

Marie Antoinette used buttermilk compresses to subdue her freckles and lighten her sallow complexion.

Lily Langtry used Jersey cream to preserve her famous complexion.

❋ Cleansing milks

Milk is nature's perfect oil-in-water emulsion. It contains lactic acid that gently dissolves away dead cells and maintains natural pH, which makes cleansing milks a great quick-fix. You can use whatever milk you have in the fridge, purchase a particular milk for your skincare or make your own kinds of milks, such as rice milk, almond milk or buttermilk. Use the different milks interchangeably in the recipes to suit you. Typically, the oilier your skin the oilier the milk you should look for, which is why cream and buttermilk are great for oily skins while almond or skimmed milks can work well for drier skins.

The simplest cleansing lotion can be made by steeping your favourite flower petals, or herb to suit your skin, in a little milk.

Overleaf are some examples of milk and herb combinations to suit how your skin feels.

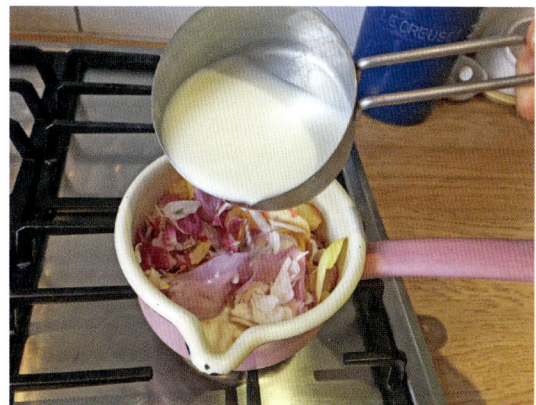

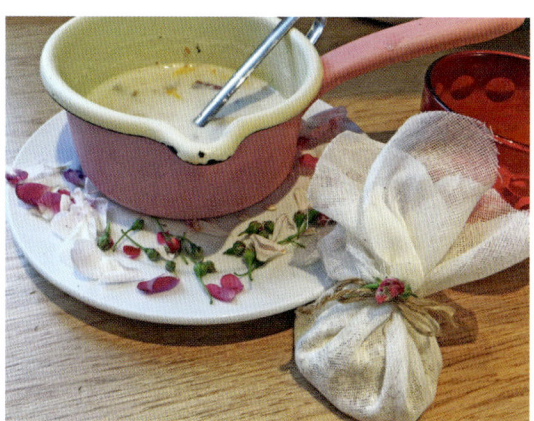

BASIC CLEANSING MILK

1 cup (237ml) milk
1 tsp (5g) of petals or leaves

MAKE Put the petals/leaves in small saucepan and pour over the milk. Leave to steep in the milk for about an hour before proceeding. Heat the milk until just boiling, then simmer for a minute before turning off the heat, covering and leaving to cool and infuse for 10 minutes. Strain off the herb and pour into a clean bottle, cap and label.

USE Wipe over your face using a cotton pad or washcloth and wash off with warm water. Alternatively, you can wrap a teaspoon of oats in a muslin, tie securely and use this to dip in the milk and wipe over your face.

STORE Keep your cleansing milk in the fridge and it should be good for a couple of days. As you make new supplies you can vary the flowers/herbs you incorporate to suit your skin.

ALMOND MILK CLEANSER FOR TIRED SKIN

To make your almond milk:

Put 50g ground almonds into a muslin bag, then place this into a bowl and pour over 150ml water.

Leave it to soak for a couple of hours, pressing occasionally with a spoon.

Lift the bag out of the water and squeeze dry. The liquid you now have is your almond milk.

(You can use the bag in the bath for scrubbing.)

Good herbs to include for tired skin: Lemon balm, spearmint.

BUTTERMILK CLEANSER FOR OILY SKIN

Buttermilk is the by-product of turning cream into butter. To make your own:

Take a large carton of fresh double cream and empty it into a bowl. Use a hand blender to whisk the cream, taking it beyond stiff whipped cream to curdling, and keep whisking. Solid clumps will form, which are butter. Once you can clearly distinguish the solid from the liquid, take out the butter and you're left with the buttermilk.

(You'll want to enjoy the creamiest, freshest butter, so continue preparing this by washing it in cold water. Continually replenish the water until it runs clear, then your butter is ready to form into pats. You can add salt if you choose. If you've made more than you need, you can freeze it.)

Good herbs to include for oily skin: Peppermint, sage, yarrow, nettle.

William Coles: "If Maids will take wilde Tansy and lay it to soak in Buttermilke for the space of nine dayes, and wash their faces therewith, it will make them look very faire."
The Art of Simpling, 1656

RICE MILK CLEANSER FOR DRY SKIN

While you can make your own rice water, this will have no fat in it. Bought rice milk typically has added thistle or rapeseed oil with the rice water. To replicate this, you can add oil to your own rice water, but it won't emulsify (see the shake-it-up lotion recipes on page 67).

To make your rice water:

Put a couple of handfuls of rice into a colander and rinse it well before putting into a saucepan and covering with water. Let it sit for about 15 minutes then drain off the rice, catching the liquid in a bowl – that's your rice water.

(Yes, you can then use the rice for cooking and eating as normal.)

Good herbs to include for dry skin: Elderflower, evening primrose.

OAT MILK CLEANSER FOR SENSITIVE SKIN

To make your oat milk:

Soak a cup (225g) of oats in water for at least 30 minutes (you can leave them overnight). Drain these, discarding the water and rinse them. Put the soaked oats in a blender with 4 cups (948ml) of clean water and blitz. Strain the liquid through a muslin cloth and you have your oat milk.

(You guessed it, the muslin full of squidgy oats can be tied – throwing in a few herbs while you're at it – and used in the bath. Alternatively, you can add the oats to a flapjack recipe, crumble topping or blend them into a smoothie.)

Good herbs to include for sensitive skin: calendula, evening primrose, rose.

Rice water has been used for thousands of years by the Japanese, and that's what they credit for their youthful, perfect complexion. Rice water contains beneficial skin properties such as vitamins B1, C, E, and minerals. These vitamins and minerals will cure acne, dark spots and scars, tighten and shrink pores, and prevent and erase wrinkles, fine lines, and crow's feet.

COW'S MILK CLEANSER FOR ALL SKINS

Feel free to substitute goats' milk, sheep's milk or whatever is your preference. Try to find full fat versions from herds that have been fed on grass.

Good herbs to include for all skins: Chamomile, calendula.

✻ Shake-it-up lotion

A 'cheat' approach to creating an oil and water blend is to cause enough friction by bashing the oil and water molecules together to temporarily combine them. The 'emulsion' you create will not be very strong, and you'll soon see the oil and water separating again, but it's handy for products you make quickly.

Use an oil with high lecithin content, such as sunflower or thistle oil, as this will help the emulsification.

Any of the cleansing milks above can be made with added oils. Add a tablespoon (15ml) of oil to one cup (237ml) of infused milk.

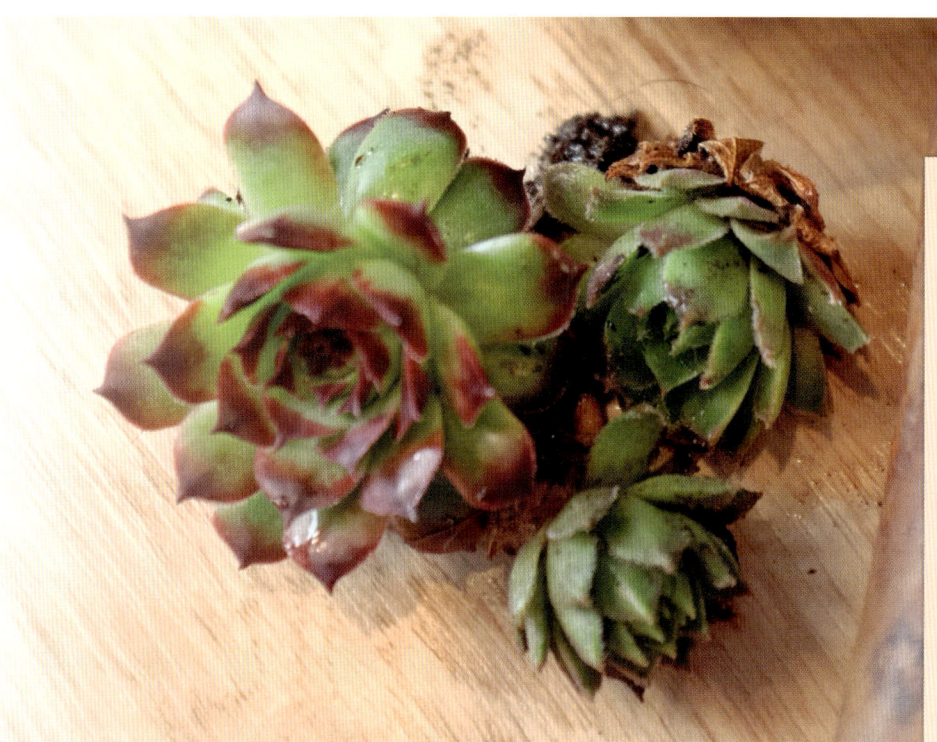

HOUSELEEK FACIAL CLEANSER

A great makeup remover, similar to the recipes known from Cleopatra's time. This has a lovely fresh scent from the houseleek and rosewater (rather like the freshness of sliced cucumber).

- 10 houseleek leaves
- 2 tsp (10ml) rosewater
- 1 tbsp (15ml) thistle oil (or olive oil, or sweet almond oil)

MAKE Combine all three ingredients in a blender. Blitz until you have a milky-looking green liquid. Then strain through a sieve and bottle.

USE Gently rub the cleanser into your skin, enjoying the fresh smell, then rinse away with warm water and pat dry.

STORE Keep your cleanser in the fridge and shake it before each use. It will last for about a week.

If you prefer a little foaminess in your cleansing routine, add about two teaspoons (10g) of grated natural soap to the blend, but stick to the basic ingredients if you have particularly dry skin.

You can make your own rosewater or substitute it for an infusion of chamomile, or use cooled green tea, which is a great skin cleanser.

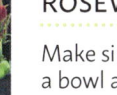

ROSEWATER

Make simple rosewater by putting a handful of rose petals into a bowl and bruising them slightly using the back of a spoon or the end of a rolling pin. Pour over ½ litre (1 pint) of boiling water then cover tightly and leave overnight. Strain through a coffee filter, being careful to remove all the petals. Bottle and keep in the fridge (or pour into an ice cube tray to freeze and defrost cubes as you need them).

For a more robust rosewater, see the 'flower waters' details in Chapter 14.

❋ Cream cleanser

Cream cleansers are beautifully nourishing to use. When making your own, unless you want to include preservatives, make in very small quantities that you can use within a week or so.

Here are some example recipes suited to dry and sensitive skin:

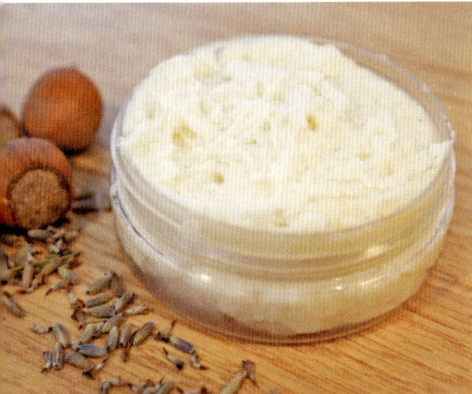

LAVENDER CLEANSING CREAM

Great for feeding and replenishing dry skin

- 2 tbsp (30ml) hazelnut oil
- 1 tbsp (15ml) sunflower oil
- 1 tbsp (15g) beeswax
- 1 tbsp (15ml) lavender water
- ½ tsp (2.5ml) witch hazel
- 1 drop lavender essential oil

MAKE Put the oil and wax into the top of a double boiler and gently heat until melted. Stir thoroughly and remove from the heat allowing it to cool slightly before whisking in the lavender water, witch hazel and essential oil. Careful, it can go lumpy as the cold ingredients are added, keep whisking until all is smooth and creamy.

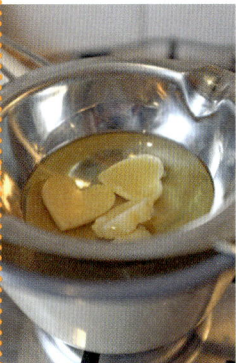

Oil and wax into double boiler

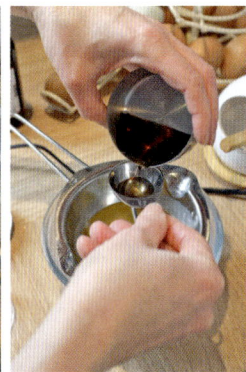

Stir in lavender water and witch hazel as cooling

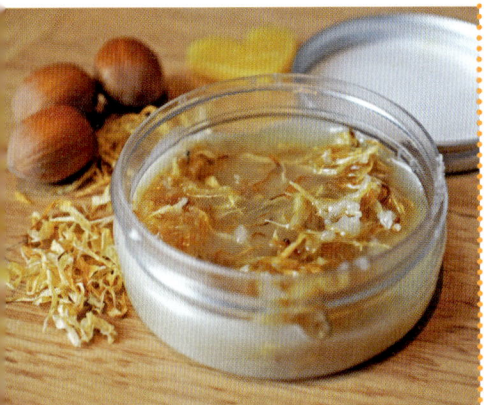

CALENDULA CLEANSING CREAM

For sensitive skin

- 1g dried calendula petals
- 1 tbsp (15ml) hazelnut oil
- 2 tsp (10ml) sunflower oil
- 5g beeswax
- 3g cocoa butter
- ½ tsp (2.5ml) witch hazel

MAKE Put calendula petals into the top of a double boiler and pour over the oils. Add the beeswax and butter and gently heat until melted, stirring with the spoon touching the base of the pan. When all has melted, turn off the heat and whisk in the witch hazel. Put in a sterilised jar and wait until it is fully cool before sealing and labelling.

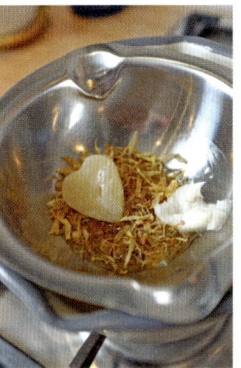

Calendula petals in double boiler

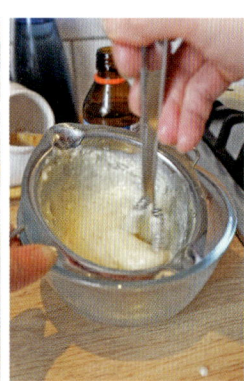

Stir in the witch hazel

For both these cleansing creams:

USE Dip a fresh washcloth into the pot to scoop up the cream and then smooth this over your face and neck. (It's best to use a cloth, rather than risk contaminating the product by putting your fingers in the pot.) Soak your washcloth in warm water then wring out and use to wipe off the cream. Moisturise within 90 seconds of cleansing.

STORE You'll be able to keep this for 2-3 weeks in the fridge.

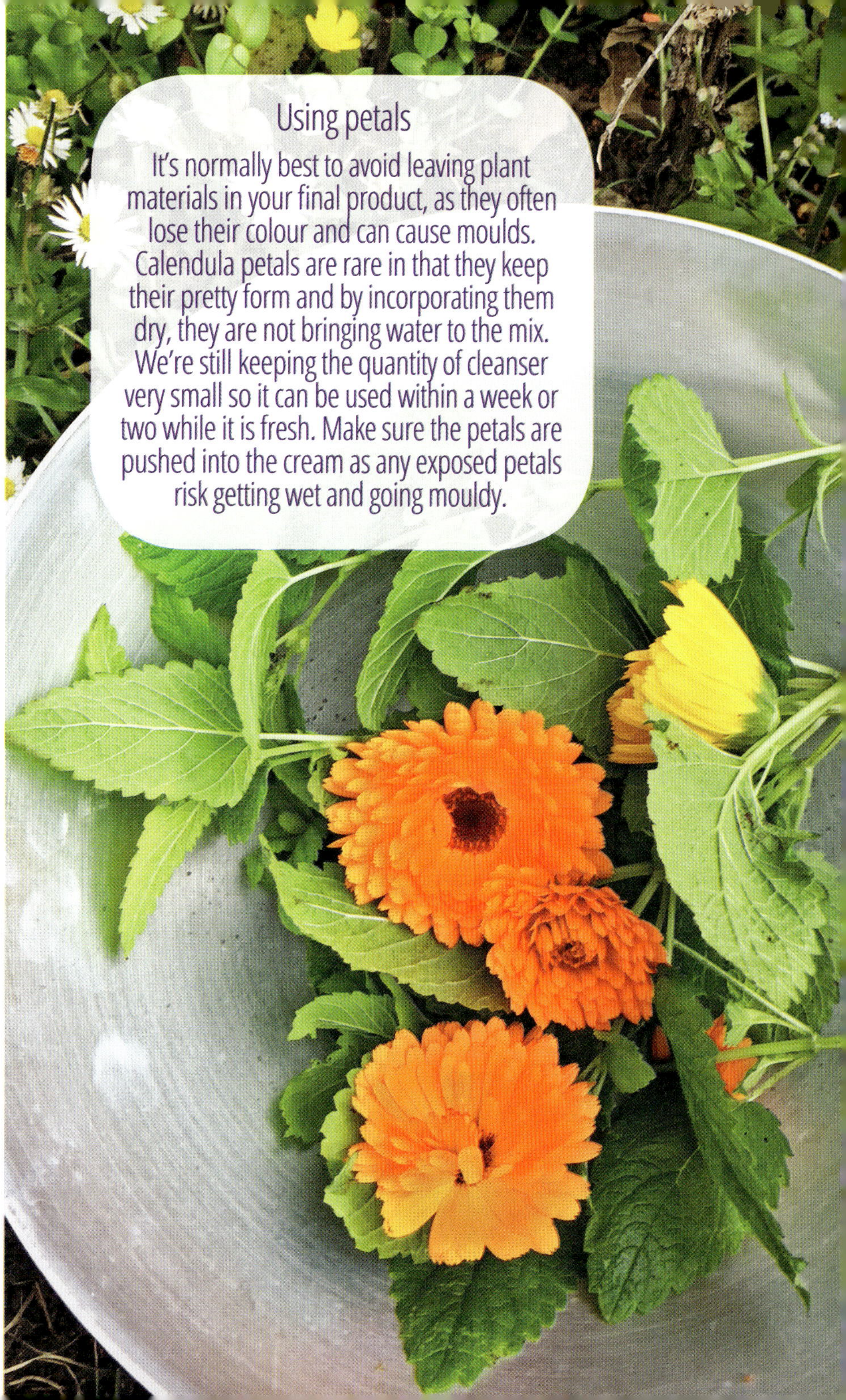

Using petals

It's normally best to avoid leaving plant materials in your final product, as they often lose their colour and can cause moulds. Calendula petals are rare in that they keep their pretty form and by incorporating them dry, they are not bringing water to the mix. We're still keeping the quantity of cleanser very small so it can be used within a week or two while it is fresh. Make sure the petals are pushed into the cream as any exposed petals risk getting wet and going mouldy.

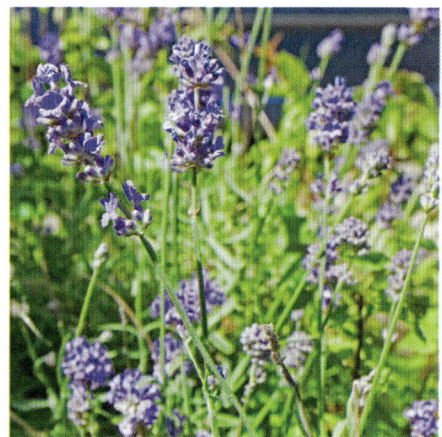

LAVENDER WATER

Make simple lavender water by infusing 1.5g of dried lavender flowers in 4 tbsp (60g) water. Bring to the boil, then simmer for 5 minutes before removing from the heat, allow to infuse for 20 minutes before straining off the lavender.

✻ Foaming cleansers

Foaming is not a necessary part of cleansing, but bubbles can play their part in encasing dirt to be washed away. To be effective the bubbles should be large enough to be able to grab hold of dirt, but not so large that they burst before being washed away (which would result in the dirt being dumped back on your skin). It's this delicate balance that makes foaming products tricky to make, and leads commercial manufacturers to often rely on sodium lauryl sulphates (SLSs), a known irritant which many people try to avoid in skincare.

If you enjoy the foamy feel, the simplest way to achieve it in your own products is by blending liquid castile soap with your skin loving oils. Here's a recipe you can try. Like the shake-it-up lotions it will separate in the bottle and need shaking before use. Keeping it in a pump-action dispenser is ideal (you can buy these online, or clean and reuse an old one). This is quite a concentrated recipe, so a little goes a long way. Don't keep this for more than a couple of weeks; discard and make fresh supplies.

GENTLE FOAMING CLEANSER

½ cup (120ml) water (omit this if using the homemade castile soap below which is less concentrated than bought castile soap)
¼ cup (60ml) liquid castile soap
10ml sunflower oil
10ml honey – this is an optional extra, nourishing and moisturising (it is humectant so helpfully draws in water to the skin) as well as antioxidant, antibacterial and skin-calming, so good in managing acne, blemishes and skin conditions. The sweetness also encourages foaming.

You can add up to 20 drops of essential oil to this. Good choices for cleansing and antibacterial properties are lavender, tea tree and rosemary.

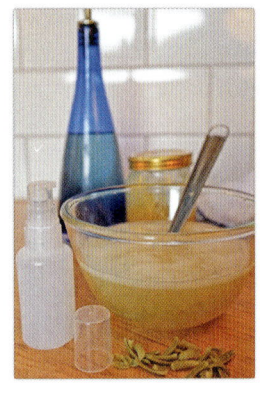
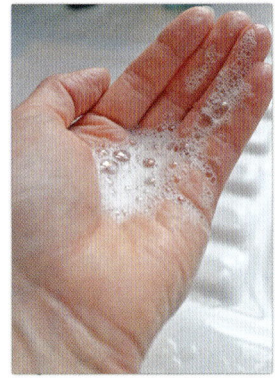

MAKE Put the water into a bowl and then add the castile soap and oil (be sure to do it in that order). Stir then add the honey and essential oils (if using) and make sure all is well combined. Transfer to a pump dispenser bottle.

USE First wet your face with warm water, then pump a little of the cleanser onto the palm of your hand and apply in small circles to your face. Splash off with more warm water.

STORE Keep this in the refrigerator and use within a week.

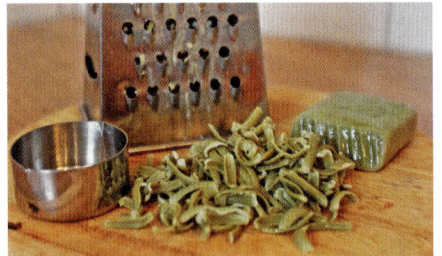

CASTILE SOAP

Traditionally, castile soap is made from pure olive oil. The liquid castile soap that you can buy is very concentrated.

If you can't find castile soap, you can make your own liquid soap by starting with the best quality natural soap you can find. Fill a ¼ cup (60ml) measure with gratings from your bar (it will probably use about ⅙ of the bar). Put this into a pan with 1½ cups (355ml) of water and heat gently until the soap dissolves (about five minutes). Switch off the heat and let it cool slowly (which could take up to four hours). Stir with a spoon or stick blender until very smooth and you're ready to use it in the recipe.

3. Soap

Making fresh skincare is a wonderful way to continually flex your products to suit your skin, but sometimes even the simplest recipes are difficult to achieve within a busy life, or when we're away from home.

A simple, long-lasting, easy-to-transport option for cleansing is a good, classic bar of soap. So why is it no longer our go-to cleanser? Soap has received bad press as it's considered to be drying, stripping the natural oils from our skin. You won't be surprised to know that this depends on the ingredients in the soap. While it's true that many of the soaps commonly available today have a list of harsh ingredients, soap itself, when made with good, enhancing ingredients, based on plant oils, can be a wonderful way to cleanse.

One of the major advantages of soap is its stability. A well made, patiently cured bar of soap can last for months in active use and is so easy to use, store and transport. There is a reason soap has endured for centuries – it works.

A caution with soap is making sure you manage your skin's pH. Soap is typically alkaline and therefore skin can need speedy rebalancing after cleansing. When using soap, always be ready with an acidic toner for afterwards to correct that balance as soon as possible. Unless you take action, it can take hours for skin to rebalance itself, and all that time your natural protective barriers are not at their most effective.

At its simplest, soap is made from just three ingredients: oil, water and sodium hydroxide. The critical cleansing ingredients of oil and water are there, but instead of relying on emulsification to combine them we have the magical process of saponification by which the oil and water combine through the introduction of sodium hydroxide.

It's one of the wonders of chemistry that sodium hydroxide – otherwise known as caustic soda – can be truly damaging in its raw form (extreme care must be taken to protect eyes and skin when handling it to avoid burns). But when combined with oils, the saponification process eliminates the caustic nature and leaves just the cleansing properties.

Making soap is a delicate business requiring accuracy in calculating and measuring the required quantity of ingredients. Each oil has its own saponification rate that enables you to calculate how much caustic soda to add. The amount of water used to dissolve the caustic soda (forming a solution known as 'lye') is related to the total weight of the oils in the recipe. If you're contemplating embarking on the wonderful process of making your own soap, you will need to research first about the oils you'd like to use and then find a soap calculator that will enable you to get the quantities right. There are a number of these available online. It's not as simple to blend your own, but offers so much scope for personalisation and creativity once you get the hang of the basic process.

Variety comes from the ingredients that can be included, the moulds you use to shape the soap and embellishments like swirling techniques, layering and decorating. For ingredients, there's the choice of different plant oils and butters, as well as herbs, essential oils and other healing, stimulating or calming ingredients. While there is little point using anything more 'special' than plain water to combine with the sodium hydroxide – so delicate rosewaters or herbal infusions would be wasted at this stage – it is possible to replace the water with other liquids. Milk is particularly popular for this but you could also use fruit or vegetable pulps or teas and coffees. All it takes is a little imagination to think what you want your ultimate bar to do, to feel like, look and smell like, plus a willingness to experiment. Some ingredients can create unexpected results, which of course is part of the fun and learning. Keep making notes of your ideas, trials and discoveries. Lots of advice is available online if you fancy getting into this.

Good soaps have a combination of ingredients to balance cleansing with moisturising and to create the right kind of foam. How you like your bar is a personal preference so it's worth looking out for ones that have the right balance for you, or mastering the art of creating your own perfect bar of soap.

4. Clay cleansers

Clay is fantastic for your skin. It is healing, cleansing and refreshing. Clay can draw out impurities and toxins through adsorption (its ability to attract impurities and toxins due to its electro negative charge) and hold them through absorption (the ability to penetrate a liquid or solid and form a transitional zone) so when we take the clay away, it takes the impurities and toxins with it.

This makes clay a wonderful ingredient for cleansing. It can be used on its own (mixed into a paste with water, infusions or oils) or incorporated into other products such as soaps, shampoos and cleansers, where it may be blended with herbs, fruit or vegetable juice, extracts or plant oils.

There are many different clays, from all over the world. They form where there has been volcanic activity and the local conditions affect the properties and mineral composition of the clay. This means there are great clays for every skin type and condition, many benefits that can be derived and many applications they can be put to.

Some clays, such as bentonite, have antibacterial properties making them great for acne-prone skin. Green clay is good for oily skin, while white clay (also called kaolin) is very gentle and suitable for sensitive, dry and mature skin. Pink clays can also be used on sensitive skin while red clays are good for facials as an efficient purifying mask. Normal and oily skin is good with yellow or green clays (which have stronger absorption qualities). French green clay is particularly absorbing and has a good, fine texture for use on the face. Mature skin also benefits from French green clay as it tightens pores, boosts circulation, reduces inflammation and evens skin tone.

Medically clay is antiseptic, anti-inflammatory and can promote healing. Cosmetically clay is an emollient, softening and soothing for the skin, and improves skin's texture. It's also a refrigerant, cooling and reducing body heat.

Clays are only active when wet which means they store well, but need to be kept moist while on your skin. You can manage this by spritzing with hydrating toners.

When working with clays, don't use metal containers or utensils; instead use glass, plastic or wood.

Here are three different ways to incorporate clays into your cleansing repertoire:

Cleansing masks
Cleansing powders
Cleansing bars

Clay cleansing masks

BASIC FACE MASK

1 tbsp (15g) clay powder
(white, pink, yellow or green for face;
don't use bentonite or rhassoul)
2 tsp (10g) warm water
1 tsp (5g) raw honey (optional)
2 drops essential oil (optional, e.g. lavender)

MAKE Mix all ingredients together in a small bowl

USE Apply the mask as soon as it's mixed, avoiding around your eyes. Leave for 15-20 minutes (hydrating periodically by spritzing), then wash off with warm water, dry face and apply a moisturiser. This can be repeated weekly, blending a new mix each time.

The following variations on this basic face mask enable you to tailor the mask to your needs by incorporating herbs in an infusion and adding further beneficial ingredients to suit your skin condition. (There are more details on how to make herbal infusions in Chapter 14).

FOR OILY OR ACNE-PRONE SKIN

1 tbsp (15g) clay
2 tsp (10ml) yarrow infusion
1 tsp (5ml) honey

FOR MATURE SKIN

1 tbsp (15g) clay
2 tsp (10ml) fennel infusion
1 tsp (5ml) honey

FOR ALL SKINS

1 tbsp (15g) clay
2 tsp (10ml) lavender and limeflower infusion
1 tsp (5g) witch hazel

FOR DRY SKIN

1 tbsp (15g) clay
2 tsp (10ml) marshmallow and comfrey infusion
1 tsp (5ml) borage oil

(Borage oil doesn't smell great so this is one combination that you'll probably want to add some essential oils to. Frankincense, geranium and lavender all work well with dry skin.)

As you experiment with masks to suit your skin, you could try adding other beneficial ingredients. Suggestions include:

Ingredient	Benefit	Quantity to add
Salt e.g. Epsom salts, Himalayan salt or table salt	Helps soften skin	About 15% of the clay amount or ratio 1:6 i.e. 2.5g salt to 15g clay
Herbs e.g. chamomile, lavender or calendula	For qualities of different herbs see Chapter 15	About 2% of the clay amount, or ratio 1:50 i.e. 0.3g herb to 15g clay
Emollient plant seed oils e.g. hazelnut oil	To stop the mask being too drying	About 30% the quantity of clay, or ratio 1:3 i.e. 5g oil to 15g clay
Essential oils	For the scent and therapeutic benefits of the oil you choose	A few drops

STORE Once you've found the combination of clays, herbs and essential oils that work for you, make a jar full of the dry ingredients and then use it a spoon at a time, mixing in the water or infusion as you use it.

❈ Clay cleansing powders

Ready-made clay cleansers are starting to appear on the market as 'cleansing powders'. They might have a combination of ingredients including powdered aloe, rice bran, pulverised pearls, and other earth ingredients, including herbs, salts and spices, but many are simple one-ingredient formulas: e.g. just Moroccan clay. These make versatile cleansers, and many of them are gentle enough to use daily.

They're simple to use as you can blend them in your palm: put a teaspoonful of the powder in your hand and then add a few drops of warm water before rubbing your palms together. You can keep adding drops of water until it feels right, and you'll soon figure out how you like it and you can vary it by incorporating more water on days when cleansing is all you need, less water for a grainier product on days when your skin could benefit from exfoliation as you cleanse.

For an even gentler and skin-feeding cleanser, you can add a drop or two of oil in with your paste.

❈ Cleansing bars

A lovely way to combine oil and clay cleansing in a simple, easy-to-travel-with form.

SKIN-SMOOTHING CLAY CLEANSING BAR

- 2 tsp (10g) kaolin
- 3 tsp (15g) cocoa butter (best to use cocoa butter for the firmest results)
- ½ tsp (2.5ml) rapeseed oil
- ½ tsp (2.5ml) pumpkin seed oil
- 1 or 2 drops essential oil (optional)

MAKE Put the rapeseed oil and butter into the top of a double boiler. Heat gently until they are melted, stirring them together. Remove from the heat, add the pumpkin seed oil and essential oil (if using) and allow to cool a little but while still liquid, whisk in the clay and quickly pour into a mould. Place in the fridge until it is firm (you're doing this quickly to give the clay minimal chance to sink to the bottom of the mould). Check after an hour to see if it has set firm; if not leave it a little longer. Once it's really firm, place a towel on your work surface and turn your bar out of the mould onto the towel.

USE Cut a small piece off the bar and take it with you to the bath or shower (it will melt quite quickly in your hand). Rub this all over your body, as you would soap, and then rinse well with water.

STORE Keep this in an airtight container in the fridge and break off pieces as you want to use them. It will keep for up to six months. The quantity in this recipe makes up enough for 2-3 uses so multiply up if you want batches to store. Making a little at a time gives you a chance to try different essential oil combinations and to use your bars fresh.

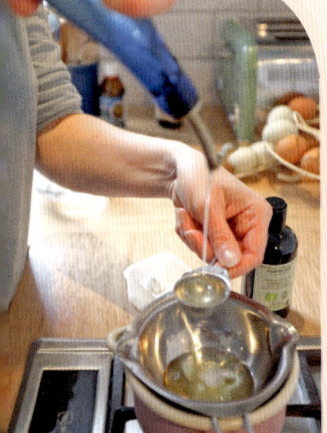
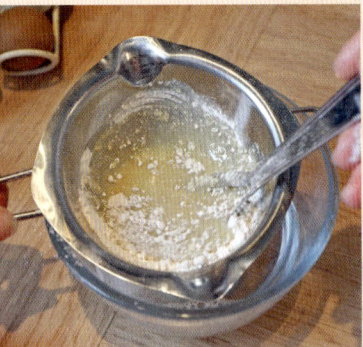
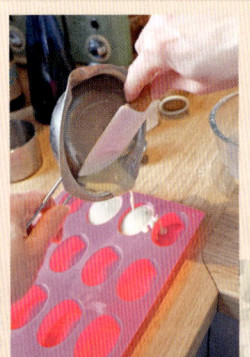

5. Oat Cleansers

Good for dry skin in particular, oats are a great alternative to soap. They are also helpful for those prone to acne. With their anti-inflammatory nature, oats are good if you suffer from redness or sore, irritable skin.

Here are two different cleansers made by combining oats with other dry ingredients. They're very simple to make and, because you only add water as you use them, you can make them in bulk and store them dry.

OATS SO SIMPLE CLEANSER

1 tbsp (15g) oats
1 tbsp (15g) dried milk

THREE IN ONE CLEANSER

1 tbsp (15g) oats
1 tbsp (15g) clay powder
1 tbsp dried herbs
Good herbs for cleansing include: Calendula, comfrey, elderflower, peppermint, sage and yarrow.

MAKE Put the ingredients into a jar, cap tightly and then shake to thoroughly combine them.

USE Put a small amount on the palm of your hand and mix with water to form a paste. You can add a few drops of oil too. Rub all over your face and neck and then rinse off with warm water.

STORE Keep in an airtight jar and store in a dry place. It will keep for about a year.

6. Cleansing masks

Cleansing masks are a relaxing way to gently draw impurities from your skin. It's worth giving over half an hour of your life at least once a month to relax and let the power of herbs do their work. We've already looked at clay masks, but there are a few other ways to benefit from an intense mask treatment using herbs.

HERBAL HEALTH MASK

Refreshing greens for your skin

2 tsp (10g) oatmeal
1 handful each of parsley, watercress and spinach

MAKE Chop the greens and put them in a pan with a cup of water. Bring this to the boil and then cover and leave to cool. Pass this through a sieve, pressing to extract all the juice. Blend your extracted green water into the oatmeal, adding a little at a time, to create a paste.

USE Apply to your face (avoiding eyes) then lie back and relax for 10-20 minutes before rinsing off with warm water and moisturising.

SEAWEED CLEANSING MASK

To open pores and cleanse skin

3 tbsp (45g) natural yoghurt
1 tbsp dried seaweed
1 tsp (5ml) honey

MAKE Mix all the ingredients together into a smooth paste.

USE Apply to your face (avoiding eyes) then lie back and relax for 5-10 minutes before rinsing off with warm water and toning.

SWEET LEAF MASK

To help reduce fine lines

6-8 lady's mantle leaves
1 tsp (5g) sugar
1 cup (237ml) rosewater (see page 67 for how to make rosewater)

MAKE Put the rosewater into a pan with the sugar and heat gently until almost boiling, stirring to dissolve the sugar. Put the lady's mantle leaves into a small bowl and pour over the hot rosewater. Leave these to soak as the rosewater cools.

USE When soft, arrange the leaves over your face. Lie down for at least 20 minutes. Then remove the leaves and tone with the rosewater.

7. Steam cleansing

Steam cleansing is an ancient means to really open up pores and enable all dirt and grease to be dislodged and removed.

Steaming isn't recommended if you have thread veins.

MAKE Gather 25g of dried herbs chosen to suit your needs, or 50g of fresh herbs (see Chapter 15 for herb suggestions). Put your herbs into a bowl and cover with 2 litres of boiling water.

USE Hanging your head over the bowl, cover your head with a towel and wrap it around the bowl to trap in the steam. Make sure you keep your face well above the hot water. Breathe deeply and calmly as you feel the steam penetrating your pores. Stay there for about 10 minutes, or as long as feels comfortable for you. Afterwards, rinse, pat dry, and spray with a toner.

8. Cleansing water

Earlier we recognised that you can't clean with water alone. However, cleansing waters have become popular recently, often marketed as micellar waters. These are not really new products, they were available before we had in-house plumbing, but they've become popular again as an all-in-one cleanser, makeup remover and moisturiser. Really useful when you haven't got access to water, such as when travelling or camping.

What makes these waters special is the addition of tiny balls (micelles) of oil. They also use very pure water and often have other supporting ingredients. The overall effect is a product that looks and behaves like water, but feels more velvety. It is very simple to make a basic cleansing water yourself. Create just a small amount and refresh every few days.

a note on cleansing wipes

It may be handy to have a pack of facial wipes in your bag for when you're travelling, but do restrict them to that occasional use and don't make them a staple in your cleansing routine. At worst all they do is smear the dirt and bacteria around your face. Even if they're effective at lifting dirt, you'll still need to wash with water (or spritz or tone) to remove the residue of the cleansing cloth ingredients. But also, they are often not biodegradable.

CLEANSING WATER

¼ cup (60ml) rose hydrosol, or rosewater
0.6ml glycerine
0.6ml thistle oil (containing useful amounts of lecithin, a help emulsifier, although the product will not fully emulsify)
0.6ml liquid soap

MAKE Put the hydrosol into a heat-proof beaker and add the other ingredients. Place the beaker into a pan of hot water to gently heat. Stir well then remove from the pan. Allow to cool a little and pour into a sterilised glass bottle. Seal and label.

USE Pour the water onto cotton wool, or a cleansing pad. Squeeze out any excess and wipe over your face, sweeping gently and avoiding rubbing. There's no need to rinse.

STORE Freshly made cleansing water will last a few days in the fridge. Make a new batch as needed or freeze extra supplies in an ice cube tray and defrost a cube at a time.

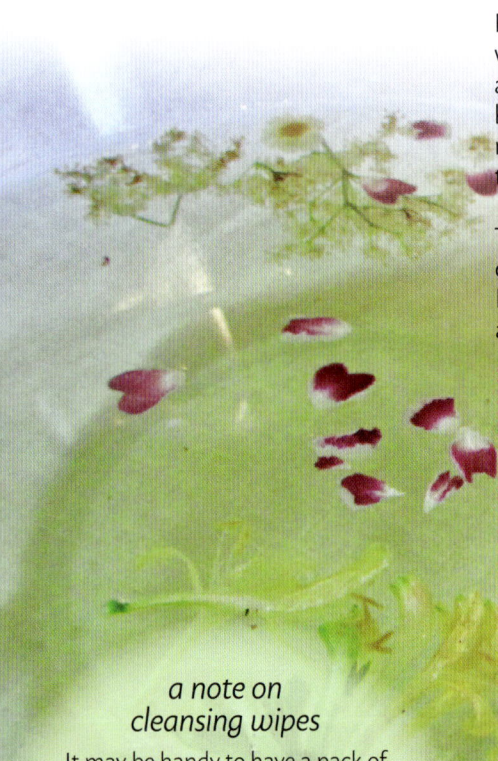
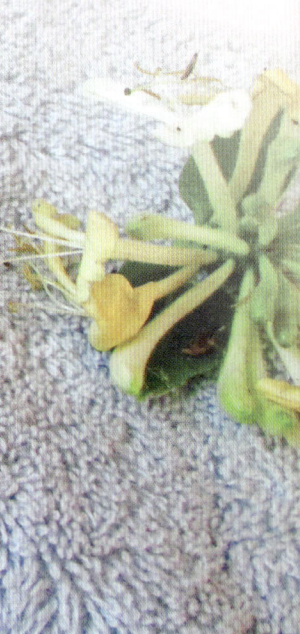

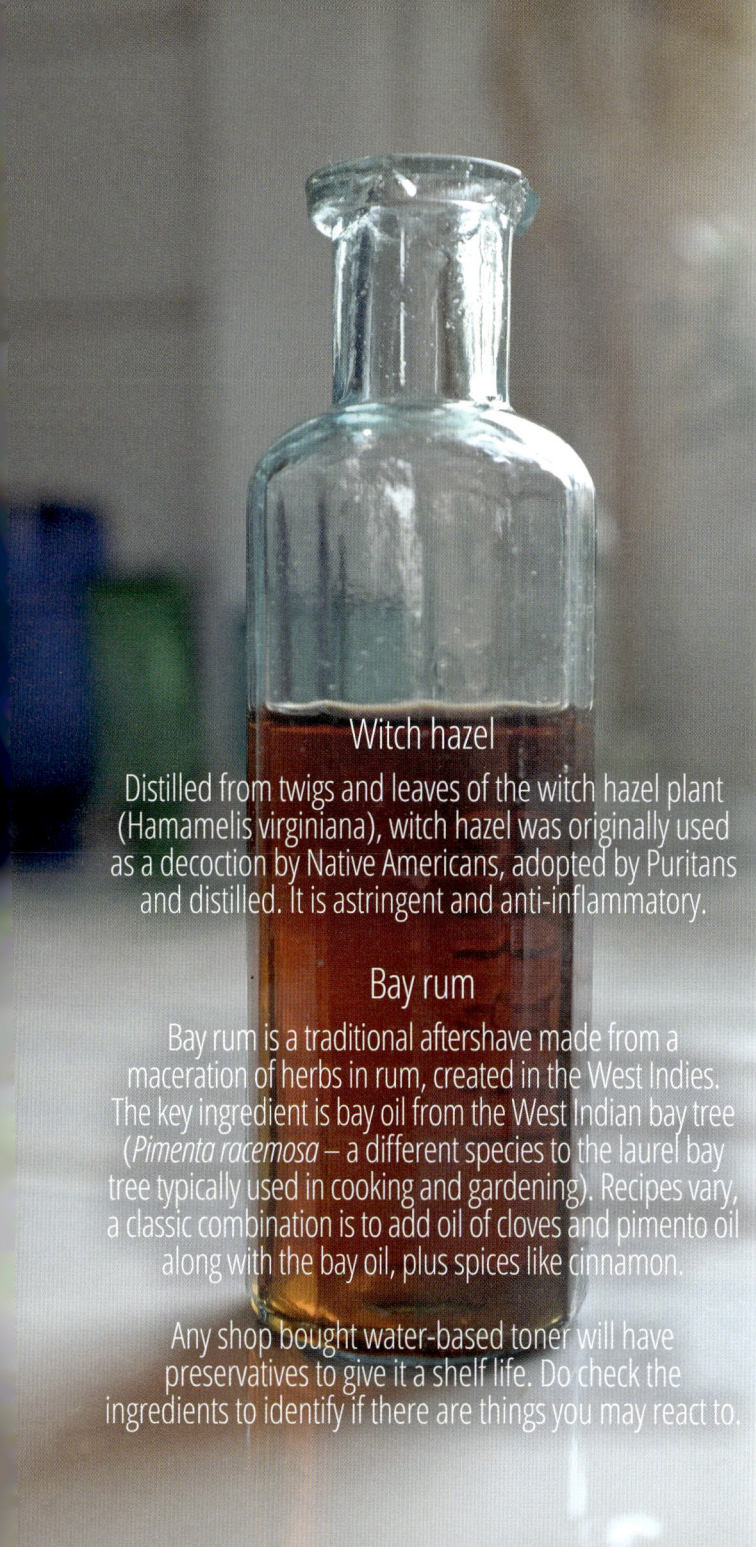

Witch hazel

Distilled from twigs and leaves of the witch hazel plant (Hamamelis virginiana), witch hazel was originally used as a decoction by Native Americans, adopted by Puritans and distilled. It is astringent and anti-inflammatory.

Bay rum

Bay rum is a traditional aftershave made from a maceration of herbs in rum, created in the West Indies. The key ingredient is bay oil from the West Indian bay tree (*Pimenta racemosa* – a different species to the laurel bay tree typically used in cooking and gardening). Recipes vary, a classic combination is to add oil of cloves and pimento oil along with the bay oil, plus spices like cinnamon.

Any shop bought water-based toner will have preservatives to give it a shelf life. Do check the ingredients to identify if there are things you may react to.

Toners

Toning should be a critical part of your cleansing routine. It's not enough to just clean away the dirt if you want to leave your skin in the best condition for its next few hours of protective work, or if you're preparing it for receiving the next product (a moisturiser, serum, sun protection or makeup).

Your toner performs three tasks: rebalancing, hydrating and conditioning your skin.

1. Rebalancing the pH of your skin

Skin's natural and best state is a pH of about 5.5, that slightly acidic environment that's good for protecting against bacteria. Often the products with good cleansing properties are alkaline (pH of above 7) so after cleansing, a toner will make the correction. For this purpose, toners need to be acidic. Many toners are therefore based on witch hazel, which has a pH of 3. A 50:50 witch hazel and water toner has a pH of 5, which is just about perfect to rebalance our skin. Other popular ingredients in natural toners are apple cider vinegar (ACV) and lemon juice, both of these are very acidic so need to be diluted with water at about 1:4.

Witch hazel is also a popular ingredient in many aftershaves. Here it is incorporated mainly for its antiseptic properties, as it is useful to counteract any grazed or nicked skin. The right aftershaves will also include ingredients that provide and lock in moisture and soothe chaffed skin.

Alcohol was a popular ingredient in commercial toners and aftershaves for its natural preservative and antibacterial properties. This is why the correct process for applying aftershave involves splashing it on the hands, rubbing them together to mix the ingredients and create a little heat and then, crucially, opening up the palms to allow some of the alcohol to evaporate, thereby reducing the burning sensation. Alcohol has a drying impact on skin that can lead to unhelpfully exaggerated sebum production, so is often avoided now. Its pH is just above neutral, meaning it's not as helpful as witch hazel in restoring the acid mantle.

You can avoid alcohol and preservatives altogether by using freshly made toners, keeping them in the fridge for no more than a few days. Given how simple they can be to make, this is an easier solution than you may think. I look forward to the day when a small fridge is standard in most bathrooms!

CLEANSING 77

2. Hydrating your skin

The more we rely on oil for cleansing, the less water reaches our faces, so we can use a toner to hydrate our skin. Oil can soften and provide nourishment for skin, but it doesn't hydrate. Drinking water is good for our skin in that it will help our bodies flush out toxins (and if they're not flushed out they could look for alternative routes which can mean open pores become spots) but it will not hydrate skin – water will go to service other organs before skin gets a look in. Therefore, for our skin to be hydrated, we need to apply water topically.

Hydrated skin is softer and more permeable, which means any products you apply to well-hydrated skin can be more effective.

Hydrating toners are different in nature to their pH-balancing sisters, often created with other properties in mind such as their vitamin and mineral content. For hydration, flower or herbal waters can be gentle, refreshing and clarifying. There's a wide choice of fragrant waters from rose, orange flower, elderflower, cucumber, lavender, parsley, mint. Making your own, you can select the herbs that best suit your skin.

There are several ways to make flower waters:

- ⇨ The simplest are infusions of herbs in water (details of how to do this are in Chapter 14).
- ⇨ Bought flower waters are often made by first creating a tincture of the active ingredient and then diluting that with water to make a suitable strength toner, incorporating a solubiliser or dispersant to achieve an even blend.
- ⇨ A luxurious form of flower water known as hydrosols are becoming increasingly popular. These are actually the by-product of the distillation process used to make essential oils. During distillation, steam is forced at pressure over the plant material that draws the volatile oils from the plant. It is then condensed and as the resulting water is collected, oil will float on the top. The oil is collected and bottled as essential oil; the remaining water is our prized hydrosol – pure water totally impregnated with the plant.

The three classic hydrosols are softening rosewater (good for mature and sensitive skin), astringent orange flower water (good for oily and dull skin) and uplifting lavender flower water (good for oily and blemished skin). Bottled witch hazel is itself a hydrosol.

3. Conditioning skin

The refreshing splash of a toner helps tighten skin, close pores and create a more even skin texture. Many are astringent, which makes them helpful in managing sebum in oily skins.

Good astringent herbs to use in toners include rose, lavender, thyme, myrtle, lemon balm, lemon verbena, calendula, chamomile, lady's mantle, chervil, parsley, sage, cornflower, yarrow, fennel, honeysuckle, ivy and walnut leaf.

You don't have to restrict their use to just after cleansing; anytime your skin needs a pick you up, reach for the toner. Putting it into a spray bottle makes it easy to apply throughout the day.

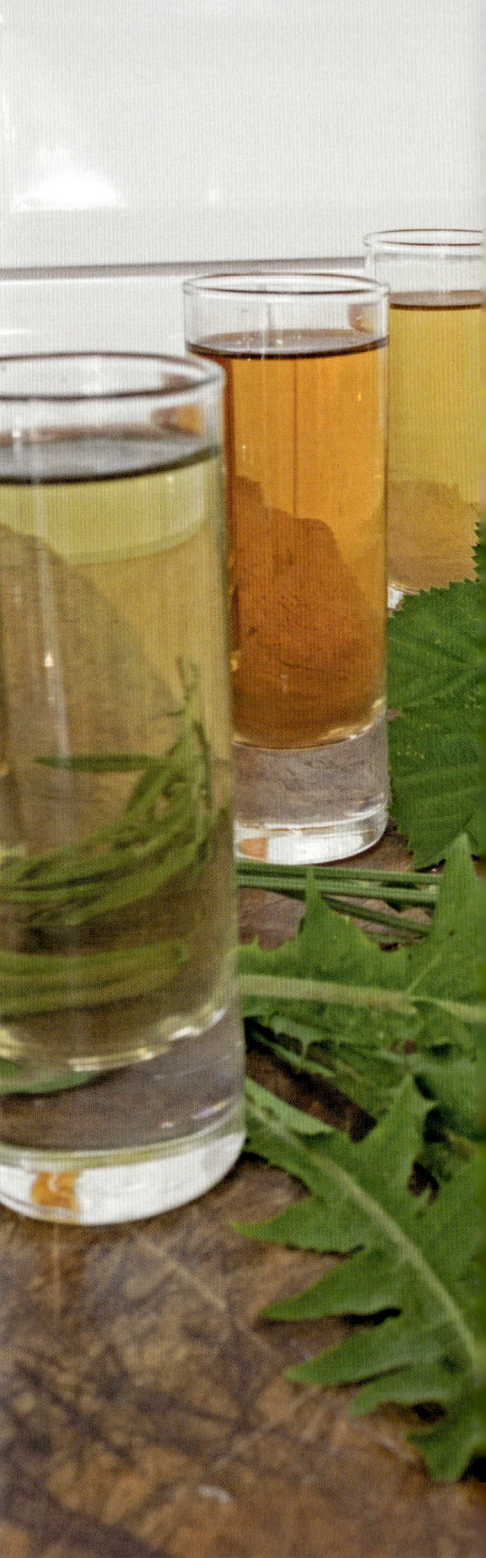

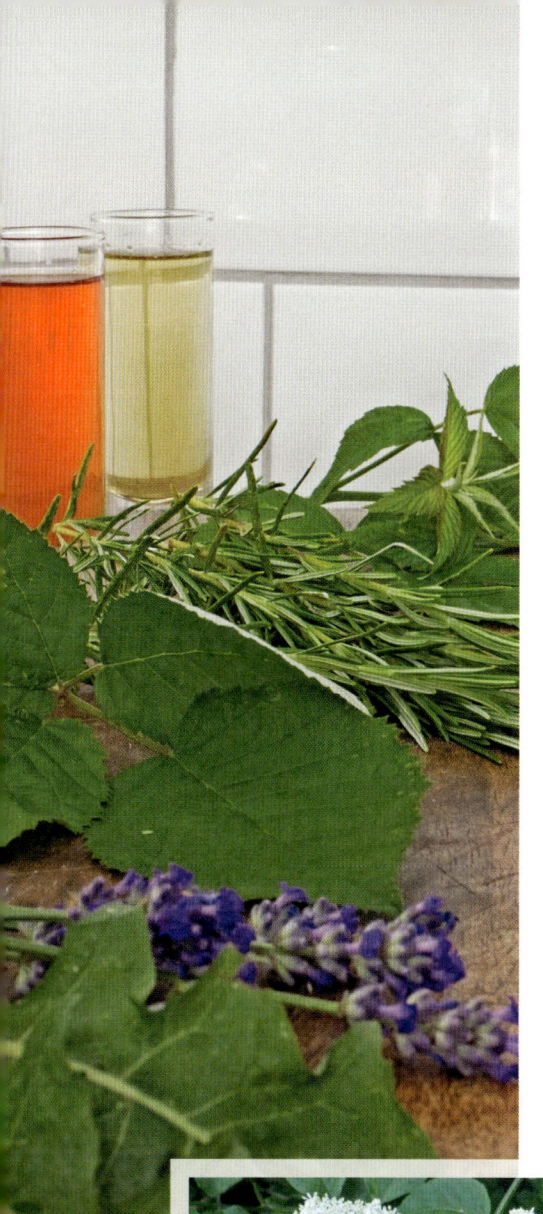

Making toners

Select your herbs to suit your skin, for example:

- For mature skin, use rose geranium (*Pelargonium roseum*) or rosemary
- For inflamed skin, use limeflower, marshmallow or honeysuckle
- For cleansing, use elderflower or parsley
- For damaged skin, use lavender or calendula
- For dull skin, use blackberry leaves, raspberry leaves or yarrow

SIMPLE HERBAL TONER

A large handful of fresh leaves or flowers
½ cup (118ml) water

MAKE Simmer the herbs in the water for 5 minutes and then cover and leave to infuse for 20 minutes before straining and bottling.

STORE Keep toners in sealed containers in the fridge, they will last for one or two days. You can freeze them in ice cube trays and handily take out one cube at a time that will last for a day or two.

make these fresh, keep them in the fridge

REFRESHING BODY SPRITZ

2 tsp fresh mint
2 tsp fresh dill
1 tsp fresh parsley
¼ cup (60ml) boiling water
1 tbsp (15ml) witch hazel

MAKE Put the herbs into a cup and pour on the boiling water. Cover and leave to infuse for 20 minutes before straining through a sieve or tea strainer. Add the witch hazel and pour into a spray bottle.

USE Spray on as needed, shaking with each use. Refill a small mist bottle each day to have by your bed, desk, sink, and in your bag. Spritz to instantly feel fresher and more relaxed. You can also use the spritz to set makeup. It can be sprayed on hair and face.

STORE Supplies will keep fresh in the fridge for about two days.

keep your cool on hot days

ELDERFLOWER WATER

Elderflowers were particularly popular in the 19th century for refining the skin, removing freckles and keeping it blemish free. Known as Aqua Sambuci, elderflower water was common on many dressing tables. Made in midsummer when the elderflower blooms, it then mellows over time.

Make simple elderflower water by infusing 100g of elderflowers in 500ml water. Bring to the boil, and then simmer for 5 minutes before removing from the heat, allowing to infuse for 20 minutes then strain off the elderflowers.

❋ Variations

The addition of **witch hazel** brings astringency to the toner for instant perkiness.

You can also add a similar quantity of **glycerine** as well as, or instead of, the witch hazel to make the toner more softening for your skin and help hold the water.

Alternatively, add the same quantity of **salt** to your toner to create a nourishing toner that is good for acne-prone skin and will leave skin feeling refreshed. Add this with the herbs so it can dissolve in the hot water.

HERBAL SKIN TONIC

Incorporate vinegar for fresh and supple skin

- ½ cup (118ml) white wine or cider vinegar
- 2 tsp dried rosemary
- 2 tsp dried lavender
- 2 tsp dried thyme
- 3 cups (711ml) rosewater

MAKE Put half the herbs (1 teaspoon of each) into a glass jar and pour over the vinegar, making sure all the herbs are covered. Seal and leave for two weeks, shaking daily. Strain off the vinegar and put the remaining half of the herbs into a clean jar then cover with the herbal vinegar. Seal and again leave for two weeks, shaking daily. Strain and combine the herbal vinegar with the rosewater. Bottle and seal.

USE Use your herbal vinegar as a toner or add a couple of tablespoons full to a warm bath.

STORE Keep your vinegar in a well-sealed bottle and store in the fridge for up to three months.

UNIVERSAL FLOWER REFRESHER

A classically simple combination of the three most common flower waters

- 2 tsp (10ml) rosewater
- 2 tsp (10ml) orange flower water
- 2 tsp (10ml) lavender water
- 1 tsp (5ml) witch hazel
- 1 tsp (5ml) glycerine

MAKE Put all ingredients into an atomising bottle and shake well.

USE Spritz yourself whenever you feel the need.

STORE Keep in the fridge when not in use. It will last for a couple of weeks.

When to cleanse

- Cleanse in the morning to remove the residue of any night time products and the salts and oils that have built up on your skin overnight. Also to give yourself a fresh start to the day.

- Cleanse in the evening to remove all the products and polluting debris that have built up during the day.

That's pretty much it. Cleanse any more and you run the risk of too much interference with your skin.

But there are certain occasions and activities when you will want to be super-clean. Do cleanse for these, but know that you're asking extra of your skin, so be especially kind to it. Use more nourishing oils, get more rest and balance out with times when you use no product and let your skin be itself.

Over cleansing, or using a cleanser that is not suited to your skin, can lead to dryness that no amount of moisturiser can replenish.

Tips for using cleansers

- When cleansing your face, start by washing your hands, before they touch your face.

- Keep your hair away from your face so you can clean thoroughly, right up to the hairline, as this is where debris can accumulate.

- Use lukewarm water for cleansing: too cold and you'll have difficulty breaking down the oily residues; too warm and it may be drying for your skin.

- To increase the efficiency of a cleanser, if you have time, apply a face cloth soaked with warm water to the skin and allow it to sit there for a minute or so before cleansing. This will open the pores and soften the skin, enabling the cleanser to penetrate the skin and remove dirt more effectively.

- Cleansers are designed to make you feel clean and fresh, so it makes sense then to use them at their freshest. To enable this, make small quantities, and keep them chilled.

- Have a stock of face cloths so you can wash each day, it's incredible how much bacteria can build up in that cloth hung over the basin – you don't want that on your skin, use a fresh one.

- Similarly, refresh your towel regularly and let it dry and air well.

- In the next chapter we look at different exfoliating tools and discover that even the softest cloths and brushes can have an impact. Remember this when choosing cleansing tools; if you only want to exfoliate once or twice a week, don't make your regular cleansing tool something that will have an exfoliating effect every day. Generally your hands, a cotton pad and a gentle washcloth should suffice for regular cleaning.

- Using your washcloth: wet it, wring it out, then gently wipe your face to remove all residue. The best washcloth is bamboo. These are soft (much more so than a terry towelling flannel), gentle (not totally drying, like a microcloth – so some water is left on your skin ready to be sealed in with moisturiser) and natural. They also have antibacterial, antifungal and odour resistant qualities and can be produced sustainably – using a crop that grows fast, requiring no pesticides, chemicals and very little water and is easy to replenish. They're also fully biodegradable and easy to wash.

- Develop a natural sweep with your cleanser that takes your skin in the direction you want it to sit (i.e. drag upwards, not downwards!). This means starting at the corners of your mouth, sweeping up the centre of your face, out across the forehead, around the eyes and onto the cheeks, pushing back towards your ears. Then single out your chin and neck for special attention. Look up to stretch out your neck and sweep your hands from its base, up to your chin. Repeat this pattern several times until you are sure all dirt is lifted. Then rinse.

- When you're super-dirty you might want to use a cleansing brush to help dislodge the dirt and grease, but make this an occasional not every day tool, and choose the softest brush you feel comfortable with.

Make sure you wash it well after use and let it air dry thoroughly.

- Know that you're aiming for clean and refreshed, but not squeaky clean. The latter is over-doing it, and you'll pay the price later as your skin pumps out more oil to compensate.
- To dry, pat your skin with a soft towel, don't rub. And if you're prone to acne or infections, use separate towels or tissues and refresh each time.
- Let your skin remain slightly damp and swiftly apply your moisturising product(s) to seal in that moisture.
- If you're in a hard water area it's worth fitting a water filter, using mineral water, boiled water or rainwater for your ablutions.
- Use any time you spend applying your cleanser to give yourself a mini facial massage.
- If you're too tired to cleanse properly when you go to bed, do it earlier in the evening. Your skin responds to the sun and moon so it begins its night time restorative work as the sun goes down. By getting in tune with this you can reap the benefits for your skin and get a relaxing evening.

Makeup removing techniques

- For eye makeup: The skin around your eyes is the finest on all your body, so take great care. It's worth having a specifically formulated gentle product to use on this area. Eyes are also prone to infection so work clean. Use a separate cotton pad for each eye and make sure your products are fresh and handled as little as possible. (You'll find an example made with calendula in Chapter 15.)
- An oil-based cleanser, or pure oil, is best for removing eye makeup that is typically oil-based. Soak your cotton pad in cleanser and hold it over your closed eye for ten to twenty seconds, there's no need to rub hard, just give it time to dissolve the oils and then gently wipe away.
- For face makeup: If light you can remove it in your standard cleansing, but if it needs a little more attention beforehand you can either use cotton pads soaked in cleansing water or a cleansing cloth.

Tips to help keep your skin clean

- Keep your pillow clean – a silk pillow is great for hair and skin
- Keep your phone clean
- Keep your hands away from your face
- Keep your hair clean and away from your face

A world of inspiration for different cleansing methods

Whatever you were taught when growing up, and whether you followed that advice or not, you can be sure that somewhere in the world people will think your ways are strange. Our methods of cleansing, and the taboos that have grown up around ablutions, are myriad.

Whichever methods you choose, clean your skin twice a day, aiming to feel cleaned, but not dried out. How intense your clean needs to be will depend on what you've experienced during the day or night, e.g. the environment you've been in, how much you've sweated, if you've been wearing makeup or other products and so on.

As you and the seasons change, recipes can be adjusted to match the formula to your skin's needs, for example, a little lighter, creamier or less scented.

So if you can't find an approach to suit in the suggestions above, take a look around the world for inspiration, find out more by following the blog at www.fieldfreshskincare.co.uk

Nature does not hurry, yet everything is accomplished

LAO TZU, CHINESE PHILOSOPHER, 6TH OR 4TH CENTURY BC

CHAPTER 10

exfoliating

Our natural cell renewal process can slow down as we get older, or may be affected by hormones, diet and weather. If you feel your skin is not looking as bright as usual, there are many ways to give it a helping hand. Don't think of this as mere vanity, your skin needs to be kept healthy through cell renewal. An accumulation of dead skin cells on the surface can contribute to clogged pores, breakouts, rough patches, wrinkles and dull skin, your skin is not working at its best then. Exfoliating is a brilliant way to work with your skin's natural processes to look your freshest and best.

There are many different techniques, tools and ingredients for exfoliation, they fall into two approaches: physical and chemical.

In physical exfoliation, the surface dead skin cells are being physically brushed, pushed and dislodged. In chemical exfoliation, the gluey web structure that holds skin cells to the surface is gently dissolved, allowing the cells to float free and be washed away.

Physical exfoliation

Physical exfoliation can be very light touch, or rather abrasive. Use the most abrasive methods only on the areas with thickest skin. Even the gentlest methods can be very effective elsewhere.

There are two approaches to physical exfoliation: using tools or using ingredients.

The tools range from a soft muslin cloth, through various grades of sponges and loofahs, to hard pumice stones. Ingredients also span the spectrum from soft oats and flours to coarse salts and shells.

Tools for physical exfoliation

Using simple tools during your cleansing process can provide sufficient friction on a daily basis to lift the dead cells and wipe them away. The process can be very gentle. Softest of all is a fine-weave muslin cloth, or slightly firmer cotton or bamboo cloths that are still very gentle. These are totally controllable, i.e. you apply the pressure you need to adjust their impact, and suitable for daily use, even with sensitive skin. A microfibre cloth is a little harsher and its large surface area provides thorough cleansing. Using a cleansing cloth is a great little and often approach for teen skin.

Alternatively, a konjac sponge provides gentle exfoliating. It's a natural product derived from yam root and has its own cleansing properties. Some sponges have added charcoal or clays to aid cleansing. Another option for the face is to use a brush, either natural, soft-bristled and hand-powered, or battery powered for an even approach (a vibrating brush will be gentler than a rotating one).

Harsher techniques such as exfoliating mitts and loofahs are best used just on the body, not the face. The truly rigorous tools such as pumice should be restricted to just the hardest areas of skin, like the feet. Dry body brushing with a soft-bristled brush is not only a great way to get the lymphatic system going, it also helps exfoliation.

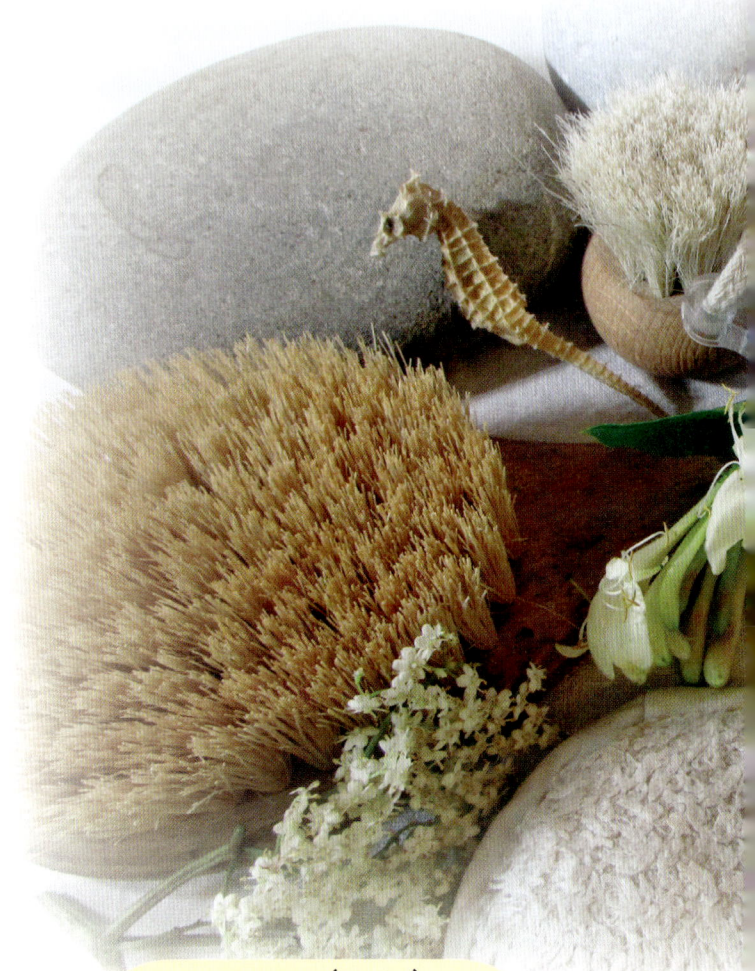

GENTLE (FACE)

TOOLS	INGREDIENTS
muslin cloth	caster sugar
konjac sponge	ground oatmeal
soft-bristled brush	jojoba beads
microfibre towel	raw sugar
flannel	coffee grounds
firm-bristled brush	apricot kernel

ABRASIVE (BODY)

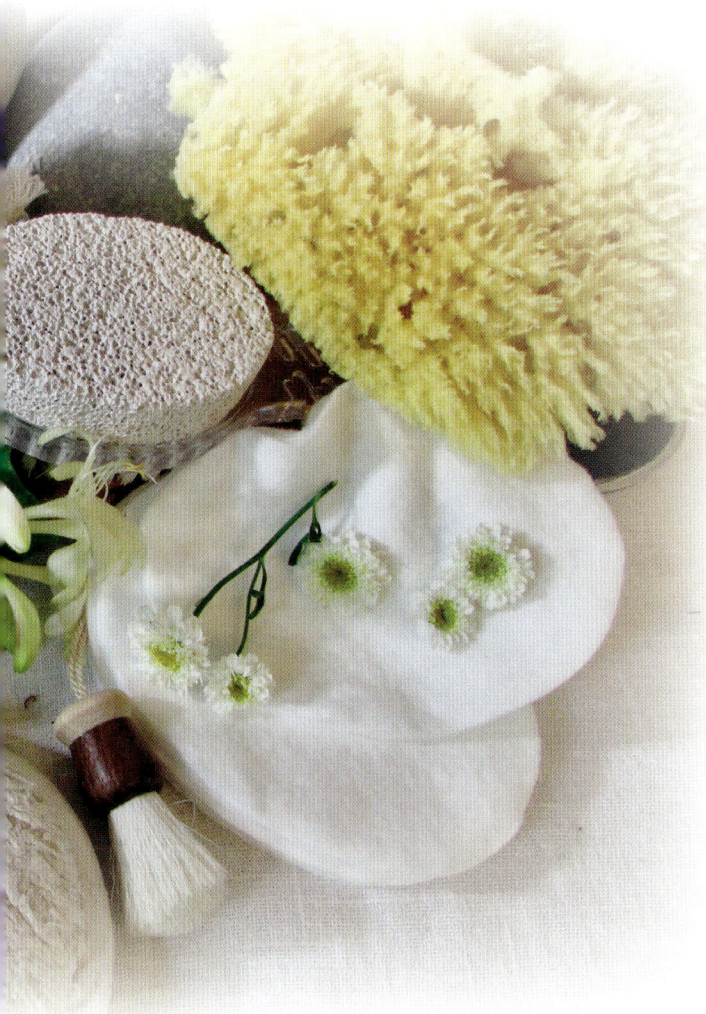

Any of the exfoliating tools can be used on their own with water or in combination with other physical or chemical exfoliants.

Whatever method you choose, keep your tools scrupulously clean. This means replacing cloths each day and washing them (without strong detergent or softener), so you'll need a small stock of cloths to circulate. Wash and thoroughly drain sponges and brushes with each use, sterilise in hot water every few weeks and replace them every few months.

All these physical methods can be carried out at home, or in a spa. In addition, spas offer microdermabrasion, a mechanical method of exfoliation using an exfoliating agent, such as crystals or flaked diamonds, along with a suction tool to remove the dead skin cells. Home microdermabrasion kits are also available.

Ingredients for physical exfoliation

Exfoliating ingredients are typically blended within various creams and scrubs. These exfoliant components are added especially to create a little abrasion on the skin to lift the dead cells. The agents may be quite fine, or much more chunky, use the finest versions for the face. Overusing physical exfoliants that are too harsh can lead to micro-tears in the skin.

The range of natural exfoliating ingredients includes salt and sugar as well as finely crushed shells, grains, nuts and oatmeal or botanical powders and flour. Men can think about using grittier ingredients than women as their skin is typically 20-30% thicker.

Microbeads are tiny beads made out of polythene or other petrochemicals that have been used for exfoliation. However, they are highly detrimental to our water systems and completely unnecessary as there are many good natural alternatives that will biodegrade. As a result, microbeads are now being phased out of skincare products. The main direct alternative to these is jojoba beads. Jojoba is a wax (often referred to as jojoba oil) and it is one of the closest natural components to the oils naturally produced in skin, which is why it is so valued in hair and skin products. It is a tropically sourced ingredient, so you may choose to look for ingredients that grow closer to home (like oatmeal, finely ground walnut shell or salt).

Coffee certainly wouldn't meet the 'closer to home' criteria and, although a popular ingredient in scrubs (added because it is cleansing too), it can be too rough for sensitive skin. Caffeine has been associated with the reduction of cellulite but the amount contained in a scrub, and the time it is in contact with the skin would not be enough to be effective.

Good options for scrubs include ground apricot kernel. Apricot, along with sweet almond and peach kernel oil, is known to be mild and therefore good for sensitive skin. However, the ground form included in scrubs is still a little large for the delicate skin on our faces, so it's best kept as a body scrub.

Ground oatmeal, which can come in various grades (from fine to medium and coarse), will soften in water so forms a gentle scrub that is suitable for use on the face. It naturally contains avenanthramides that have hydrating and anti-irritant properties.

Salt and sugar also come in various grades. These can be too harsh for facial skin (although may be used to slough the rough skin on lips). When using these, take advantage of the fact that they dissolve in water by bringing them into contact with moisture (either blending the scrub a little before you intend to use it, or by applying to damp skin and waiting a minute before rubbing it in). This way they will dissolve just a little, becoming finer, softer and gentler for your skin. Sugar and salt are a good option for a scrub because they dissolve after, so there are less messy bits to clear up in the bath or shower.

Finely ground adzuki beans have been used by Japanese women for centuries in their skincare routines. They're gentle enough to be used on the face and include enzymes that provide chemical breakdown when activated by water.

All these ingredients can be used easily by creating your own scrubs. To do this, add them to a natural oil, blend them with your normal cleanser, or combine them with water (or an infusion) to make a really simple scrub. Typically work with a 1:1 ratio (e.g. 1 tablespoon salt to 1 tablespoon oil) but adjust to suit and experiment to find the consistency you like best, which will vary according to the absorbency of your ingredients and the thickness of your chosen oil.

Scrubs are very simple to make and use, but can be a little messy, so use them in the shower or bath and be aware that the oil may make surfaces slippy.

Physical exfoliation scrubs and creams are always designed to be rinsed off. The ingredients will only stay in contact with your skin for a short period of time. It can be a good idea to

Quick physical exfoliators for the face

When exfoliating your face, don't forget to include your neck.
Make it easier by looking upwards, extending your neck so the skin is taut.

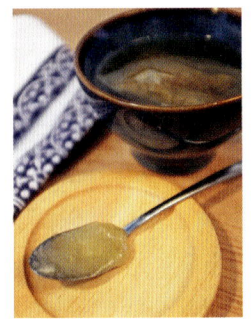

CHAMOMILE AND HONEY FACE SCRUB

1 tsp dried chamomile (or a chamomile teabag)
1 tsp (5ml) honey

MAKE *Infuse the chamomile in a cup of water then strain (or take out the teabag and open it) and put the petals in a small bowl. Blend with the honey.*

USE *Apply to your face in small circular movements. Then wash off with warm water. You can either use the warm chamomile tea to rinse and tone your face, or you can drink it and relax.*

Chamomile is great for all skin types, but you can use alternatives too:
- For oilier skin, replace the chamomile flowers with lavender flowers
- For older or sensitive skins, replace the chamomile with rose or calendula petals

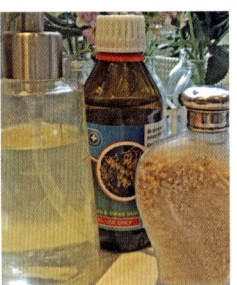

OATMEAL, WITCH HAZEL & THISTLE FACE SCRUB

1 tsp (5g) fine oatmeal
½ tsp (2.5ml) witch hazel
½ tsp (2.5ml) thistle oil

MAKE *Simply blend the three ingredients together in a small bowl or, for real ease, in the palm of your hand.*

USE *Apply to your face in small circular movements. Then wash off with warm water.*

Thistle oil is great for all skin types but you may want to ring the changes with some other oils, for example:
- For dry skin use hemp seed oil which will penetrate quickly and moisturise
- For sensitive skin use comfrey oil which will help it become more resilient
- For acne prone skin use pumpkin seed oil to repair damaged skin.
- For oily skin use hazelnut oil which is dry, light and astringent
- For older skin, use mullein oil, a natural wrinkle-fighter with its vitamins, minerals, tannins and elastin

use a scrub prior to shaving as it will lift and loosen the dead skin cells, leaving the razor free to do its work. Make sure this is of the gentlest kind or skin will need recovery time before you begin to shave.

Always choose the mildest, gentlest form of physical exfoliation you find effective, and don't overdo it. Work lightly in small circles; gently buffing is a lot kinder and more effective than using pressure to scrub hard, even if it takes a few moments longer, you can enjoy the process and take care over it.

If your skin is dry, keep scrubs gentle (as harsh scrubs will remove dry flakes and damage your skin, which will make the problem worse) and think about their moisturising properties. Oatmeal is particularly good for dry skin as it is a humectant (so it will hold water to your skin) and is naturally moisturising.

There is another type of physical exfoliating method that may appear a little more like chemical exfoliating. These are the peeling gels and gommages. Their special property is the cellulose or carbomer they contain. When this meets with your skin it has a tendency to roll up and form little fibres that scrub the skin. In this remarkable way, they provide a very gentle, while also thorough, exfoliating experience. These may take a little getting used to, especially in getting the right amount of water to make them truly effective. Too much and they become runny, and you'll find it slipping away before they take effect.

Quick physical exfoliators for the body

Using the tougher scrubs on hips, thighs and areas of harder skin can get the circulation going. This encourages the lymph system to maximise the beneficial flow of skin nutrients and minimises cellulite.

SALT BODY SCRUB

A handful of fine sea salt
A handful of olive oil
A few drops of essential oils (optional)

MAKE Simply blend the three ingredients together in a small bowl or, a little at a time, in the palm of your hand.

USE Best used in the shower – massage into dry skin then shower off (just be careful as the oil may make the shower floor a little slippy).

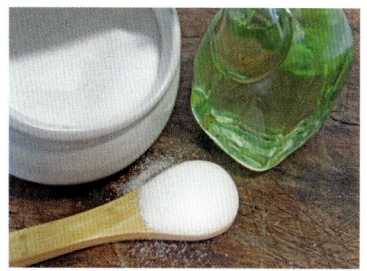

QUICK EXFOLIATOR FOR HANDS, FEET OR LIPS

2 tbsp (30ml) light oil, e.g. sunflower, thistle or rapeseed
2 tbsp (30g) granulated sugar
A few drops of essential oil (optional)
A drop of food colouring (optional)

MAKE Mix the oil and sugar in a small bowl, add the essential oil and food colouring (if using) and then pack into a jar with a lid.

USE Rub into skin as required, then rinse with warm water and pat dry.

STORE Packed tightly in an airtight jar this will keep for up to a year. It's great to have handy by the sink so you can apply it whenever you think about it.

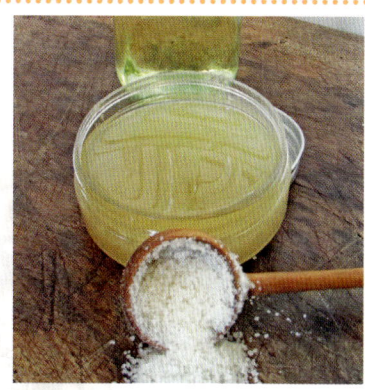

Indulgent physical exfoliators for face

When you have time to spare, or if you could benefit from making yourself sit down and relax, a herbal mask will exfoliate and calm, leaving you radiant.

Many masks are based on clays, but as these are generally quite fine, their exfoliating effect is minimal. If you want the clay to act as a physical exfoliator, use the larger textured green clays such as green zeolite clay, which is best for oily skin.

The new skin exposed following an exfoliating mask should be treated gently and moisturised. This makes it a great evening-in or pre-bedtime treat giving skin plenty of restorative time to settle afterwards.

- When your skin is **oily** it is more likely to have blocked pores. Dead skin cells are one of the things that block pores so exfoliating is an important way to look after oily skin
- If your skin is **dry** it may look dull. An exfoliating mask formulated for dry skin can bring back a healthy glow
- If your skin is **thin or sensitive**, it's best to avoid exfoliating masks

'ME THYME' FACE MASK

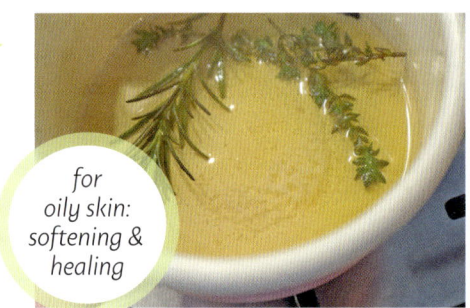

for oily skin: softening & healing

2 tsp (10g) oatmeal
1 tsp each of dried lavender, rosemary and thyme
2-4 houseleek leaves (depending on size)
A few tsps (up to 10ml) of thyme infusion, or plain water

MAKE Grind the oatmeal, dried herbs and houseleek leaves (optional) together using a pestle and mortar (or blitz them in a blender). Add the infusion (or water) a little at a time, stirring to form a spreadable consistency.

USE Apply to your face (avoiding the eye area) and leave for 15 minutes. Then wash off with warm water. If you have any thyme infusion left, you can splash or spritz your face with this before moisturising.

GREEN CLAY MASK

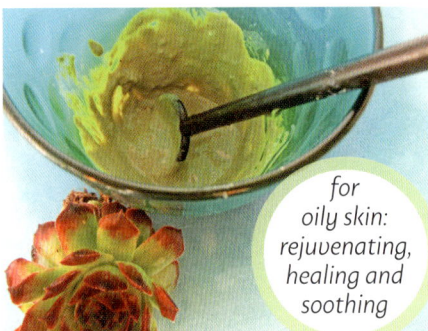

for oily skin: rejuvenating, healing and soothing

2 tsp (10g) green clay
10 houseleek leaves
1 tsp (5ml) witch hazel
1 drop lavender essential oil (optional)

MAKE Pound the houseleek leaves in a pestle and mortar then add the witch hazel. Put the clay into a separate (non-metal) bowl, and gradually add your houseleek liquid, stirring until blended. Add the lavender essential oil and mix thoroughly.

USE Gently apply over the face, avoiding the eyes, and leave for 10 minutes before washing off with warm water.

HONEY SALT MASK

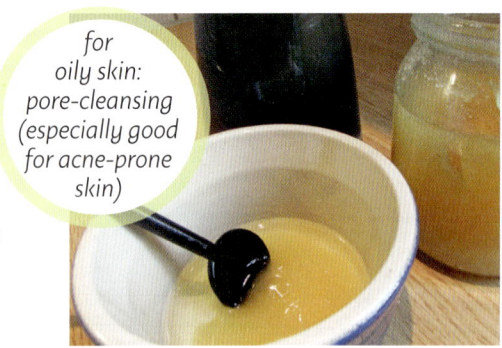

for oily skin: pore-cleansing (especially good for acne-prone skin)

1 tbsp (15ml) honey – to help settle and protect inflamed skin
1 tsp (5g) salt – to help tighten the skin
1 tsp (5ml) sunflower oil
A few drops of lavender essential oil

MAKE Simply blend all the ingredients together.

USE Soak a face cloth in warm water and then place over your face to open up the pores and moisten your skin. With the skin damp, apply the mask in very gentle, small circular motions. Leave for 15 minutes and then rinse off with warm water and moisturise well. Use once or twice a week.

STRAWBERRY SKIN FOOD

1 tbsp (15g) kaolin clay
1 tbsp (15ml) clear honey
1 tbsp (15ml) natural yogurt
4 fresh strawberries
Rosewater (optional)

MAKE Mash the strawberries with a fork and then add to the other ingredients and mix well.

USE Gently apply the paste over your face, avoiding the eyes, and leave for 15 minutes.

For added pink indulgence, soak cotton pads in rosewater and rest them on your closed eyes as you lie back. Rinse off the mask with warm water and then splash with rosewater.

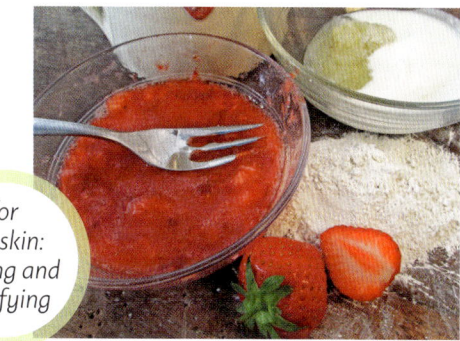

for dry skin: firming and clarifying

ELDERFLOWER EARTH MASK

1 tbsp (15g) diatomaceous earth (a gentle abrasive)
1 tbsp fresh elderflower or 1 tsp dried elderflower
1 tbsp (15ml) honey
4 tbsp (60ml) water

MAKE First, prepare your infusion. Put the elderflower into a pan and add four tablespoons (60ml) water, gently bring to the boil then turn off the heat, cover and allow to cool. Strain off the elderflowers using a fine sieve, muslin or tea strainer, and return the infused water to the pan. Add the honey and heat gently, stirring to combine. To blend your mask, put the diatomaceous earth in a (non-metal) bowl and gradually add the honeyed elderflower infusion, stirring to make a paste.

USE Apply this to your face in small circles, avoiding the eyes and let it set (which will take a couple of minutes). Remove with warm water and use a cotton pad dipped in any remaining honeyed elderflower infusion to wipe over skin to tone before moisturising.

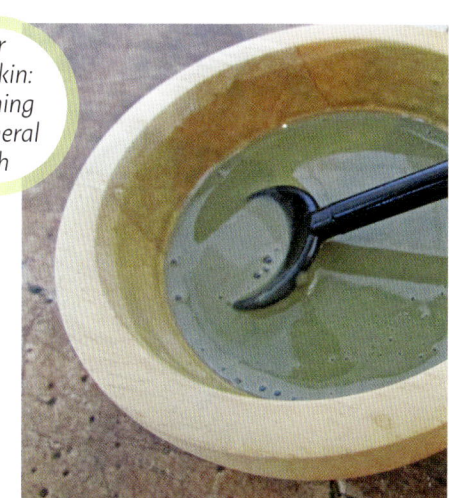

for dry skin: soothing & mineral rich

ALMOND, ROSE AND MARSHMALLOW MASK

A handful of almonds
1 tbsp fresh marshmallow leaf or 1 tsp dried marshmallow leaf
1 tbsp (15ml) rosewater

MAKE First prepare the almonds by immersing them in boiling water, leaving them to soak for a few minutes, then draining and, one-by-one, squeezing them between thumb and forefinger to slip off their skins. Next, blend: Put the skinned almonds with the marshmallow leaf in a blender and pulverise (do use a covered blender or grinder, not a stick blender to contain the nut smithereens). Add a little rosewater to the almond and marshmallow mixture to make a paste.

USE Massage gently into the skin using small circles, avoiding the eyes. Leave for 10 minutes, then wash off and tone with remaining rosewater.

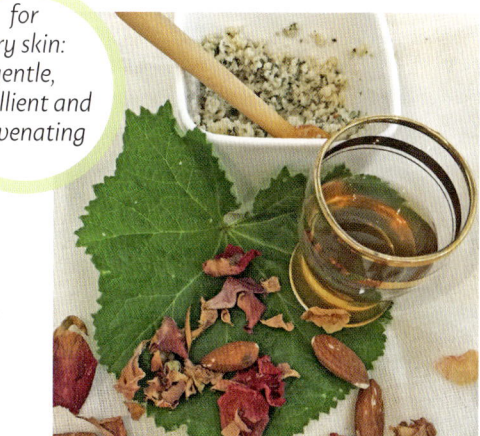

for dry skin: gentle, emollient and rejuvenating

Indulgent physical exfoliators for body

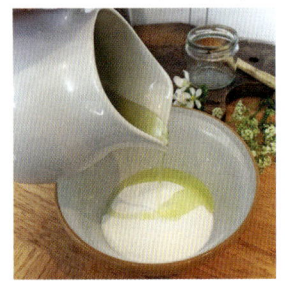
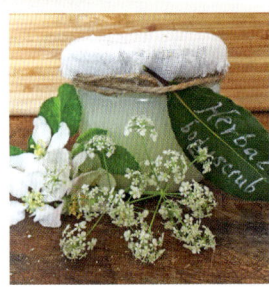

HERBAL BODY SCRUB

⅔ cup (158ml) sunflower oil
4 tbsp herbs – select the herbs for their beneficial properties, using the guidance below
400g fine grain salt

MAKE First prepare by macerating the herbs in the oil. Put them together in a pan and heat gently for five minutes. Cover and allow to cool, then strain through a muslin. Next, to blend your scrub, put the salt into a large bowl and gradually add the macerated oil, mixing thoroughly. Reserve a tablespoon of oil. Pack the salt into a sterilised jar and pour the remaining oil on top to create an air lock.

USE Apply to wet skin in the bath or shower. Scoop a handful of the herbal salt out of the jar and rub in small circles over your body. Leave for a minute before rinsing off thoroughly with warm water.

STORE Your scrub will keep in the jar for up to a year. Ensure the herbs are continually covered by the oil.

Herbal blends to use in the maceration:
- For post-sport restoring and deodorising: lovage, parsley, spearmint and borage
- For ache relieving: bay, borage, hyssop and St John's Wort
- For conditioning oily skin: yarrow, spearmint, plantain and parsley
- For conditioning dry skin: comfrey, chamomile, elderflower and marshmallow leaf

SWEET MUD FLOWER SCRUB

A gentle but effective cellulite fighter

2 tbsp (30g) fine grain salt
2 tsp lavender flowers
2 tsp chamomile flowers
5 tbsp (60g) sugar (you can use caster or granulated; the finer the sugar, the smoother the scrub)
2 tsp (10g) green clay
1 tbsp (15ml) sunflower oil

MAKE First, prepare by putting the flowers in a bowl and covering them with the salt, turning them to ensure they are fully covered. Leave for a few hours (or overnight). Next, to blend your scrub, put the sugar and clay into a bowl and add the salt and flowers before gradually pouring in the sunflower oil. Mix thoroughly. Once all is well combined, pack into a jar, seal and label.

USE Apply to wet skin in the bath or shower. Scoop a handful of the herbal salt out of the jar and rub in small circles over your body. Leave for a minute before rinsing off thoroughly with warm water.

STORE If kept free of water, your scrub will keep in the jar for up to a year.

HERBAL BATH BAG

Use your bathtime to rejuvenate, stimulate and soothe

1 tbsp (15g) bran
2 tbsp (30g) oats
1 tsp rosemary
1 tsp lavender
1 tsp bay

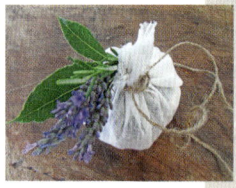

MAKE Tie all the ingredients inside a muslin bag.

USE Hang over the bath taps as you run a warm bath. Let the water run through the bag and turn cloudy. Once in the bath, use the bag to scrub your skin.

Chemical exfoliation

Chemical exfoliation involves using products that help dissolve the 'glue' that holds the dead cells together so they can be more easily lifted away. This offers more even results than achievable with physical exfoliation, and all with a simple wipe on/wipe off action, with no scrubbing or abrasion required.

Quite often there is more than one action taking place in chemical exfoliation, making the methods more complex and something worth taking your time to experiment with and understand your skin's response to. Proceed with caution as there are more likely to be undesired reactions with chemical approaches. For example, some ingredients may cause photosensitivity so are better saved for use in the evening. If you do have AHAs (Alpha Hydroxy Acids) in daytime products, be sure to moisturise with a good SPF factor afterwards, and keep up the SPF for at least a week (SPF use is likely part of your normal routine anyway, if you spend a lot of time outdoors).

All the blend it yourself options offered here for chemical exfoliation are ones to take your time over, allowing for trial and error. Understand the ingredients, gradually try out new things, or increase the concentration levels of active ingredients (and therefore their intensity) to a level that suits your skin. Always work within the suggested pH and concentration levels. Make your chemical exfoliation part of a full routine, preceded by cleansing and toning and followed by nurturing serums and moisturisers (see the next chapter to know how to layer these together for best effect).

Introducing chemical exfoliants into a natural, blend it yourself skincare routine requires thought and dedication. Start simple and see how you get on. Think of it as an occasional foray, not a regular staple.

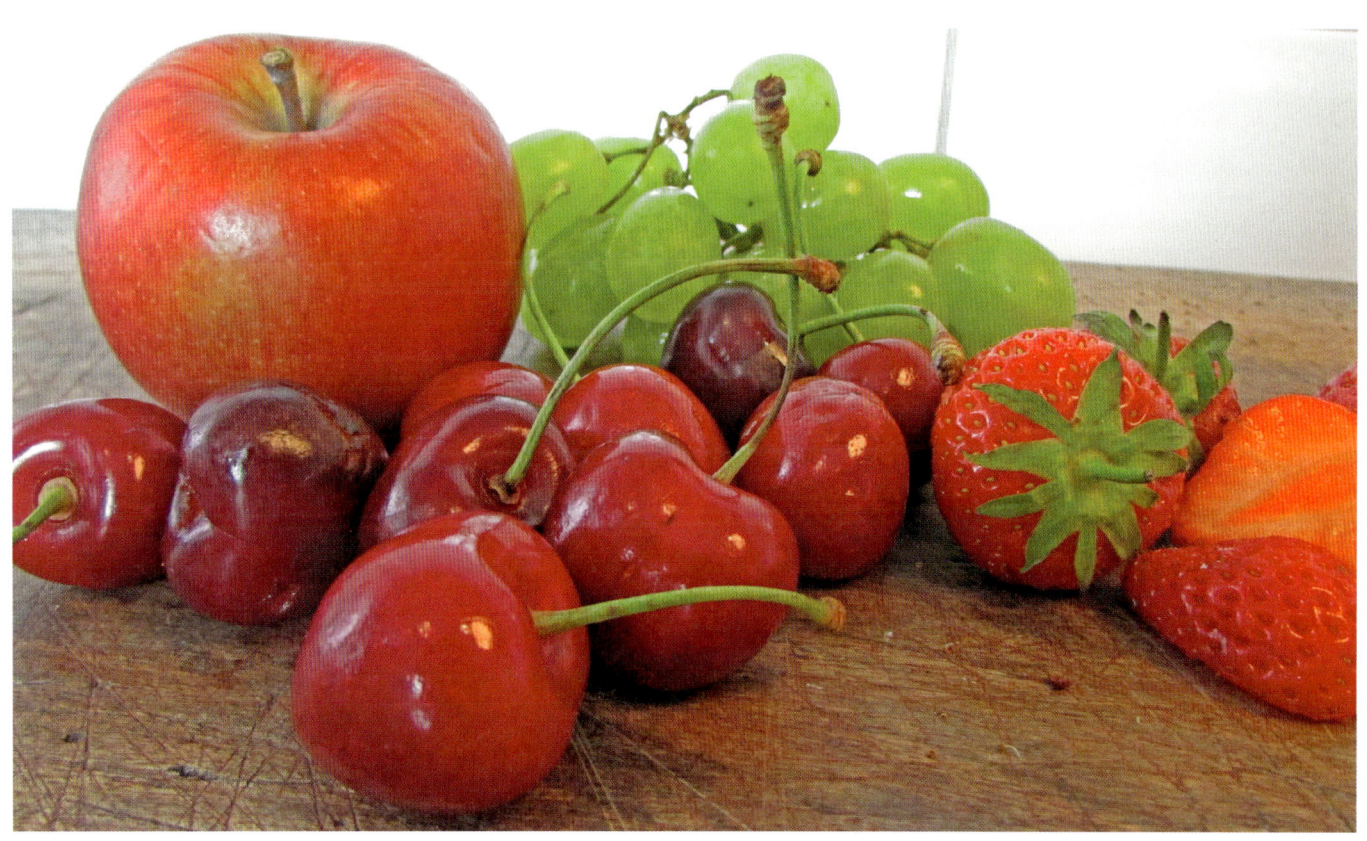

Ingredients for chemical exfoliation

Alpha Hydroxy Acids (AHAs)

The most common chemical exfoliant ingredients are alpha hydroxy acids (AHAs). These are found naturally in many fruits, notably papaya, pineapple and apples (malic acid), as well as in almonds (mandelic acid), milk (lactic acid), wine (tartaric acid), sugarcane, beets, cantaloupe melon, pineapple and unripe grapes (glycolic acid). Their exfoliating role is to loosen dead skin cells but AHAs also help in cell renewal, evening out skin tone and reducing wrinkles.

They are often used in the form of scrubs and peels or included as active ingredients in exfoliating creams. These can be used on the body and face; just use milder treatments on your face, and not more than once a week. A typical range for the AHA component in a product is 4-10%. Use the lower concentrations on the face. The body can tolerate higher concentrations. It's important to keep the pH below 4 for the AHA to work effectively.

Beta Hydroxy Acids (BHAs)

Beta hydroxy acids (BHAs) are sometimes used as exfoliators, mostly in the form of salicylic acid, useful for oily skin as it is oil-soluble (its antibacterial properties also make it a favoured option for those who suffer from acne). Salicylic acid penetrates deep into pores, effectively unblocking them. It is affected by pH, preferring conditions even lower than AHAs. A pH of 3.5 or less is ideal, however such an acidic product can be quite irritating for some skins. If this is a problem for you, you can still benefit from salicylic acid, but try it at a higher pH. It will still work anywhere in the acid range (i.e. up to pH 7) but just not quite as effectively. Keep concentration levels for salicylic acid below 2%. Betaine salicylate is another oil-soluble BHA that is sometimes used while butyric acid is rarely used (if you've smelt rancid butter, you've encountered butyric acid, not something you want to put on your skin).

Polyhydroxy Acids (PHAs)

We also have polyhydroxy acids (PHAs) such as lactobionic acid and gluconolactone. It is possible that these may provide a less irritating alternative to AHAs and BHA, more suited to sensitive skin, but they are such new ingredients to be used in skincare, there is not much research or evidence as yet.

Retinoids (forms of vitamin A: Retinol, Retinol A, Retin-A)

Retinol A has become a very popular skincare ingredient, with signs that it can slow down the breakdown of collagen and help reverse the effects of long-term UV. It also helps with exfoliation and cell renewal. The effects of retinol (such as smaller pores and fewer lines) tend to result from use over an extended period rather than the quick effects achieved with other forms of exfoliation.

Retinol is light and air sensitive, so most applications restrict it to night creams and serums, and packaging keeps it well protected. Retinol can be very irritating, so use it with caution. It can cause redness, photosensitivity, dryness and itching or burning and is not recommended for use during pregnancy. Thankfully, retinol can be effective at very low concentrations so never needs to be above 2%. Stronger forms are available only on prescription.

Enzymes

It's often not just the AHAs but also the enzymes in fruit that can have a powerful exfoliating effect.

Enzymes also act on the bonds that hold dead skin cells together as they digest the protein. They are gentle and using them does not require scrubbing, so they are good for sensitive skin. Enzymes work on the surface of the skin, in contrast to acids that penetrate deeper. While acids can be applied to dry skin, enzymes are activated with water, so should be applied to damp skin. As a gentler option, enzymes can be used more regularly than acids and are a good alternative if you find your skin is too sensitive for acid exfoliators.

The fruit most often used for their enzymes are pineapple (bromelain), papaya (papain), pomegranate, pumpkin and kiwifruit (actinidin). To benefit from these fruits in blend it yourself skincare, either use the fresh fruit in a mask, or simply rub the peel over your skin before taking a shower. Don't use fruit that has been heat treated (e.g. tinned fruit) as the heat affects the enzymes so they won't work.

'No' to citric acid and baking soda

Citric acid and baking soda (sodium bicarbonate) may be included in online exfoliating recipes, but are best avoided. Both disrupt pH; citric acid brings it too low (at best irritating, at worst burning skin) and baking soda takes pH too high, thereby destroying the protective acid mantle. During exfoliation skin needs protection, not exposure like this. Better to use a few applications of an exfoliant with mild ingredients than to wreak havoc with something too strong.

Chemical exfoliation methods

❈ Cleansers

Ingredients packed with AHAs can be included in cleansers – whether in lotion, cream or gel-based form. They'll take effect as these are massaged into the skin. However, because chemical exfoliants need a little time to do their work, rinsing off the cleanser too quickly can minimise their effectiveness. So if you're wanting chemical exfoliation through a cleanser, slow down your routine.

❈ Toners

A toner is typically wiped on and evaporates quickly, so any active ingredients don't get long to do their work. However, if you simply want a freshening, light exfoliation, the tingle of wiping on a toner is swift and easy. It's also good preparation for whatever goes on top – lotion, cream or serum – as you'll have exposed fresh cells receptive to the new ingredients which will therefore penetrate well and be most effective.

❈ Serums and creams

Serums and creams differ in their molecule size. Serums have smaller molecules that are therefore more able to penetrate into pores. For this reason, serums have become a very popular way to apply chemical exfoliation, especially when working with BHAs. Salicylic acid is more effective in a serum than in a cream.

Creams are a good way to incorporate AHAs for working on the surface, as they do not penetrate the pores so much.

❈ Lotions

Chemical exfoliating lotions generally contain AHAs. Once these have got to work dissolving the glue around dead skin cells, they can be washed away. It's best to use exfoliating gloves when applying these to ensure the effect is where you want it, not on your hands. By using slightly abrasive gloves you can combine the benefits of physical and chemical

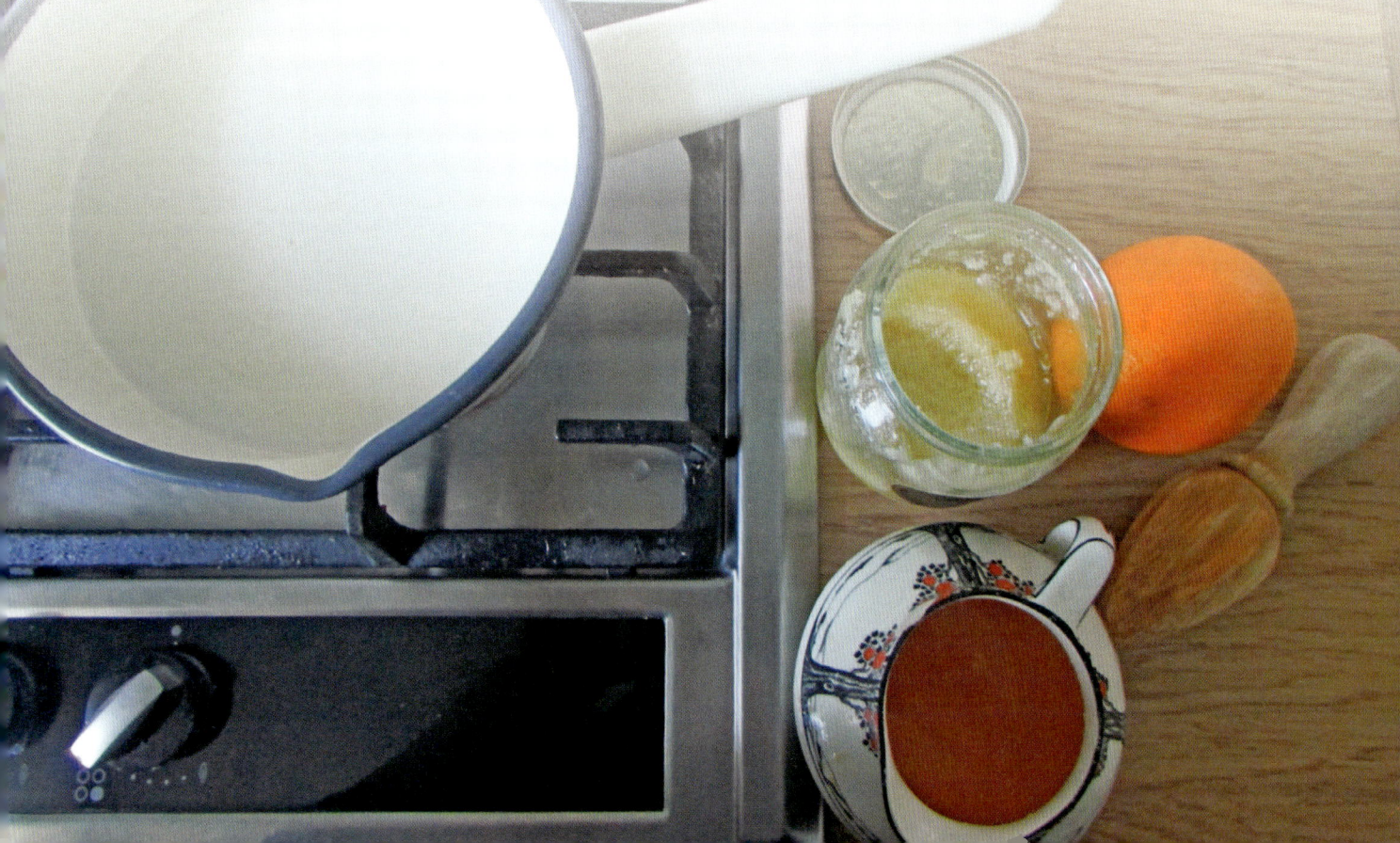

exfoliation. You can buy a lotion or make one fresh yourself.

Papaya and pineapple are classic exfoliating fruits, packed with AHAs and enzymes, but if you want things grown closer to home, use apple, cherries, pumpkin (also containing vitamins A, C and zinc, all of which can help combat acne) or tomatoes (which are full of vitamin C and lycopene, which has antioxidant benefits).

Milk products are good for chemical exfoliation lotions as the lactic acid they contain activates the breaking down process. Options include goats, cows or sheep milk, buttermilk, cream or yoghurt, depending on your preference and the consistency you're looking for (but of course you won't get lactic acid in any of the lactose-free 'milks' such as almond, rice, oat, etc.).

❋ *Splashes*

Less talked about these days, but very much advocated in times gone by, wine splashes were a popular way to cleanse and, given the liberal dose of tartaric acid they offer, it could be an exfoliating cleanse.

❋ *Masks*

Masks used for chemical exfoliation should typically be left on for between 5-15 minutes, no longer. All traces should then be rinsed off with lukewarm water. Often people experience a tingling sensation with chemical exfoliation and equate this to effectiveness. In reality, the tingle is a sign of your skin's natural barriers being compromised. Over time, your skin may become more used to the exfoliant and therefore not react in the same way. That doesn't mean it's stopped being effective: many AHAs perform skin cell healing too, so used in moderation they can develop a good relationship with your skin, making it healthier, hence the tingling lessens, but the effectiveness continues. To know whether your approach is working, look at the end results. If your skin is healthy, fresh and glowing, you're getting it right.

❋ *Scrubs*

Exfoliating scrubs that include AHAs help smooth skin and manage dryness. They may also help treat the small bumps associated with keratosis pilaris (KP). A body scrub can be done 2-3 times a week, followed with lavish applications of moisturising lotion.

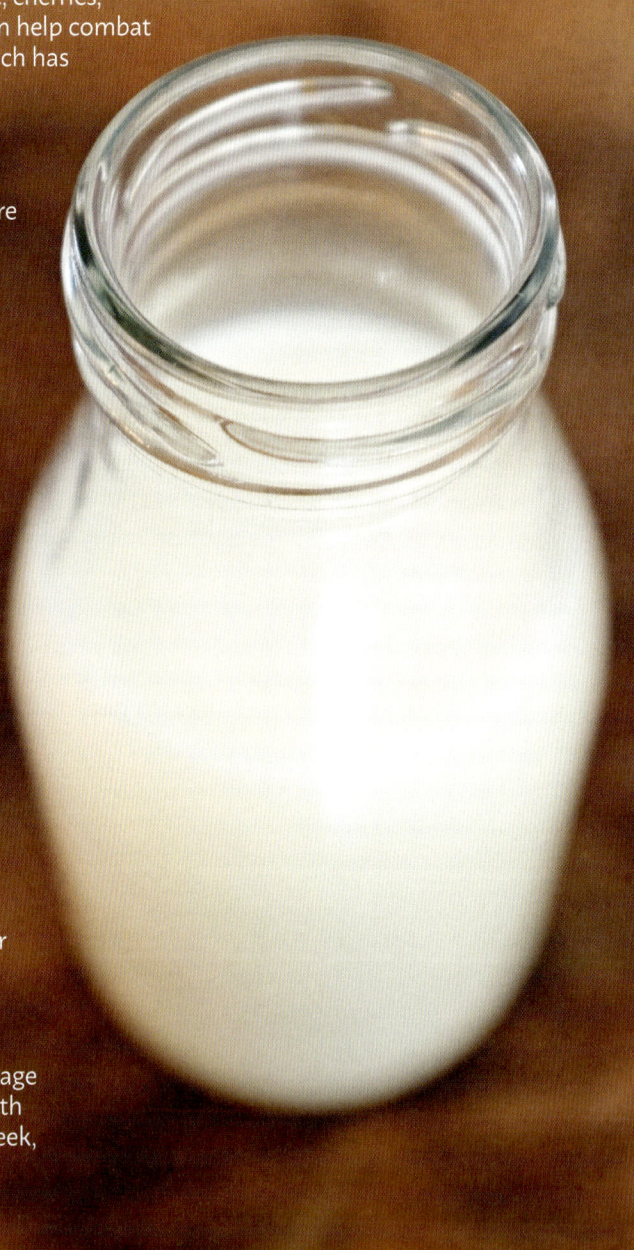

Chemical exfoliation recipes

When your skin feels dry:

- Use gentle exfoliation with AHAs
- Look for those that are also humectant
- Avoid retinoids (they're drying)
- Moisturise well after exfoliating

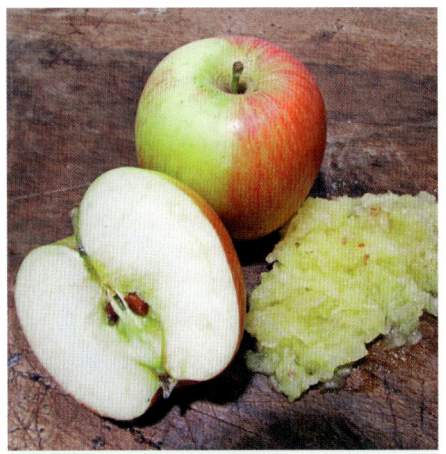
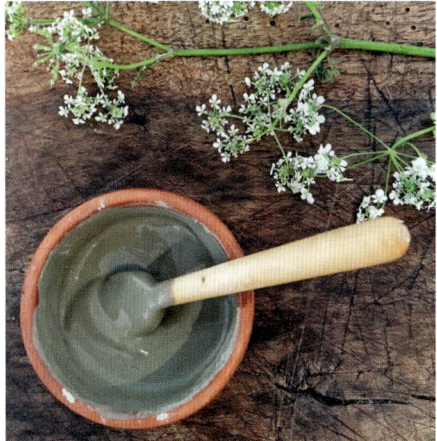
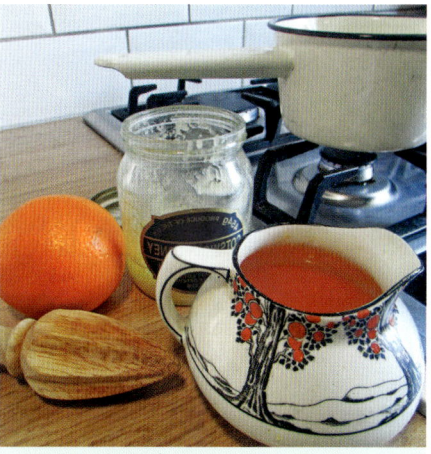

APPLE MASK

1 apple
2 tsp (10ml) hazelnut oil
1 tsp (5ml) glycerine

MAKE Peel, core and grate the apple. To the grated apple, add the hazelnut oil and glycerine and mix to form a smooth paste.

USE Apply to your skin and leave for 15 minutes then wash off with warm water.

HONEY CLAY MASK

1 tbsp (15ml) honey
1 tbsp (15ml) water
1 tsp (5g) green clay

MAKE Blend the water with the honey to thin it down. Put the clay in a separate bowl and gradually add your honey water, bit by bit, stirring to make a paste. You may not need it all.

USE Apply to your face and leave for 15 minutes then rinse with warm water and tone with any remaining honey water.

MILK SPONGE BATH

1 cup (237ml) milk
1 tbsp (15ml) honey
Juice of 1 orange

MAKE Warm the milk and honey together in a saucepan until the honey has dissolved. Then allow to cool to room temperature and add the orange juice and pour into a bowl ready to use.

USE Stand in the bath or shower and use a sponge to pat the orangey milk all over your body. Give it a few moments to dry and then wrap yourself in a large towel and rest for 15 minutes. Shower off the milk, pat dry and moisturise.

For this it's best to use full fat cow's milk as you want to benefit from the lactic acid. Orange is a traditional skin softener (brought to fame in the 17th century by the Duchess of Neroli) and, combined with the milk, it will leave your skin feeling silky and smooth.

When your skin feels oily:

> You can probably tolerate medium exfoliation, but start with just once a week
> Gently try introducing salicylic acid

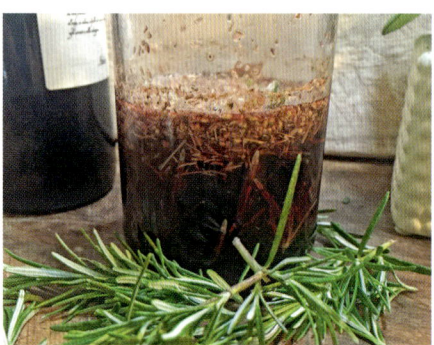

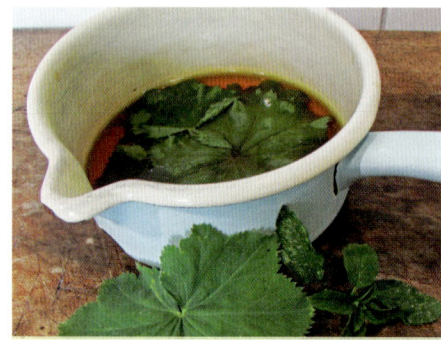

This is a type of 'eau sedative'. It will help with fatigue by boosting circulation and instilling calm. You can make an equivalent for dry skin using white wine that will have the calming effect, but red wine is best for exfoliating because it contains more tannins.

HERBAL WINE RUB

1 tsp yarrow
1 tsp rosemary
1 tsp thyme
1 large glass (250ml) of red wine
½ cup (115g) salt
5 drops camphor essential oil

MAKE First prepare by macerating the herbs in the wine using the sun method (see Chapter 14). Allow about three days on a sunny windowsill. Put your herbal wine into an empty screw top wine bottle (or similar) with the salt and essential oil and top up with boiling water. Screw on the cap and shake vigorously. Allow to cool to room temperature, then pour into a bowl ready to use.

USE Stand in the bath or shower and dip your washcloth into the wine. Gently rub it all over the body (except for nipples and genitals). Once you're done simply rub dry with a towel.

MINT LEAF FACE MASK

1 handful peppermint leaves
1 handful lady's mantle leaves
1 tbsp witch hazel

MAKE Put the peppermint leaves in a saucepan and pour over a cup of water. Gently bring to the boil then remove from the heat, cover and allow to infuse. When cool, strain the peppermint leaves from the water and return the minty water to the pan. Add the witch hazel and heat gently. As it approaches the boil, add the lady's mantle leaves and turn off the heat, leaving them to soak until soft (about 5-10 minutes).

USE Arrange the leaves over your face and lie down to relax for 15 minutes. After removing the leaves, tone with any remaining mint water.

For skin troubled with acne:

> Use minimal exfoliation to avoid inflaming skin
> Gently try introducing salicylic acid
> Introduce retinoids but in very low concentrations

HONEY NUT FACE MASK

2 tsp (10ml) honey
2 tsp (10ml) hazelnut oil

MAKE Blend the honey and hazelnut oil together in a small bowl.

USE Apply in small circles, rest for 5-10 minutes and then wash off with warm water.

The honey in this mask is a humectant, locking in moisture. It also helps the natural skin regeneration process by promoting new tissue growth. The honey will protect newly exposed skin due to its antibacterial and anti-inflammatory properties. Hazelnut oil is astringent, its dryness is counteracted by the honey.

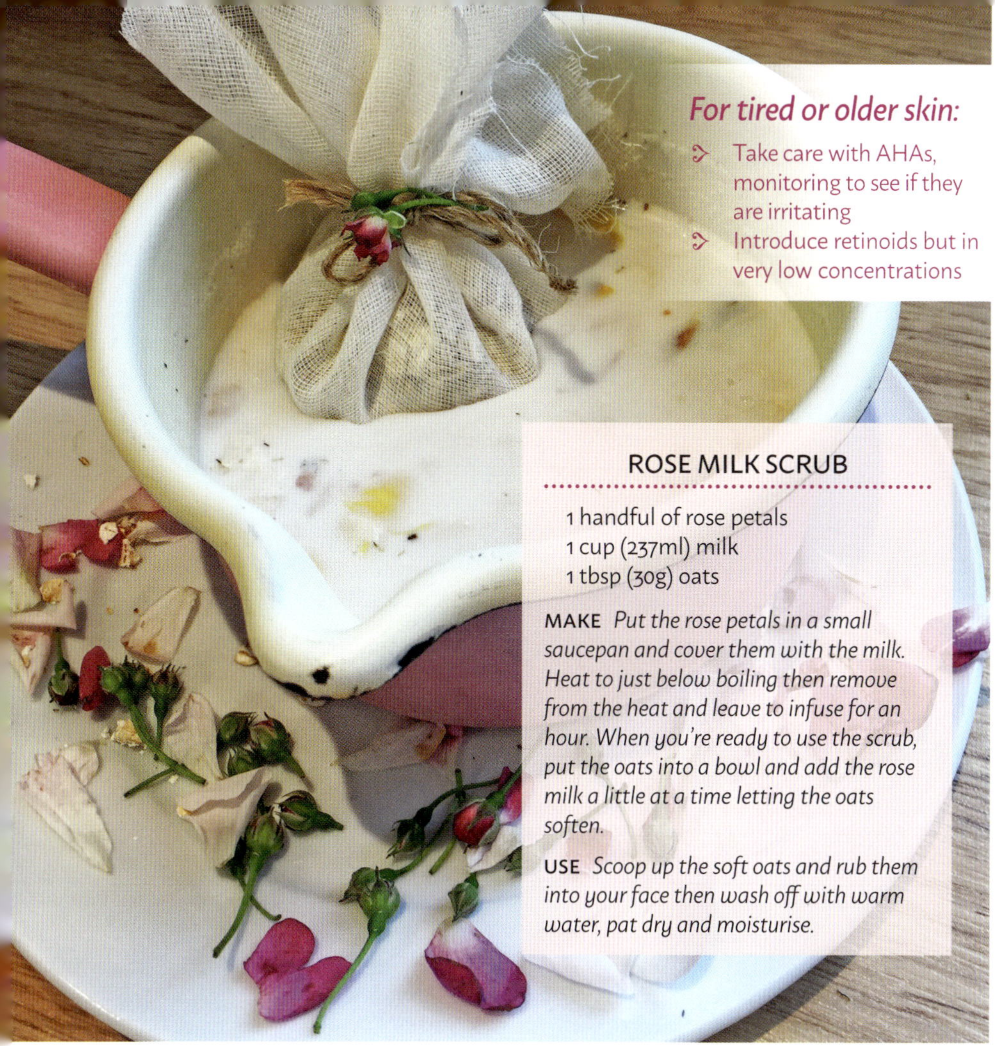

For tired or older skin:

- Take care with AHAs, monitoring to see if they are irritating
- Introduce retinoids but in very low concentrations

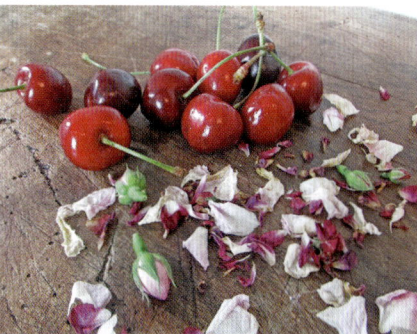

ROSE MILK SCRUB

1 handful of rose petals
1 cup (237ml) milk
1 tbsp (30g) oats

MAKE *Put the rose petals in a small saucepan and cover them with the milk. Heat to just below boiling then remove from the heat and leave to infuse for an hour. When you're ready to use the scrub, put the oats into a bowl and add the rose milk a little at a time letting the oats soften.*

USE *Scoop up the soft oats and rub them into your face then wash off with warm water, pat dry and moisturise.*

CHERRY RIPE SUMMER FACE MASK

A handful of rose petals
A handful of cherries

MAKE *First prepare your rose petal infusion as a post-mask toner by putting the rose petals in a bowl and pouring over a cup (237ml) of boiling water. Leave to infuse for 10 minutes then strain, letting the rosewater cool ready for use. Next, remove the cherry stones, catching all the juice in a bowl. Crush the cherries in the collected juice and then immediately spread them over your face.*

USE *Relax for 10 minutes, then wash off with warm water and tone using the rosewater.*

▮ Cherry juice can stain so best to cover up before making this mask. You'll want to use it right away so be sure you have everything you need ready (towel, flannel, post-mask toner and moisturiser).

CUCUMBER SKIN BRIGHTENING MILK

¼ cucumber
¼ cup (60ml) of milk

MAKE *Peel the cucumber and put the flesh in a blender to pulverise. Add the milk and keep blending.*

USE *Apply to your face using cotton wool and leave for 5 minutes before cleansing with a warm, damp cloth and applying a soothing oil.*

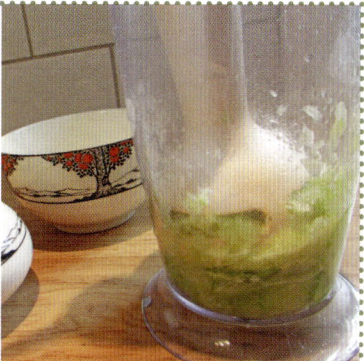

If your skin is sensitive:

- Exfoliate only very infrequently
- Use gentle exfoliants with a soothing quality, for example milk

EXFOLIATING 97

When to exfoliate

With exfoliation you can work with natural processes and natural ingredients and turn them to your advantage. If you're not exfoliating, you're missing a trick in getting your skin to look its best. Just a little caution, if you're trying out new products or techniques, you will want to find out how your skin reacts to them at a non-critical time. The eve of a big occasion is not the time to start experimenting. Whenever trying something new on your skin, test just a small patch first so you can be aware of any reaction (see the advice on patch testing in Chapter 7). Find the methods you like and use them at the times to suit you, and enjoy feeling your best.

Anything beyond the mildest exfoliation should only be done once or twice a week. Any more and you may find your skin cells can't keep up with the regeneration process. That would mean cells coming to the surface that aren't ready, which could lead to over-sensitivity, redness and soreness. So be gentle with your skin giving it just the occasional refresh when you'll most appreciate it. This is particularly so for those with sensitive skin as one gentle physical exfoliation is potentially all this skin can take. The skin on your body should be able to cope with more exfoliating than the delicate and highly exposed skin of your face. Exfoliate your face once a week, maybe twice a week for your body. Make sure you listen to and observe your skin so you know what's right for you.

Certainly, the harsher the form of exfoliation, the less often you should do it. It's always better to under, rather than over-exfoliate. If your skin becomes sensitive, red, tight and shiny you're doing too much.

It's good to vary or combine exfoliants in your routine, but remember if you're using two different approaches together, that can be equivalent to exfoliating twice. Be careful that you're not exfoliating too much this way.

Introduce any new elements in a gradual and controlled way or it will be hard to isolate what, if anything, you have a reaction to, or respond well to. If you're using some of the stronger chemical exfoliants, such as retinol, it may be too much to also use a physical exfoliant so go carefully.

Occasionally you may find an exfoliation technique a little too harsh for your skin. If this happens, stop immediately and take some remedial action. Something simple like a few drops of soothing oil (olive oil or another favourite for your skin type), or perhaps a more intensive option of a serum or restorative face mask that you know works well for you.

After exfoliating

Take care of your new skin: always moisturise after exfoliating. Your skin will be highly receptive to moisture so take advantage by slathering on oil, cream or lotion. Choose something with nourishing natural plant oils and other health-enhancing ingredients that your body will absorb readily and get a good boost from. The sooner you apply moisturiser the better, especially if you are prone to dry skin. Hydrate your skin and quickly seal to prevent water evaporating.

Also, if you are in the habit of exfoliating, know that you have young, freshly exposed skin cells at the surface. These will need protection from UV so make sure you use an appropriate SPF outdoors.

Getting exfoliation right is a real balancing act as we search for the sweet spot between refreshed, rejuvenated skin and the sore, redness of overdoing it. The plethora of different ingredients and methods add to the complexity, but means there are sufficient options and variety that enable you to find what's right for you. Develop your range of go-to tools and recipes and flex them as your skin cycles and flows through the seasons.

Your goal is to enjoy the glow of your fresh, new skin.

Nature, time and patience are the three great physicians

H.G. BOHN, BRITISH PUBLISHER, 1796-1884

CHAPTER 11

moisturising

Supple, glowing skin has plump, moist cells. Our skin's moisture is hydrolipid i.e. a combination of oil and water. Keeping cells moist and skin in best condition requires sufficient supplies of both oil and water. Moisturisers will have a combination of oil and water: oil to keep skin supple, water to hydrate.

Great moisturisers are a combination of the right ingredients in the right texture. Knowing the job you want your moisturiser to do will ensure you get this combination right.

Why use moisturisers?

Getting the right oils is easier using a moisturiser. Diet can help enormously in getting oils into your body, but will not hydrate your skin. Getting water to your skin has to be done with a moisturiser: drinking water is vital for your internal organs, but is not likely to have much impact on hydrating your skin. Our skin's need for moisture is constant, the variety comes in how we moisturise, and what we use.

When to moisturise?

The vital functions moisturisers provide can necessitate use throughout the day. Moisturise all over after a shower or bath to lock in moisture. Top up moisturiser on exposed skin as required whenever you need to.

Night time moisturising

We have separate day and night moisturisers because our skin behaves differently through these times. Our skin is responsive to the sun and moon. At dusk it will begin its restorative processes and we can help by providing antioxidants or other skin repairers like retinol and peptides. At night your skin is resting and not being exposed to environmental stresses, so it can concentrate on reparative work.

Your evening skincare routine can begin as soon as it's dark, it doesn't have to be just before bed. By bringing your self-care forward to when the sun goes down, you can take your time over it (before you're too tired to bother), you have opportunity to enjoy your lovely products (and the beautiful, relaxed feeling they give you) and your creams have time to sink into your skin before you hit the pillow.

Seasonal moisturising

Change your moisturiser as you move through the seasons, and respond to the different requirements your skin has for moisture.

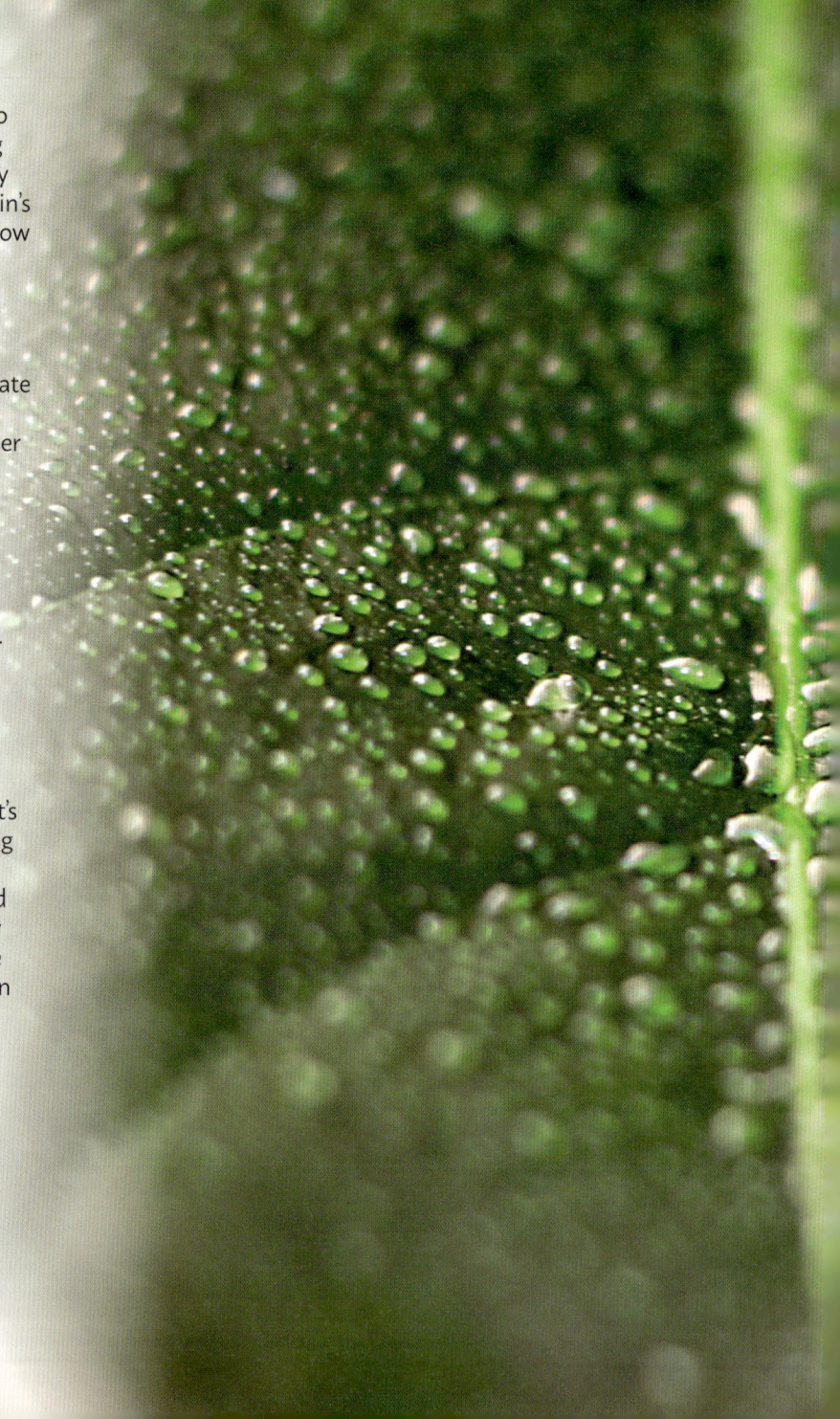

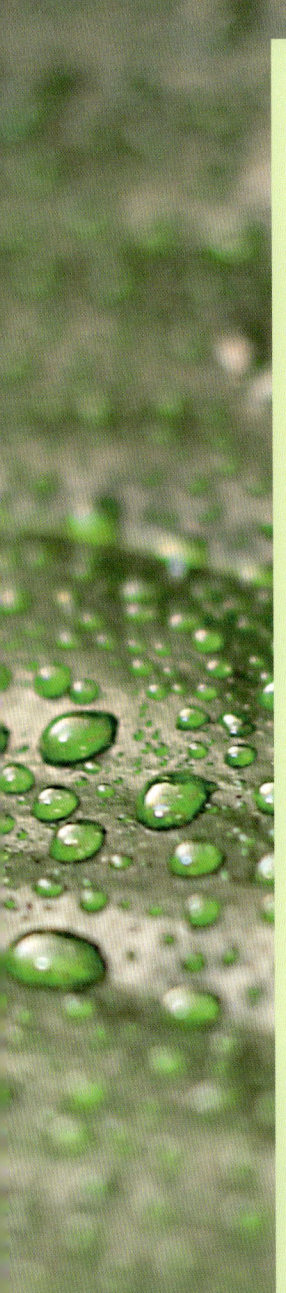

What do moisturisers do?

A good moisturiser will:

- Rehydrate the skin
- Keep it feeling supple
- Not be greasy
- Not clog pores
- Provide a barrier against pollutants and irritants
- Protect against the sun
- Penetrate the surface of the skin (making it a good vehicle for therapeutic ingredients)

Products are formulated to work with skin on specific areas of the body, for example:

- Those for use on a small area (face or hands) should have short, controllable oils, while ones for the whole body benefit from long oils that allow the product to stretch along limbs, back and torso
- Hand creams will be the most regularly applied and need to be swift to use and sink into the skin
- Foot creams need to be able to penetrate thicker skin
- Face, neck and eye creams need to be kind to delicate skin and provide protection to these exposed areas

Moisturiser functions

Moisturising products can perform their role in three different ways:

1. *By providing moisture:* **emollient** *ingredients help soften skin so products can sink in.*

Many light oils are emollient. Used in a moisturiser, they will help replace natural oils and also bind skin cells together, making skin smoother.

Other emollients that are found in moisturisers include: castor oil, glyceryl, stearate, cholesterol, silicones including cyclomethicone and dimethicone, isopropyl isostearate, isopropyl palmitate, jojoba oil, panthenol and vitamin E.

2. *By drawing in moisture:* **humectant** *ingredients attract water to them.*

Humectants are often added to products in a gel form, they include glycerine/glycerol, hyaluronic acid, propylene glycol, sorbitol, honey, urea and polyethylene glycol (PEG).

3. *By sealing in moisture:* **occlusive** *ingredients help slow down evaporation by creating a sealing effect.*

Occlusives can be greasy and difficult to dissolve in water. They include petroleum jelly, mineral oil, lanolin, silicones, olive oil, carnauba wax, candelilla wax, beeswax, some vegetable oils, cetyl alcohol, stearyl alcohol, stearic acid, lecithin and cholesterol. Make sure skin is thoroughly clean before applying occlusives as they seal everything in.

Some ingredients perform more than one of these tasks so may have multiple classifications.

Most shop-bought moisturisers will blend oils to provide all three functions in varying quantities. When you blend your own skincare you can be quite specific about what you want to include and which ingredients suit you and your purpose best.

Which moisturiser should you use?

To know what moisturiser or moisturising ingredients to use, you first need to know whether your skin is in need of oil or water. Without oil your skin is 'dry'; without water your skin is 'dehydrated'. These are different conditions with different causes and treatments.

❄ Dry skin

Dry skin needs more oil. If your skin is dry and flaky it lacks oils and needs repairing. Start by gently exfoliating to rid the old skin cells, and follow immediately with emollient oils that will penetrate into your skin, replenishing supplies. Humectants can help but don't solve dry skin.

Occlusive oils may feel soothing to apply but don't tackle the root problem as effectively.

Applying water to dry skin, without oil, will only make it dryer. Keep your bath or shower water temperature as low as you can bear to minimise the oil-stripping effects of higher temperatures. You can add oils to your bath and apply pure oils as soon as you step out of the bath or shower. While your skin is still warm and damp to create your own instant oil and water mix.

Dry skin can't hold onto water, so can lead to dehydrated skin. You'll need to tackle the dryness and the dehydration separately.

❄ Dehydrated skin

Dehydrated skin needs more water. Skin is losing water all the time; the technical term is transepidermal water loss (TEWL). This is something we can take steps to manage. It's most effective to apply moisturiser to your skin where and when it needs to rehydrate.

Take care to protect your skin against the drying elements: sun and wind, and central heating.

Avoid harsh products when your skin is dehydrated, as these can strip oils, giving the impression of dry skin, which can be confusing when you really need to be tackling your dehydrated skin.

Dehydrated skin is a temporary situation, it may even fluctuate through the day for you. Your skin can be oily and yet dehydrated (it can't however, be oily and dry, as dry skin is that which doesn't produce enough oil). You may often notice your dehydrated skin in particular areas, such as on your upper cheeks, or flaking skin on your chin, nose or mouth. Or maybe it's just all over dull and lacklustre, though sometimes it can look tight and shiny. You'll notice dehydration by the wrinkles when you pull the skin. Often it's a result of using harsh, drying cleansing products. It can improve quite quickly with a switch to gentler products and careful moisturising.

To replace water we need to offer it to our skin in a hydrolipid format (combined with oils). Emollient, humectant and occlusive ingredients all play their part in helping manage water content in our skin.

To start, hold onto the water on your damp body as you step out of the shower or bath by applying a humectant-rich lotion to draw in the water. Follow this with a watery lotion, including emollient oils, to introduce more hydration. Moisturising sprays are great for applying these quickly. End with an occlusive cream to seal the moisture in.

This trio of humectant, emollient and occlusive moisturisers can be used together for three-step hydration.

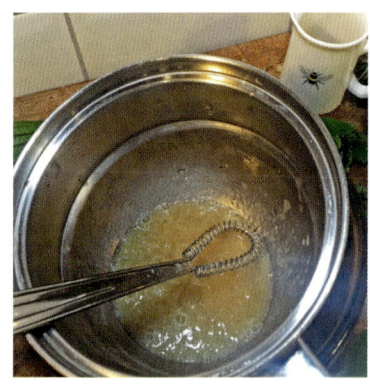

Using oils with high proportions of essential fatty acids, such as borage oil and evening primrose oil, helps create water-resistant membranes for cells, making them better able to retain moisture.

MARSHMALLOW AND CHAMOMILE LOTION

1g dried marshmallow leaves (about 1½ tsp)
1g dried chamomile flowers (about 1 tsp)
6g thistle oil
4g borage oil
2g emulsifier L
1g cetyl alcohol
1g honey
0.5g glycerine
0.5g hyaluronic acid gel
0.3g Preservative Eco

OPTIONAL:
4 drops geranium essential oil
4 drops lavender essential oil
1 drop cedarwood essential oil

a humectant-rich lotion – with borage oil, honey and hyaluronic acid

MAKE First prepare an infusion by putting the marshmallow leaves and chamomile flowers into a pan and adding 4 tablespoons (60ml) of water. Bring to the boil and then simmer while you prepare the oils. Put the oils, emulsifier and cetyl alcohol into the top of a double boiler. Heat and stir until the waxes melt, then strain the infusion and add 2 tablespoons (30ml) of it to the oils, little by little, stirring all the while. Replace the water in the bottom of the double boiler with cold water and stir as you add the honey, glycerine, hyaluronic acid gel and essential oils (if using). Keep stirring until it is completely cool and then transfer to a wide-necked bottle.

USE Apply immediately after getting out of the shower or bath.

STORE Keep in the fridge for up to 2 weeks.

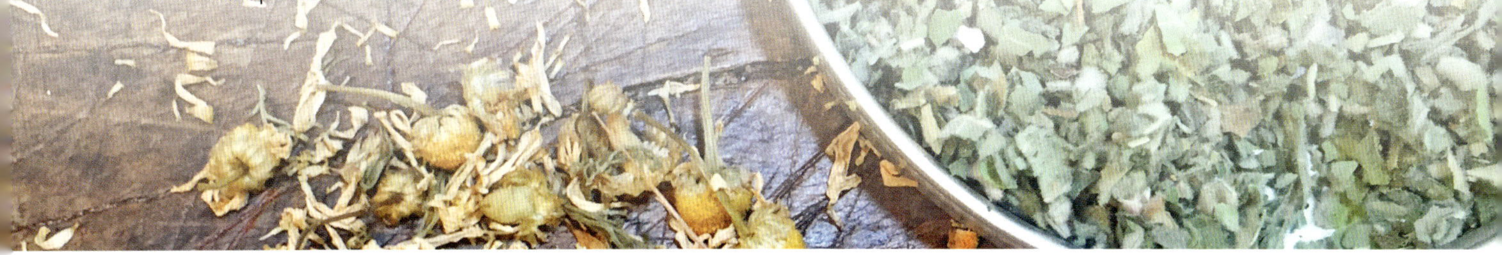

SPRAY OF ROSES AND VIOLETS

an emollient watery lotion spray – with rosehip oil for its fatty acid content

0.5g violet leaves
0.5g rose petals
0.5g plantain
0.5g ivy leaves
½ tsp (2.5g) hazelnut oil
½ tsp (2.5g) borage oil
½ tsp (2.5g) rosehip oil
1g emulsifier L
0.5g glycerine
0.5g vitamin E

OPTIONAL:
6 drops geranium essential oil
6 drops lavender essential oil
4 drops lemon essential oil

MAKE First prepare an infusion by putting the violet flowers, rose petals and plantain and ivy leaves into a pan and add 8 tablespoons (120ml) of water. Bring to the boil and then simmer while you prepare the oils. Put the hazelnut and borage oils with the emulsifier into the top of a double boiler. Stir well to combine them together as the wax melts. Strain the infusion and add 4 tablespoons (60ml) of it to the oils, little by little, stirring all the while. Replace the water in the bottom of the double boiler with cold water and stir as you add the rosehip oil, glycerine, vitamin E and essential oils (if using). Keep stirring until it is completely cool, then transfer to bottle with a spray top.

USE Shake well and apply post-shower or bath or whenever your skin needs rehydration.

STORE Keep in the fridge for up to 2 weeks.

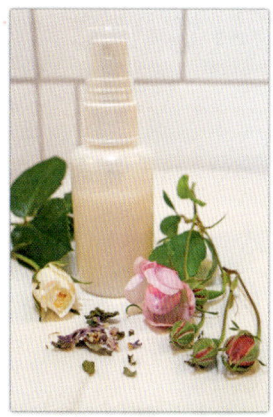

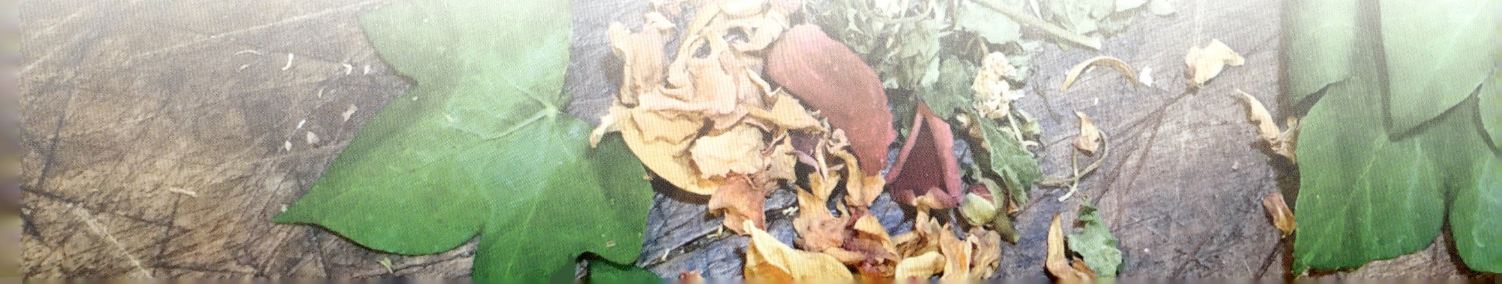

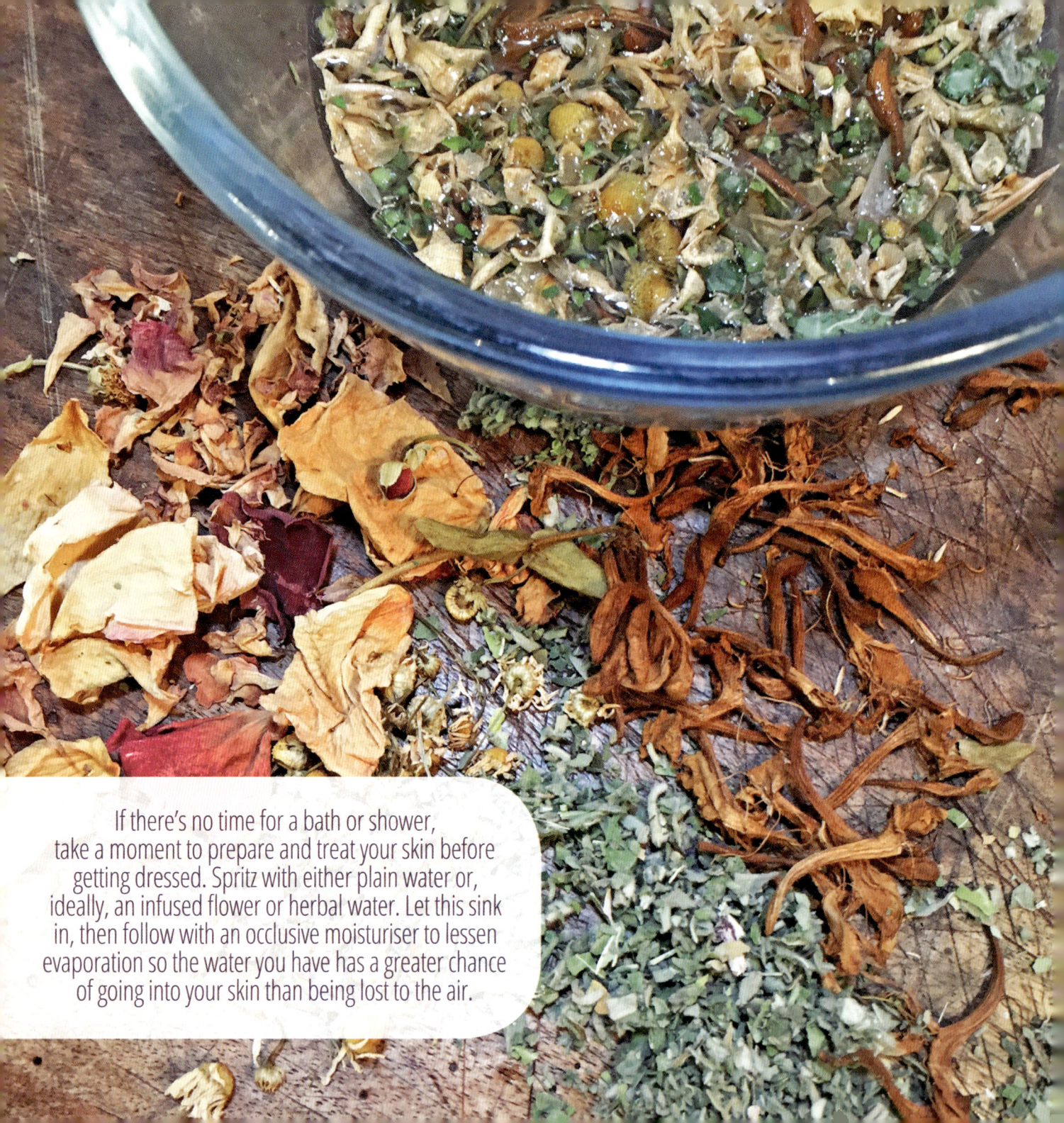

If there's no time for a bath or shower, take a moment to prepare and treat your skin before getting dressed. Spritz with either plain water or, ideally, an infused flower or herbal water. Let this sink in, then follow with an occlusive moisturiser to lessen evaporation so the water you have has a greater chance of going into your skin than being lost to the air.

LAVENDER BODY PROTECTING CREAM

an occlusive moisturiser with hemp seed oil and lavender

4g lavender
2 tbsp (30g) sunflower oil
1 tsp (5g) beeswax
½ tsp (2.5g) cetyl alcohol
4g walnut butter
6g rapeseed oil
6g hemp seed oil
3g rosehip oil
0.3g Preservative Eco
0.5g vitamin E
OPTIONAL:
5 drops geranium essential oil
5 drops lavender essential oil
2 drops clary sage essential oil

MAKE Prepare by impregnating your oil and water with lavender. Put half the lavender into a pan, pour over the sunflower oil and gently heat to macerate. Put the other half in a bowl or cup and cover with 4 tablespoons (60ml) of boiling water, and leave to infuse. Meanwhile, melt the beeswax, cetyl alcohol and walnut butter in the top of a double boiler and then add the lavender macerated sunflower oil, rapeseed and hemp seed oils. Strain the infusion and stir a tablespoon (15ml) of this into the oils. Replace the water in the bottom of the double boiler with cold water and stir as you add the rosehip oil, Preservative Eco, vitamin E and essential oils (if using). Stir until cool and transfer to a wide-necked pot.

USE Apply to clean, moist skin as a final protective layer.

STORE Keep in the fridge. It will last for up to three months.

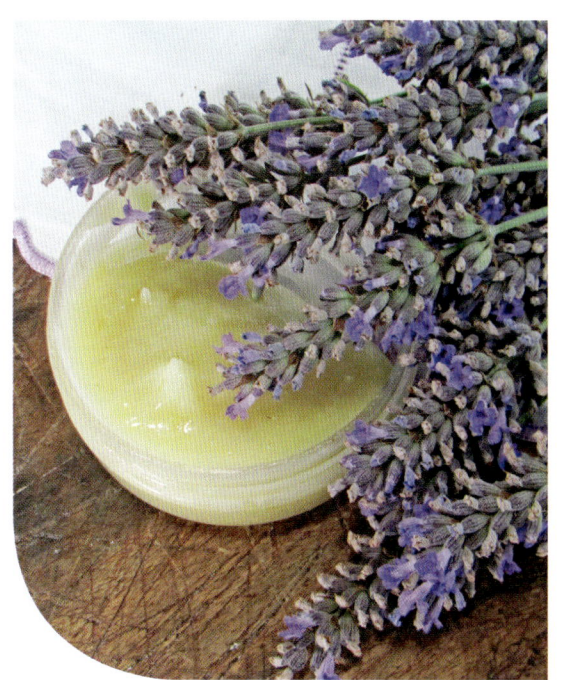

FLORAL BODY SPRITZ

using humectant herbs

2g marshmallow leaves
2g chamomile flowers
2g honeysuckle flowers
2g rose petals
4 tbsp (60ml) rosewater
1 tsp (5ml) apple cider vinegar

MAKE Put 1g of each herb in a bowl or cup and pour over ½ cup (118ml) of boiling water. Leave to infuse for 30 minutes before straining into a pan. Add the remaining herbs to the infused water in the pan and bring to the boil, then simmer for 20 minutes. Switch off the heat and leave to cool completely, then strain (ensuring all the herbs are removed) and stir in the rosewater and apple cider vinegar. Transfer to a bottle with a spray top.

USE Spritz over the body before getting dressed and follow with an occlusive moisturiser.

STORE Keep in the refrigerator. It will only last a short while, 2-3 days, but surplus supplies can be frozen in ice cube trays and defrosted as needed to replenish the bottle. Always wash and sterilise the bottle before adding new supplies.

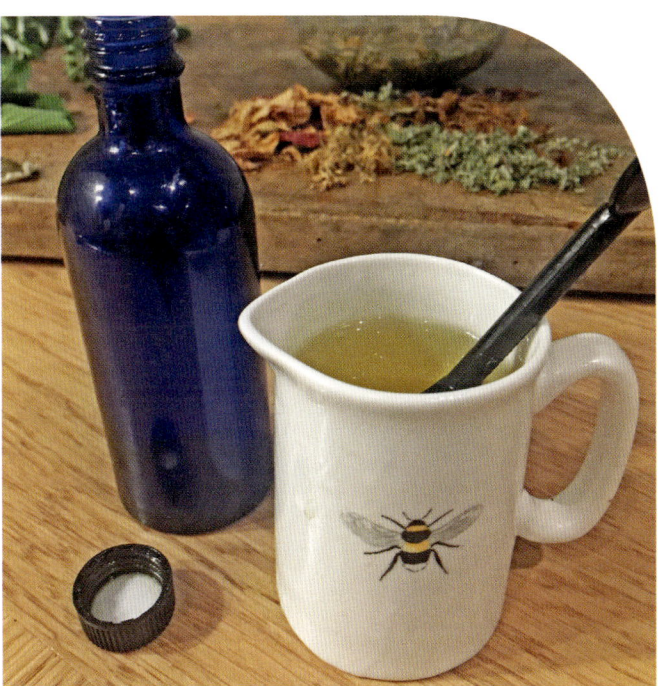

How to moisturise when ...

... your skin is damaged

Rich, comforting creams can provide relief, but you also want to solve the underlying problem, heal your skin and restore its protective properties. Before smothering with heavy oils, apply a layer of gentle emollient oil such as camelina.

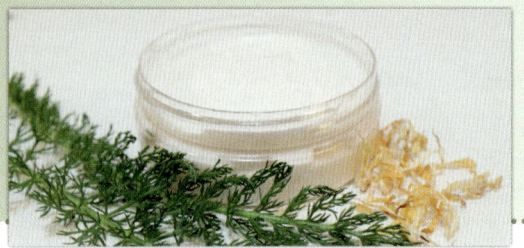

RESTORATIVE LOTION

with camelina oil and walnut oil

1g dried yarrow
0.5g dried calendula flowers
1 tsp (5g) camelina oil
1 tsp (5g) walnut oil
2g emulsifier L
1g cetyl alcohol
0.5g glycerine
0.3g Preservative Eco
0.5g vitamin E

OPTIONAL:
5 drops mandarin essential oil
2 drops chamomile essential oil
1 drop cedarwood essential oil

MAKE First prepare an infusion by putting the herbs in a pan and adding 4 tablespoons (60ml) water. Bring to the boil and then turn down and simmer. Meanwhile, put the oils, emulsifier and cetyl alcohol into the top of a double boiler and heat, stirring, until they are melted and well combined. Strain the herbal infusion and slowly stir 2 tablespoons (30ml) of this into the oils. Replace the water in the bottom of the double boiler with cold water. Stir as the lotion cools and then add the glycerine, Preservative Eco, vitamin E and essential oils (if using). Keep stirring until it is cold, then pour into a wide-necked bottle.

USE Apply wherever there are signs of damaged skin in need of protection.

STORE Stored in the fridge this will keep for three months.

... your skin is dull

First exfoliate to loosen and wash away any dead skin cells, encouraging a fresh flush of youthful cells to come to the surface. Then take immediate steps to protect and nurture fresh cells with nutrient-rich natural oils. Apply the oil neat or in a serum. Rosehip oil is wonderful for this as it is packed with vitamin A that naturally brightens skin.

HEDGEROW BRIGHTENING SERUM

with rosehip oil, broccoli seed & borage oil

2g dried blackberry leaves
1g dried elderflowers
2 tbsp (30ml) sunflower oil
1 tsp (5ml) borage oil
1 tsp (5ml) broccoli seed oil
1 tsp (5ml) rosehip oil

OPTIONAL:
6 drops geranium essential oil
3 drops clary sage essential oil

MAKE First macerate the blackberry leaves and elderflowers in the sunflower oil, it's best to use the sun method with small quantities of oil (page 141). Strain and blend the macerated oil with the borage, broccoli seed and rosehip oils plus the essential oils (if using). Stir to combine well then transfer to a bottle.

USE Massage gently into skin as needed, or it can be used as a spot treatment.

STORE Keep in a cool, dark place. It will last for six months.

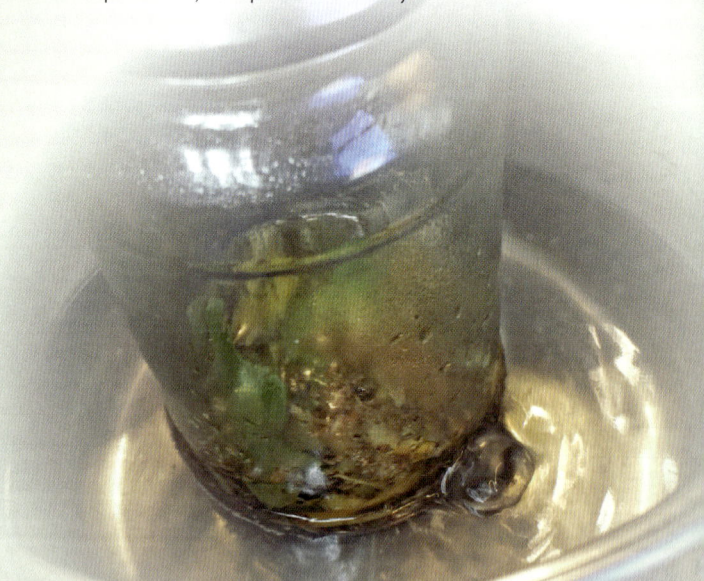

... your skin is oily

You are producing enough of your own oils, but you may still lack moisture due to dehydration. Use water-based moisturisers containing dry oils. These are lightweight, emollient and non-greasy, so they won't clog pores but will nourish and can encourage skin to reduce overproduction of oil. Focus on humectants (to draw in water) and avoid the more occlusive oils.

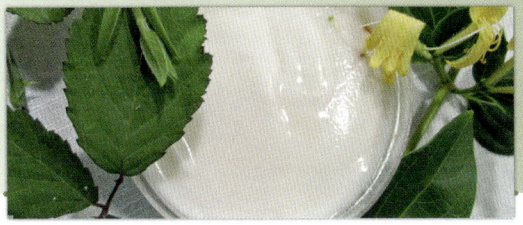

BLACKBERRY AND HONEYSUCKLE LOTION

1g dried blackberry leaves
1g dried honeysuckle flowers
2 tsp (10g) thistle oil
2 tsp (10g) hazelnut oil
2g emulsifier L
1g cetyl alcohol
1 tsp (5g) witch hazel
1g honey
0.3g Preservative Eco
0.5g hyaluronic acid gel

a non-oily body lotion with hazelnut oil, thistle oil & humectants

MAKE First prepare an infusion by putting the blackberry leaves and honeysuckle flowers into a pan and adding 4 tablespoons of water. Bring this to the boil then leave to simmer. Meanwhile, put the oils, emulsifier and cetyl alcohol into the top of a double boiler and stir to combine. Once the wax has melted, strain the herbs from the infusion then gradually add 2 tablespoons (30ml) of the infusion to the oils, stirring continually. Add the witch hazel and honey, still stirring. Replace the water in the bottom of the double boiler with cold water, stir some more, then add the Preservative Eco and hyaluronic acid gel. Keep stirring until it cools and then transfer to a wide-necked bottle.

USE Apply to oily skin after a shower or bath to help bring it back in balance.

STORE Keep in the fridge. It will last for three months.

... your skin is sensitive

Sensitivity and dryness often come hand-in-hand because dry skin is often more sensitive. So tackling the dryness, or dehydration could help reduce sensitivity.

Sensitivity is a sign that your body is trying to cope with more than it can handle. This may be toxins from the environment, foods or medication that your body finds hard to tolerate or physical and emotional stresses. Always seek the root cause of your sensitivity so you can take steps to eliminate it. Meanwhile, take gentle care of your skin to minimise discomfort.

Plant oils can help nourish and reinforce skin cells with the potential to gradually reduce sensitivity. Use the simplest combination of ingredients possible. Making fresh products little and often will avoid the need for potentially irritating preservatives. Incorporating herbs such as chamomile and lavender can help soothe, calm and fortify. If your skin is sensitive, be wary of including humectants in your products.

SERUM FOR SENSITIVE SKIN

1.5g dried lavender flowers
1.5g dried chamomile flowers
2 tbsp (30ml) camelina oil
1 tsp (5ml) rosehip oil
OPTIONAL:
  5 drops lavender essential oil
  2 drops clary sage essential oil

MAKE First macerate the herbs in the camelina oil, it's best to use the sun method with small quantities of oil (page 141). Strain off the herbs and blend the macerated oil with the rosehip oil and essential oils (if using). Stir well to ensure all is combined, then transfer to a bottle.

USE Massage gently into skin as needed, or use as a spot treatment.

STORE Store in a cool, dark place. This will last for six months.

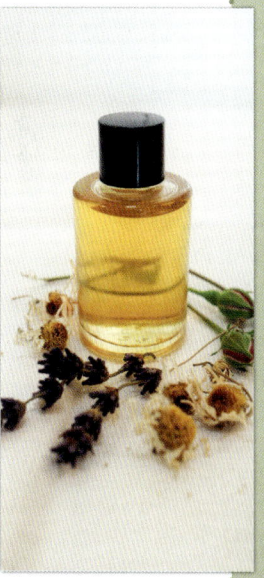

MOISTURISING

Moisturising in your teens and twenties...

Skin can go through big changes during our teenage years as it adjusts to changing hormones, sleep patterns, stress levels, foods and environments. Often this involves more natural oil production. It's good to start introducing plant oils that will help balance out your skin's own oils. Lightweight, emollient plant oils can nourish, hydrate and keep skin healthy. Just avoid heavier oils, and certainly anything petroleum-based, as these may clog pores and exacerbate spots. Good oils to try include hazelnut, camelina and sunflower.

Enjoy massaging your face and body as you moisturise, and don't forget to moisturise hands and feet too – plant oils can really help look after and strengthen your nails. Adding oils to the bath is a gentle way to introduce them into your routines. You could make your own blend of light oils to use at night; these will help calm and settle your mind. A weekly moisturising face mask can help soften skin and tone and balance your own oil production. This acts as a good defence against acne.

NAIL STRENGTHENING BALM

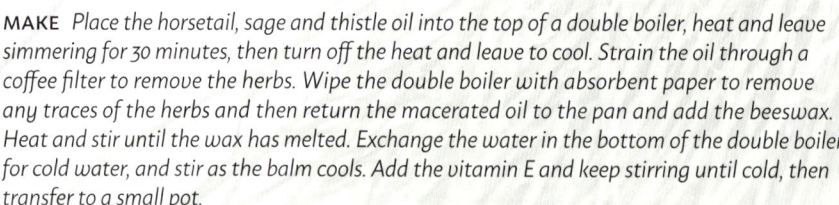

3g dried horsetail – contains silica to help healthy nails (silica promotes mineral balance of calcium and magnesium and is required for the body to properly utilise calcium, which means strong bones and nails)
2g dried sage – to guard against fungal infections
60ml thistle oil
5g beeswax
5 drops vitamin E oil (or one capsule)

MAKE Place the horsetail, sage and thistle oil into the top of a double boiler, heat and leave simmering for 30 minutes, then turn off the heat and leave to cool. Strain the oil through a coffee filter to remove the herbs. Wipe the double boiler with absorbent paper to remove any traces of the herbs and then return the macerated oil to the pan and add the beeswax. Heat and stir until the wax has melted. Exchange the water in the bottom of the double boiler for cold water, and stir as the balm cools. Add the vitamin E and keep stirring until cold, then transfer to a small pot.

USE Gently massage into each nail in turn.

STORE Keep in a cool dark place. This will last for six months.

❋ Bath Oils

Luxuriating in an oil-enriched bath can be a wonderful way of soaking much-needed oils and water into your skin. Simply adding oil to the bath water is quick and easy (as well as enabling you to incorporate essential oils of your choice) but it will not disperse in a useful way; instead you'll see it film on the surface. To benefit from this floating oil, scoop handfuls of the oily film and massage yourself with it. Beware, the bath can become slippy, and the tell-tale ring of oil will need cleaning from the bath afterwards. There is one special type of oil that will disperse when added to bath water. This is sulphonated castor oil and it is known as Turkey Red Oil (traditionally associated with the classic red headgear, a Fez).

FLOATING OIL BATH

10 drops essential oil
1 tbsp (15ml) sunflower oil

DISPERSING OIL BATH

10 drops essential oil
1 tbsp (15ml) Turkey Red oil

Draw the bath and then add your tablespoon of oil to ensure you benefit from the fragrance.
(Note, always combine essential oils with a carrier oil before adding to the bath.)

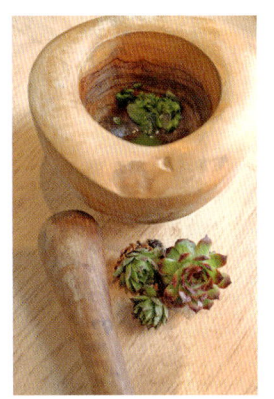

MOISTURISING FACE MASK

1.5g mint leaves (or a peppermint teabag)
1 cup (237ml) boiling water
10 houseleek leaves
1 tbsp (15g) green clay
OPTIONAL:
2 drops lavender essential oil

MAKE Infuse the mint leaves in the boiling water. Meanwhile, use a blender or pestle and mortar to blitz the houseleek leaves and then sieve to extract the juice, you want about a tablespoon. Put the green clay in a small bowl, add the houseleek juice and then take a tablespoon of the mint infusion and add a little at a time (you may not need it all). Keep stirring as you combine the ingredients into a thick paste. Add the essential oil (if using).

USE Apply the mask thinly to your face, using a brush or your fingers. If you have areas that are particularly prone to congestion, perhaps the central panel of your face, or chin, add a double layer. Leave for 10 minutes, or until it starts to dry, then rinse off with warm water. It's good to spritz with a refreshing spray afterwards.

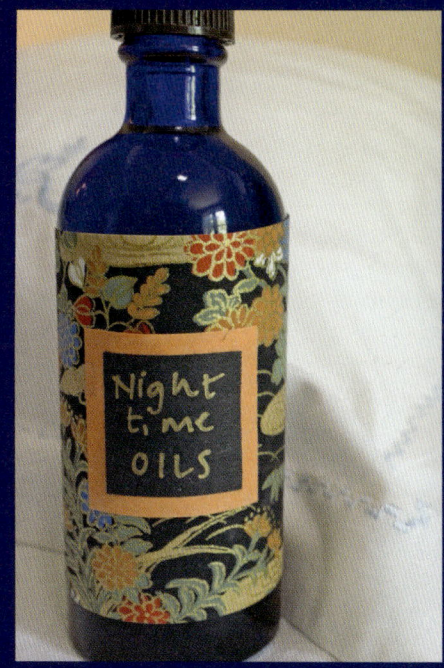

NIGHT TIME OILS

4 tbsp (60ml) thistle oil
2 tbsp (30ml) hazelnut oil
1 tbsp (15ml) hemp seed oil
Splash of rosewater
OPTIONAL:
12 drops lavender essential oil
5 drops frankincense essential oil
4 drops bergamot essential oil

MAKE Blend the oils and essential oils (if using) together and pour into a bottle.

USE At night time, pour a little of your oil blend into the palm of your clean, warm hand and add a splash of rosewater. Blend them together in your hand and apply to your face for simple moisture. Enjoy taking your time massaging them in.

STORE The blended oils will keep for 12 months.

MOISTURISING 109

Moisturising in your thirties, forties and fifties ...

George Orwell is attributed with saying that 'at 50 everyone has the face he deserves' – it applies to women too. Days of dewy plumpness and puppy fat are long gone; years of characteristic facial expressions and environmental stresses take effect. We are by now intimately connected with the reflection we see in the mirror, as it shapes our psyche and self-belief. Rejoice in seeing your true character shine through your facial shape and skin condition, and take steps to maintain your natural vibrancy.

Look after the window to your soul by applying eye cream in the morning, including UVA protection to guard against ageing crow's feet wrinkles. Make sure you extend your face cream down onto your neck. Look up as you do so and take your strokes upward as a daily inducement against saggy skin. Give your neck as much attention as your face, not just the leftovers.

Be more vigilant about applying body lotion after your shower or bath and incorporate oils with a high GLA count, such as borage oil.

If you spend a lot of time in air-conditioned spaces make sure to hydrate your skin well. If you're rushing from one environment to the next, give your skin a defensive barrier with occlusives to create your own protective bubble.

Take particular care of your hands, as they show the first signs of ageing. They can be constantly exposed to all environments, conditions and potential pollutants. Prevention is better than cure with all skincare, especially hands. Thorough cleansing using natural oil-rich soaps, plenty of nourishing creams and gloves should be daily staples. Treat yourself to a weekly hand-spa, taking care of your nails at the same time with natural oils and herbs.

EYE CREAM – LOVELY AND LIGHT

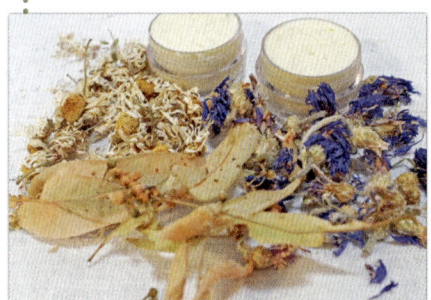

1g dried chamomile flowers
1g dried cornflowers
1g dried lime flowers
10 houseleek leaves
12g rosehip oil
2g carrot oil
1.5g emulsifier L
1g cetyl alcohol
0.3g Preservative Eco
0.25g vitamin E

MAKE First put the flowers in a pan and pour over 4 tablespoons of water, bring to the boil and then leave to simmer. Meanwhile, put the emulsifier and cetyl alcohol into the top of a double boiler and heat gently to melt. Next, crush the houseleek leaves and strain the juice. Then strain the flowers from their infusion. Add the houseleek juice to the melted wax, along with 1 tablespoon (15ml) of the strained flower infusion and the oils, stirring well. Replace the water in the bottom of the double boiler with cold water and keep stirring as the cream cools. Add the Preservative Eco and vitamin E and keep stirring until cold, before putting into a jar.

USE Apply around and under your eyes each morning using your ring finger to ensure you work delicately.

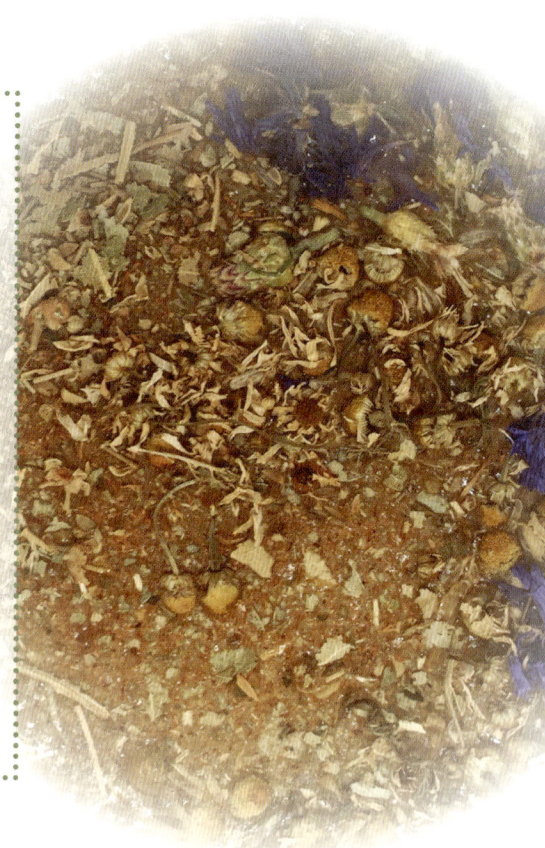

CALENDULA AND ROSE EVERY DAY CREAM FOR FACE AND NECK

1g rose petals
1.5g calendula flowers
2 tsp (10g) rapeseed oil
2 tsp (10g) camelina oil
4g beeswax
4g walnut butter
2g cetyl alcohol
4g borage oil
0.4g Preservative Eco
0.25g vitamin E

OPTIONAL:
4 drops rose de mai essential oil
4 drops lavender essential oil
2 drops sweet marjoram essential oil

MAKE Place the dried petals in a saucepan and pour over 4 tablespoons (60ml) of water and heat to infuse. Put the rapeseed oil, camelina oil, beeswax, walnut butter and cetyl alcohol into the top of a double boiler and heat gently to melt. Once the beeswax has melted add 1 tablespoon (15ml) of the strained petal infusion to the oils and stir well. Exchange the water in the bottom of the double boiler for cold water and keep stirring as the cream cools. Add the Preservative Eco and vitamin E along with the borage oil and essential oils (if using) then continue stirring until cold. Pour into a wide-necked jar and allow to settle before putting the lid on.

USE Apply to face and neck using upward strokes. Your skin may look shiny when you first put it on, so give it time to sink in and nourish.

STORE Keep in the fridge. This will last for three months.

HERBY POST-SHOWER TONING & FIRMING BODY LOTION

1g dried rosemary
1g dried thyme
2 tsp (10g) pumpkin seed oil
2 tsp (10g) hazelnut oil
2g emulsifier L
1g cetyl alcohol
1 tsp (5g) glycerine
0.4g Preservative Eco
0.5g hyaluronic acid gel

OPTIONAL:
10 drops neroli essential oil
2 drops cedarwood essential oil

MAKE Put the herbs into a pan and pour over 4 tablespoons (60ml) of water. Bring to the boil and then let simmer to infuse. Meanwhile, put the oils, emulsifier and cetyl alcohol in the top of a double boiler and heat, stirring to combine well. Once the wax is melted, strain the herbal infusion and gradually add 2 tablespoons (30ml) of this and the glycerine into the oils, stirring continuously. Replace the water in the bottom of the double boiler with cold water, then add the Preservative Eco, hyaluronic acid gel and the essential oils (if using). Keep stirring until it cools then transfer to a wide-necked bottle.

USE Apply all over your body while still damp from the shower.

STORE Keep in the fridge. This will last for three months.

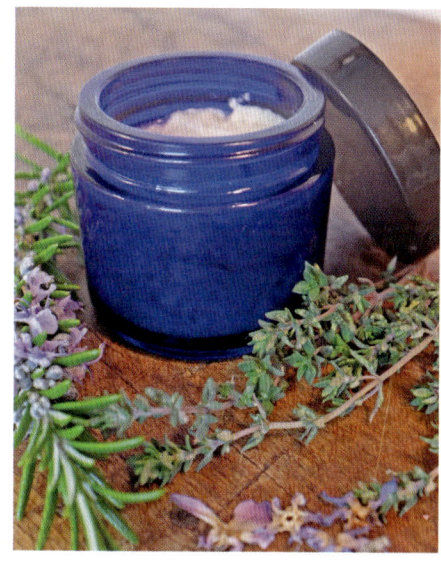

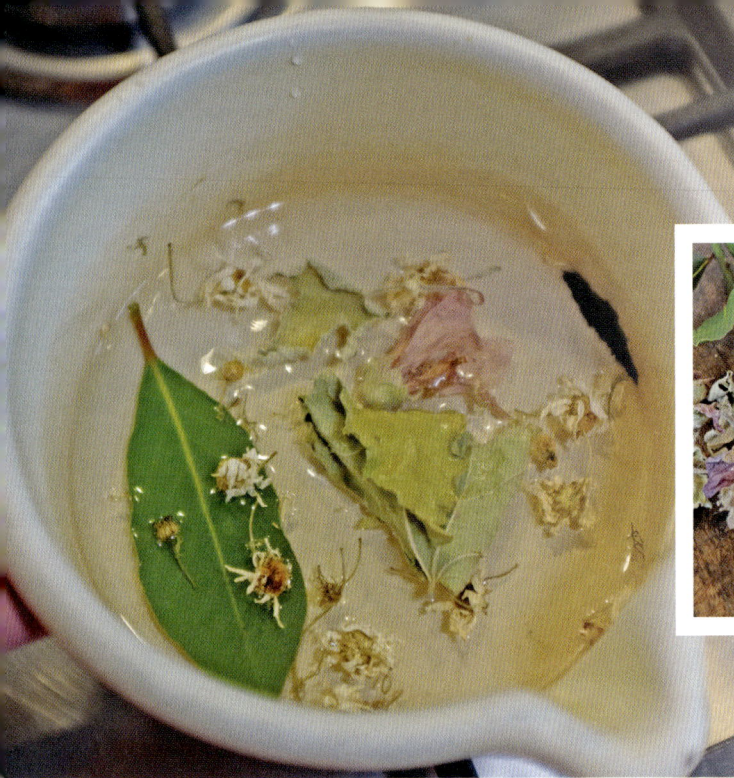

BAY, CHAMOMILE AND MARSHMALLOW NOURISHING BODY CREAM – WITH BORAGE OIL

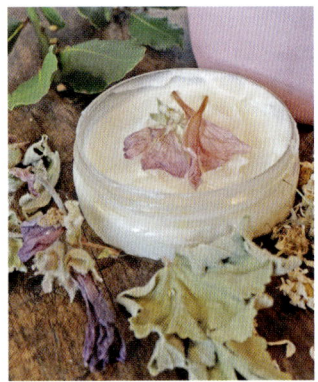

    0.5g dried bay leaves
    0.5g dried chamomile flowers
    0.5g dried marshmallow leaves
    8g thistle oil
    8g camelina oil
    4g hemp seed oil
    5g beeswax
    4g walnut butter
    2g cetyl alcohol
    4g borage oil
    0.4g Preservative Eco
    0.25g vitamin E

OPTIONAL:
    6 drops geranium essential oil
    2 drops clary sage essential oil
    2 drops chamomile essential oil

MAKE Place the dried herbs in a saucepan and pour over 4 tablespoons (60ml) of water, bring to the boil then simmer to infuse. Put the thistle, camelina and hemp seed oils with the beeswax, cetyl alcohol and walnut butter into the top of a double boiler and heat gently to melt. Once the beeswax has melted, strain the infusion and gradually add 1 tablespoon (15ml) of this to the oils, stirring well. Replace the water in the bottom of the double boiler with cold water and keep stirring as the cream cools. Add the Preservative Eco and vitamin E along with the borage oil and essential oils (if using). Keep stirring until cold. Pour into a wide-necked jar.

USE Apply all over your body.

STORE Store in the fridge. This will last for three months.

LEMON, LAVENDER AND CHAMOMILE HYDRATING SPRAY

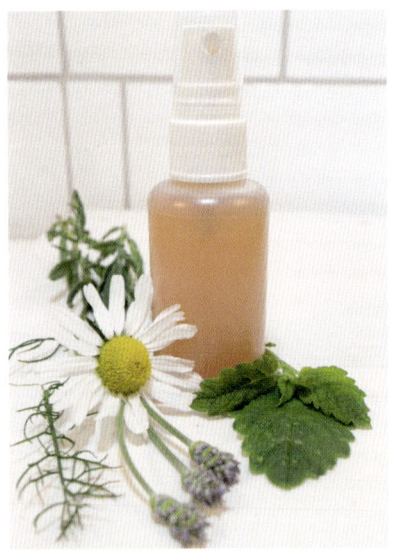

    4g lemon balm leaves – soothing, restorative, relaxing, reviving
    4g lavender flowers
    4g chamomile flowers
    50ml elderflower water – conditioning, emollient, soothing
    1 tbsp (15ml) glycerine

MAKE First take half the quantity of each of the flowers and leaves (2g of each), put in a pan and pour over 100ml of water. Heat to boiling then cover and leave to infuse for 30 minutes. Strain off the liquid and then return to the pan with the other half of the herbs; heat these and leave again to infuse. Strain the infusion and combine with the elderflower water and glycerine, then transfer to a bottle with a spray top.

USE Spray all over whenever you need to add moisture.

STORE Keep in the refrigerator. This will only last a couple of days. You can freeze the infusion in an ice cube tray and bring out cubes at intervals to replenish supplies. Always clean and sterilise your spray bottle before refilling.

1 INTENSIVE HAND TREATMENT

2g lady's mantle leaves
2 tbsp (30g) fine oatmeal
1 tbsp (15ml) hazelnut oil
1 tsp (5ml) glycerine

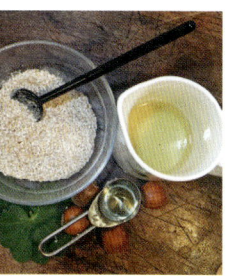

MAKE First prepare an infusion by placing the lady's mantle leaves in a pan and pour over 4 tablespoons (60ml) of water. Bring this to the boil, then switch off the heat, cover and let it cool and infuse before straining off the leaves. Put the oatmeal into a bowl and add the hazelnut oil and 1 tablespoon (15ml) of the lady's mantle infusion, along with the glycerine. Mix well to form a smooth paste.

USE Apply the paste to your hands and leave for about 30 minutes before washing off and moisturising. You can wear cotton gloves over your hands while the treatment sinks in, or use it as an excuse to spend half an hour doing very little.

2 NAIL SOAK

2 tbsp (30ml) pumpkin seed oil
2 tsp (10ml) broccoli seed oil

MAKE Put the oils into a heatproof jar or high-sided bowl and place this in a pan with a little water, making sure the water does not go over the edge of the jar. Heat to warm the oils and then carefully remove the jar from the pan.

USE Soak your nails for 5 minutes in the warm oil then gently push back the cuticles with an orange stick. You'll find it easier to remove nail varnish after soaking like this. Clean under the nails with a natural bristle brush.

hand spa

3 ELDERFLOWER AND COMFREY NOURISHING HAND CREAM

2g St John's Wort
12g sunflower oil
1g dried elderflowers
1.5g dried comfrey leaves
8g camelina oil
5g beeswax
4g walnut butter
2g cetyl alcohol
2g broccoli seed oil
2g hemp seed oil
0.4g Preservative Eco
0.25g vitamin E

OPTIONAL:
4 drops clary sage essential oil
4 drops rosemary essential oil

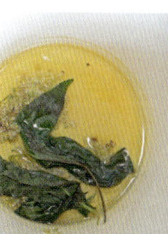

MAKE Macerate the St John's Wort in the sunflower oil, it's best to use the sun method when working with small quantities (page 141). Once this is ready, place the elderflowers and comfrey leaves in a saucepan and pour over 4 tablespoons (60ml) of water, bring to the boil, then simmer to infuse. Meanwhile, put the infused sunflower oil, camelina oil, beeswax, cetyl alcohol and walnut butter into the top of a double boiler and heat gently. Once the beeswax has melted, gradually add 1 tablespoon (15ml) of the strained elderflower and comfrey infusion to the oils, stirring well. Exchange the water in the bottom of the double boiler for cold water and keep stirring the cream as it cools. Add the broccoli seed and hemp seed oils, Preservative Eco, vitamin E and essential oils (if using) and keep stirring until cold. Pour into a wide-necked jar.

USE Apply as the final part of your hand treatment and then repeat several times a day, each time allowing it to soak in and nourish.

STORE Keep in the fridge. This will last for three months.

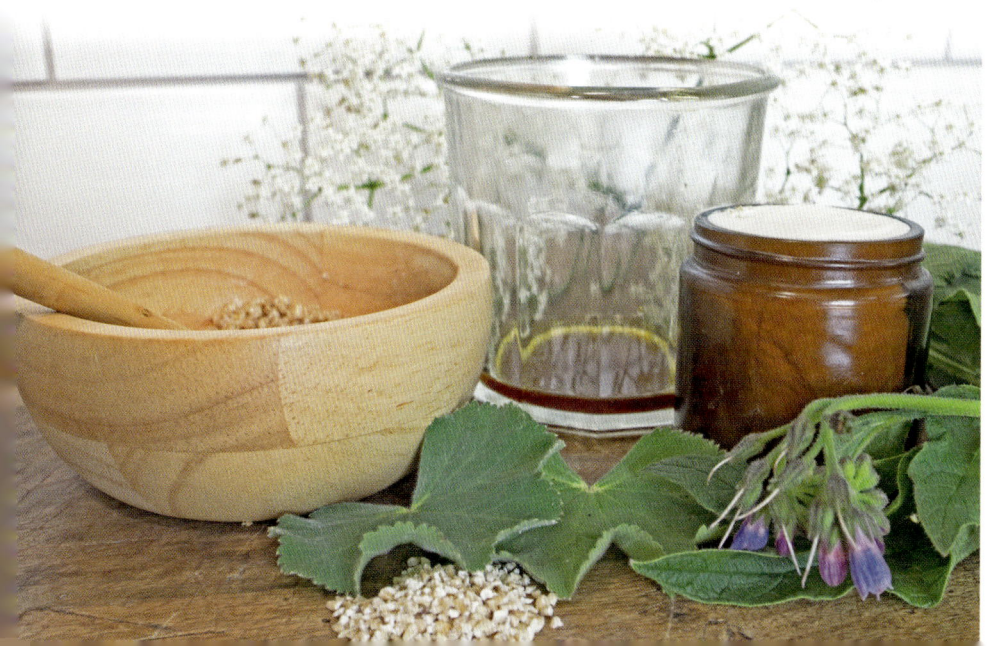

Moisturising forevermore ...

As we age, natural oil production typically slows down so we find ourselves needing to be more generous in our applications. Make daily top to toe applications of pure oils or rich body butters and creams, as the seasons dictate, to keep skin soft and supple.

At night apply serums as spot treatments to your most affected areas and use a rich face and neck cream packed with nutrients and penetrating oils to deliver deep into your skin.

TONING BODY OIL

1g fennel seeds
1.5g raspberry leaves
4 tsp (20ml) sunflower oil
2 tsp (10ml) walnut oil
2 tsp (10ml) hazelnut oil

OPTIONAL:
5 drops mandarin essential oil
5 drops fennel essential oil

MAKE Prepare by macerating the fennel and raspberry leaves in the sunflower oil – it's best to use the sun method with small quantities of oil (page 141). Once this is ready, blend with the walnut and hazelnut oils and add the essential oils (if using). Pour into a dark glass bottle.

USE Apply daily as an all over body toning and moisturising oil.

STORE This will last for six months.

FLOWER FILLED BODY BUTTER

1g evening primrose flowers
1.5g calendula flowers
4 tsp (20ml) sunflower oil
2 tbsp (30g) walnut butter
2 tsp (10ml) borage oil

OPTIONAL:
8 drops geranium essential oil
2 drops lemon essential oil
2 drops sweet marjoram essential oil

MAKE Begin by macerating the evening primrose and calendula petals in the sunflower oil – it's best to use the sun method with small quantities of oil (page 141). Once this is ready, put the macerated oil with the butter in the top of a double boiler and heat to melt, stirring all the while to blend them together. Exchange the water in the bottom of the double boiler for cold water and add the borage oil and essential oils (if using), stirring all the while. When well incorporated, put the pan into the fridge until it firms up but is still soft (about half an hour to an hour). Once cold and firm, whip the butter by hand or with an electric beater until it resembles fluffy butter then put into a pot.

USE Apply all over.

STORE Keep in the fridge. This will last for three months.

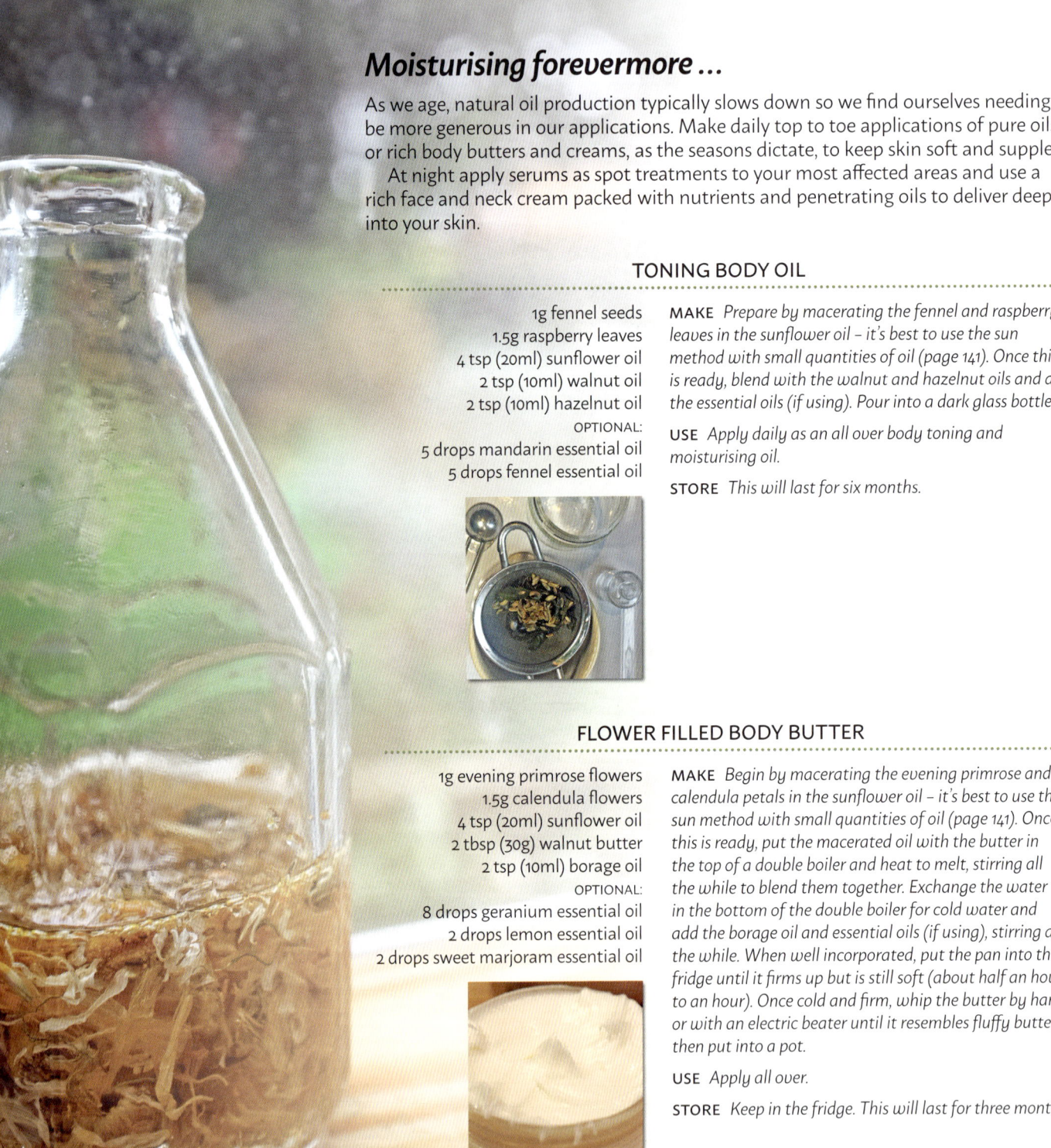

CALMING SERUM

good for sensitive skin

2g dried chamomile flowers
1g dried calendula flowers
3 tbsp (45ml) thistle oil
2 tsp (10ml) hemp seed oil
2 tsp (10ml) rosehip oil

OPTIONAL:
4 drops lavender essential oil
2 drops chamomile essential oil

MAKE Prepare by macerating the chamomile and calendula in the thistle oil, it's best to use the sun method with small quantities of oil (page 141). When ready, strain off the macerated oil and blend 2 teaspoons (10ml) with the hemp seed, rosehip oils and essential oils (if using), then transfer to a bottle and label.

USE Massage gently into skin as needed, or use as a spot treatment.

STORE This will keep for six months.

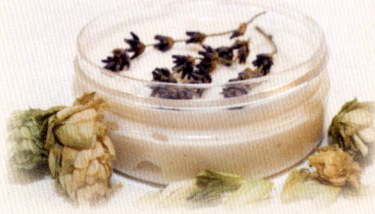

LAVENDER AND HOPS NIGHT CREAM

with hemp seed and thistle oils

1g dried lavender
1.5g dried hops
2 tsp (10g) thistle oil
1 tsp (5g) camelina oil
1 tsp (5g) hemp seed oil
5g beeswax
4g walnut butter
2g cetyl alcohol
4g borage oil
0.5g hyaluronic acid gel
0.4g Preservative Eco
0.25g vitamin E

OPTIONAL:
5 drops lavender essential oil
3 drops bergamot essential oil

MAKE Place the lavender and hops in a saucepan and pour over 4 tablespoons (60ml) of water. Bring to the boil and then simmer to infuse. Meanwhile, put the thistle oil, camelina oil, hemp seed oil and beeswax, cetyl alcohol and walnut butter into the top of a double boiler and heat gently. Once the beeswax has melted, gradually add 1 tablespoon (15ml) of the strained infusion to the oils and stir well. Exchange the water in the bottom of the double boiler for cold water and keep stirring as the cream cools. Add the hyaluronic acid, Preservative Eco and vitamin E along with the borage oil and essential oils (if using). Keep stirring until it is cold, then scoop into a wide-necked jar.

USE Apply to your face and neck at night time using upward strokes.

STORE Keep in the fridge. This will last for three months.

REJUVENATING SERUM

1g dried rose petals
1g dried chamomile flowers
1g dried valerian
3 tbsp (45ml) camelina oil
2 tsp (10ml) pumpkin seed oil
2 tsp (10ml) borage oil
1 tsp (5ml) rosehip oil – for its vitamin A and skin-brightening qualities

OPTIONAL:
3 drops rose de mai essential oil
2 drops chamomile essential oil
2 drops frankincense essential oil

MAKE Begin by macerating the rose petals, chamomile flowers and valerian in the camelina oil, it's best to use the sun method with small quantities of oil (page 141). When ready, strain off the macerated oil and blend 2 teaspoons (10ml) with the pumpkin seed, borage and rosehip oils and essential oils (if using). Transfer to a bottle.

USE Massage gently into skin as needed, or use as a spot treatment.

STORE This will keep for six months.

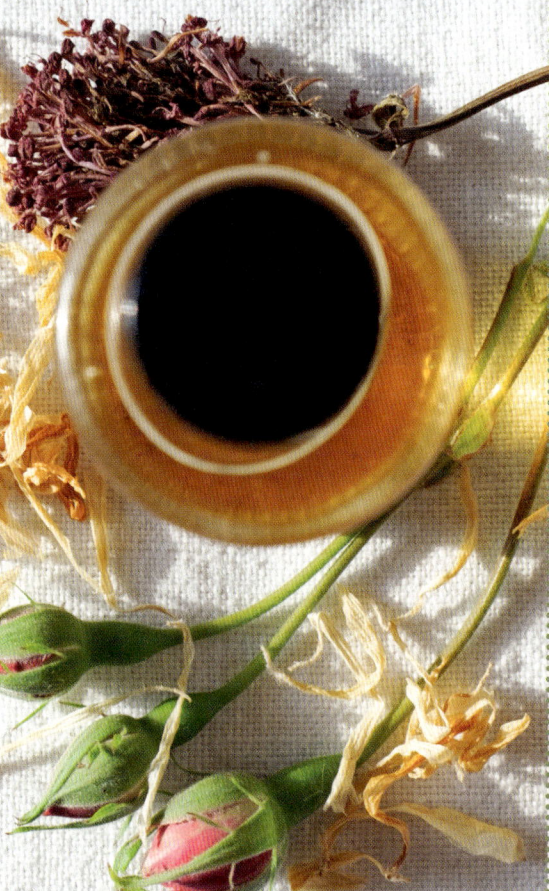

Product form

The spectrum of products that enable you to add moisture to your skin ranges from very light and simple floral waters to serums, lotions, light to heavy creams and balms and waxes. We will typically all need a selection of products from this range to provide for our skin at different times. Our skin's needs will depend on the strains it is under due to the seasons, our lifestyle and our environment.

The drier your skin, the richer the moisturiser you should apply. It's no good putting lots of layers of thin lotion on, as this will just waste product. When your skin is dehydrated, adding the wrong type of oil or cream could be detrimental. You need to use products that will help your skin retain water.

All products are formed using varying combinations of four main ingredients: wax, butter, oil and water.

Beeswax keeps skin hydrated and protected, and it has a lovely scent. I choose to use it in my skincare products as it can be sourced locally (the alternative plant-based waxes all come from tropical regions of the world). This potentially has therapeutic benefits, which are enhanced further by very local sourcing. I am a beekeeper, wanting to do what I can to nurture our essential pollinators. The beeswax used in skincare is essentially a waste product for bees. It's the wax cappings that they use to seal the honey into the comb. This is chewed through and deposited at the bottom of the hive when they want to access the stored honey. It's the cleanest form of wax available to us. The majority of wax made by the bees forms their wonderful hexagonal structured combs, which stays with the bees. They clean and reuse their combs multiple times to store each season's honey. I consider using the wax cappings in skincare to be part of the complex symbiotic relationship between ourselves, the plants and other creatures living in our environment.

Wax   Wax gives the product firmness. The typical wax used in natural skincare is beeswax, but other plant-derived waxes are available (such as candelilla, carnauba, jojoba, hemp and rice bran wax) mostly from tropical grown plants.

Butters   The butters used in skincare are not the dairy-produced type. They have a totally different origin being extracted from the seeds and kernels of plants, and are more akin to peanut butter. Some nuts yield butter quite easily (such as cocoa and shea), others require a process of extraction and then mixing with hydrogenated oil from the same plant to create the butter. These plant butters vary in hardness, so which butter is used will make a difference to the texture of the final product. Incidentally, some can be good to spread on toast just like peanut butter, (have you tried almond butter, or walnut butter?) but the cosmetic grade versions are processed to be very fine and smooth.

   Butters have different levels of firmness but this will vary depending on ambient temperature. For example, cocoa butter is one of the firmest butters with a relatively high melting point (34-36°C), so at room temperature it can be quite hard. Interchanging butters in recipes will likely create a different product consistency. Most butters will melt on contact with the skin.

Oil   Plant oils are the superfood of skincare. They are pressed from the seeds of plants so contain all the vitality needed to fuel and sustain new plants. They're so important that Chapter 13 is dedicated to looking at them in detail.

Water   The water used in skincare should be from the purest, cleanest sources available. In many old recipes they suggest gathering rainwater, as this can be naturally soft (have you ever felt the softening effects of washing your hair in rainwater?). Spring water is a good option, or bottled water (so long as it is a newly opened bottle) but types do vary so this could make a difference to your product. It's absolutely fine to use tap water; if concerned you can boil and cool this first, but many recipes require you to boil the water anyway within the making process.

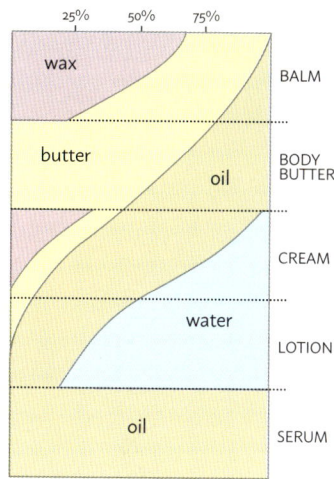

Moisturising skincare products all have a variant on the blend of oil and water. Some contain more oil, others water. Butters and waxes are added to vary the texture of the product and bring their own lubrication or protection too.

   Overleaf are basic recipes for the simpler products giving you the relative quantities of wax, butter and oil. Once you're comfortable with a product type, try adding your own herbs (in macerations) or essential oils to personalise your products. There are details on how to do this in Chapter 14.

Balms

Balms are rich and soothing. They are created for use on small areas, often for healing or protective purposes, such as a lip balm. At their most basic, balms are a blend of butter and wax, and oils can be added too. The greater the proportion of wax, the firmer the balm. Balms are often made with herbal infused oils and added essential oils for their therapeutic properties.

Body Butters

A body butter is a means to provide intense, caring moisture. Its density means it will take longer to sink in, so give it time and enjoy it. Be careful to apply just enough, but not too much, or it will not be absorbed and will feel greasy. Listen to your skin to know how much it needs, often just small dabs are adequate.

Use a body butter when you want to increase protection for your skin, such as in cold or dry weather, or when you need an intense softener for dry or rough skin. Butters are greasy and can clog pores so keep them away from your face and don't make it an every day staple.

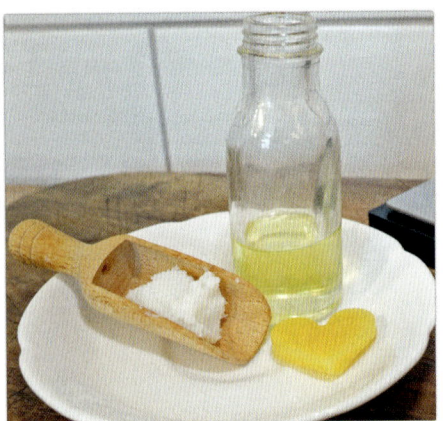

BASIC BODY BUTTER RECIPE

60g shea butter
40ml sunflower oil – a light, non-greasy oil balances out the heavier butter, the softer the butter you use, the less oil you will need to add
20 drops essential oil (optional)
0.5ml vitamin E (optional) – revitalises and fights wrinkles, and can prevent the oils in the product from oxidising and going rancid, meaning your product lasts longer.
1 tsp (5g) cornflour, rice flour or arrowroot (optional) – reduces the greasiness of the butter

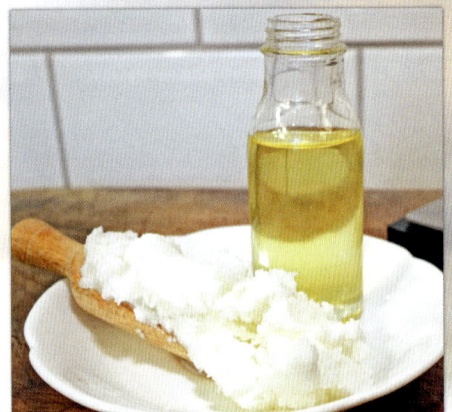

BASIC BALM RECIPE

1 tsp (5g) beeswax
1 tsp (5g) cocoa butter
1 tbsp (15ml) oil (can be herbal infused)
OPTIONAL:
  5 drops essential oil
    – add as the liquid cools

MAKE Put the wax and butter into the top of a double boiler and heat until melted, then add the oil. Exchange the water in the bottom of the double boiler for cold water and keep stirring until the balm cools. If using, add the essential oils and stir in well.

USE Apply as necessary to soothe skin.

STORE Keep in a cool dark place. It will last for 12 months.

MAKE Put the butter and oil into the top of a double boiler and heat to melt, stirring well to combine them. Replace the water in the bottom of the double boiler with cold water and continue stirring as the butter cools (this prevents it from feeling grainy on use). If using, add the essential oils, vitamin E and flour. Transfer to the fridge for at least 30-60mins until it is quite cold, then whip by hand or with an electric beater until it is fluffy. Scoop into a wide-necked jar.

USE Apply sparingly, allowing the butter to sink in.

STORE Keep in the fridge. Your butter will last for six months.

Lotion bars

Lotion bars make it easy to carry moisturiser. Strictly speaking they're balm bars as they contain no water.

Creams

A huge variety of products come under the basic banner of 'creams'. They can be rich, with just a few droplets of water blended in to lighten what would otherwise be classified as a balm or butter, or much lighter (mostly water). They are quick to sink in and deliver instant softness, but with shorter-lived impact.

Creams and lotions are more complicated to make as they combine oil with water, which requires creating an emulsion. There's much more about this in Chapter 12. The inclusion of water means they can go mouldy very quickly (within a few days) so they will need a preservative if you want the product to last more than a few days.

Lotions

Lotions are light, typically non-greasy and should absorb quickly into the skin. Being more water than oil, they're best for dehydrated rather than dry skin. Some will have a little butter added to make them richer.

In blend it yourself skincare, a lotion-like product is often created using ingredients that have their own natural emulsions, especially dairy products like milk, buttermilk and cream. This will naturally have a short shelf life and needs to be kept in the fridge. However, as they are so simple to make, it is easy to create small batches and refresh your supplies on a regular basis.

Serums

Serums are designed to penetrate well into the skin. They are packed with beneficial ingredients intended for deep delivery and maximum impact. This is achieved by using oils with small molecule sizes so they can travel swiftly and far. To maximise their potency, apply serums onto bare skin (before any other products). Be especially vigilant about any sensitivities you may have to the ingredients.

Oils

Oils on their own are good for dry skin, but not for dehydrated skin.

BASIC LOTION BAR RECIPE

40g shea butter
30ml sunflower oil (less with a softer butter)
15g beeswax
17 drops essential oil (optional)

MAKE Put the butter, oil and beeswax into the top of double boiler and heat until melted, stirring to combine well. As it cools, add the essential oils. Pour into a mould and put in the fridge, leaving overnight to set. Once set, bars can be wrapped in paper for storage and travel.

USE Rub the bar over your warm body and let your own heat melt just enough of the moisturising bar to care for your skin.

STORE Keep your bars in a cool, dark place. They will keep for six months.

Benefit of combining

It's apparent why we often accrue a plethora of jars and bottles, potions and lotions when you recognise the different needs of your skin at different times. Often you'll be switching between products from morning to night, day to day or season to season. But what if you want to benefit from several different products at the same time?

To use products in combination, think in layers. Understand the impact one product will have on your skin's ability to receive the next.

So, for example, if you have a product that is packed with active ingredients that need to penetrate deep into your skin, this will likely be one of the first things to apply in order to give it best contact with the skin. By contrast, an occlusive product, which forms a seal, will be the last thing to apply, as nothing you put on top of that will penetrate through to be of benefit.

A lot is influenced by the molecule size of your product. In general, the more delicate or water-based the product, the smaller the size of the molecules it contains. Serums are formulated to benefit from very small molecule sizes, which means they can penetrate well while lotions and creams will have increasingly large molecules. Naturally, once you've applied something with large molecules, these will cover your skin making it difficult for anything you put on top to have an effect. To benefit from both, apply the small molecule product first, give it a few moments to sink in and settle, then apply the product with larger molecules. Be patient and use a light touch (dabbing not smearing) so each product retains its integrity and function.

Make sure you consider your sun protection and where this needs to sit in your layering. You'll need to know the active properties of your product to get this right. If your product is designed to work through a chemical reaction, it will need to be as close to the skin as possible, so use it as a base layer. If your product provides a physical barrier to UV, it will be the top layer you apply. Many sun creams are occlusive, so you should apply moisturiser underneath them.

Some moisturising tips:

- ⇒ Apply moisturiser evenly, don't let it build up (e.g. around the hairline as you push it outwards) or you'll get clogged pores
- ⇒ Push upwards as you apply (don't drag your skin down)
- ⇒ Work quickly to apply moisturiser and seal in water before it starts evaporating
- ⇒ Check in with your skin regularly to see what it needs, don't just use the same thing day-in/day-out; rotate your products
- ⇒ Use arrowroot brushed onto the face to remove excess oils

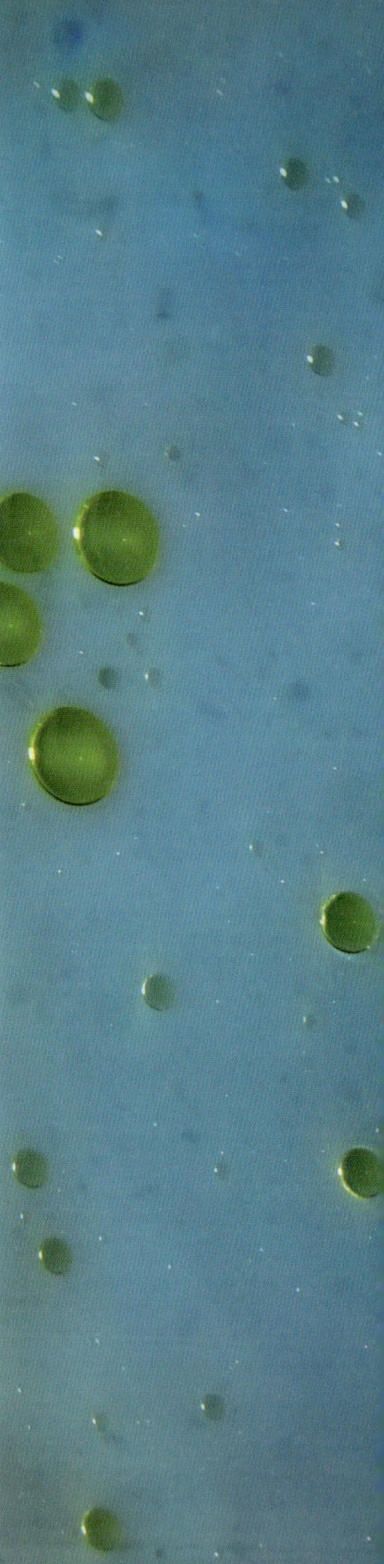

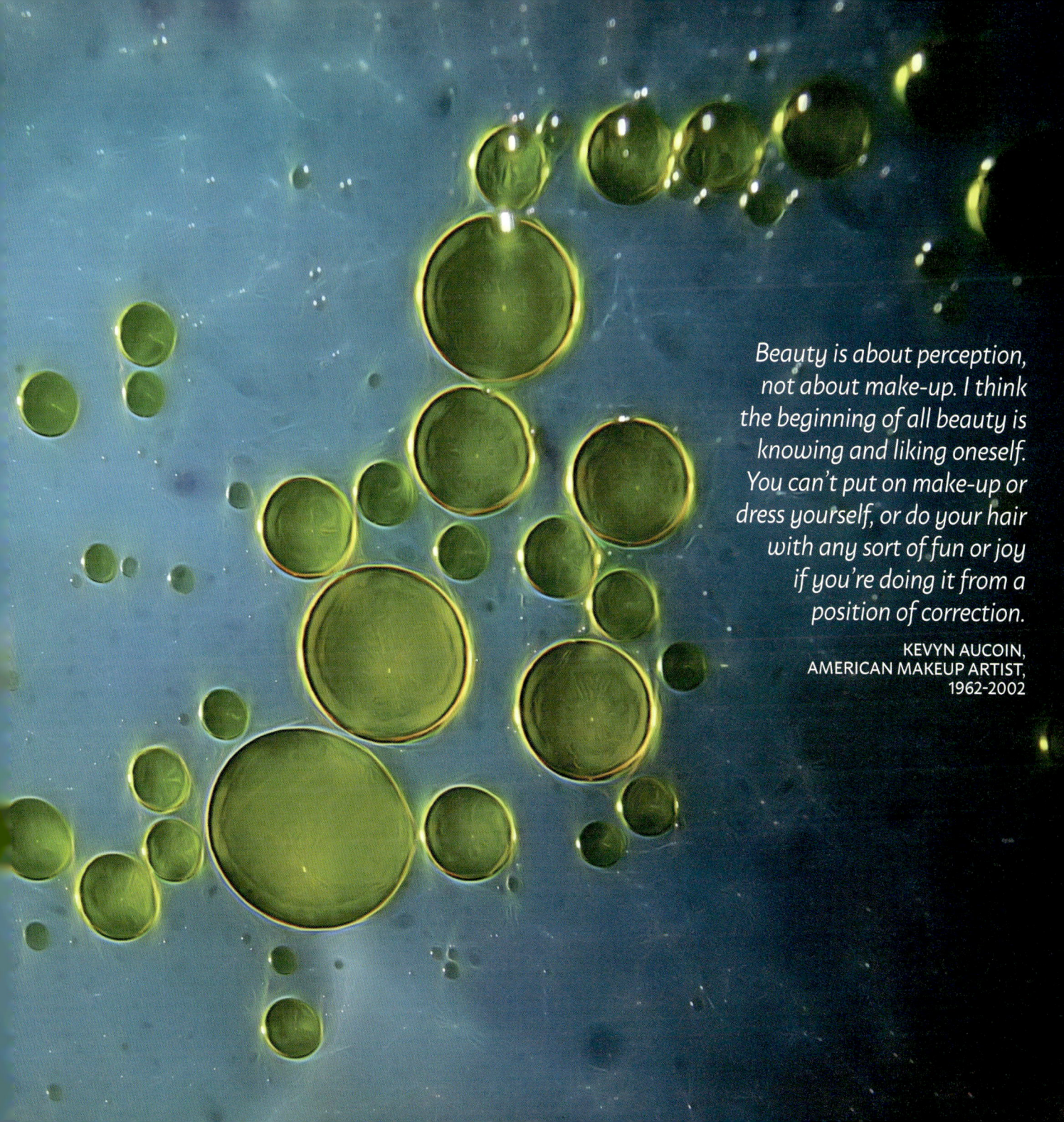

Beauty is about perception, not about make-up. I think the beginning of all beauty is knowing and liking oneself. You can't put on make-up or dress yourself, or do your hair with any sort of fun or joy if you're doing it from a position of correction.

KEVYN AUCOIN,
AMERICAN MAKEUP ARTIST,
1962-2002

Part 4
Vital Techniques

CHAPTER 12

learn to blend like a pro

Whatever skincare function you buy products for, you can make an equivalent yourself, be it creams, butters, serums, masks, scrubs, cleansers, lotions etc. When making your own, it's more important to focus on the function of the product than on trying to replicate the form of the bought product. Many homemade products can look and feel quite different to off-the-shelf versions, just as a plastic-wrapped sliced loaf is different to the bread that comes out of your oven when you bake your own.

The skills of making your own skincare have largely been lost to modern generations but are very easy to re-learn. The simpler products can be created as easily as making a cup of tea. As with many traditional skills, it's great to learn from someone, so look out for skincare making workshops in your area; they're a brilliant way to get used to the terms and techniques, handle the equipment and meet others interested in doing the same. There's nothing quite like getting hands-on with the ingredients yourself.

If you don't want to splash out on stocking up with ingredients, you can buy kits that provide just what you need to have a go at making products. As your confidence and experience grows, you'll become familiar with the ingredients you like to work with and try more recipes and techniques. You'll begin to know where and how to alter recipes to suit your needs and make the most of the ingredients that grow around you.

Using this book, you can begin to approach skincare recipes with wisdom, know which ingredients you can trust, and minimise the error rate in your trials.

Start by knowing:

- What you want from a product, how it needs to help your skin
- How you expect the product to work and good ingredients you expect to see in it
- How much you want to make at a time (particularly depending on the likely shelf life). Tot up the ingredients in the recipe to get an idea of the quantity it will make

There are very few requirements to get started: gather some useful tools around you and utilise a couple of basic techniques.

Kit and Caboodle

1. Cleanliness

A golden rule in skincare making is to work as cleanly as possible. Be meticulous about hygiene and sterile equipment. No one wants germs or dirt in their skincare, and contamination can massively shorten its lifespan.

So, thoroughly clean your hands, put on an apron and tie up your hair.

Wipe down surfaces using an antibacterial cleaner. Use your normal one, or you can make your own by blending 3 cups of water and ½ cup vinegar in a spray bottle; add 15 drops lavender essential oil, shake and spray-away.

Make sure all your equipment is scrupulously clean: pans, spatulas, whisks and spoons all need to be spotless to avoid fungus spores, bacteria, dust and dirt. Metal, glass and china are easy to sterilise using boiling water. First wash them in hot soapy water, as normal, then place them in a bowl or suitable container and pour boiling water all over them. Leave to stand for a few minutes and then lift out and allow to drain. Either air dry (you can use a hair dryer to speed this up) or use clean paper towel. If you're using oils, make sure your kit is absolutely dry because you don't want water getting into your product (that would severely shorten its lifespan).

If any equipment is plastic, or won't take kindly to being immersed in boiling water, use sterilising fluid instead (available in supermarkets – look among the baby products. Milton is the most common brand.) Buy this in a bottle or as tablets and dilute as directed. The same fluid can be used to rinse several pieces of equipment, or you can have a large bowl of prepared fluid in which you leave items to soak for half an hour or so.

One of the simplest ways to sterilise is with an alcohol spray. You can make your own easily by filling a bottle with a fine spray nozzle (such as a perfume atomizer) with the strongest proof vodka you can find. Use it on surfaces, equipment and hands. After spraying, either leave to dry naturally or wipe with a clean paper cloth.

Sterilise the container you'll be putting your product into in a similar way. Containers bought new from skincare suppliers should be good to use right away. But if you're using a pot purchased elsewhere, reusing pots, or opting to store your products in pretty china or glass, make sure these are sterilised using one of the methods above. It only takes a few moments. Once your container is sterilised, be careful to handle just the outside. Don't put your fingers inside your nice clean pot.

When the making is done, get your product into the pot as quickly as possible, and leave to cool for a few minutes before securing the clean cap or lid, ideally with a waxed card insert.

Clean any equipment you've used while it is still warm, or warm it again briefly to loosen any waxes and butters. The simplest method is to wipe around with an absorbent paper towel (if necessary pushing it into corners with a wooden spoon or similar implement) to remove all oil and wax residue. Then you can immerse in warm, soapy water to wash up as normal.

To maximise the life of your finished product, be aware of cleanliness whenever you're using it. Only have the lid off the product while it is in use, replacing it as quickly and securely as possible. Ensure your fingers are clean before touching the product, or don't touch it at all. Instead, use a spatula or clean cloth to take what you need. Try to touch as little of the surface area as possible. Treat it with gentle love and care.

If there are signs of your product 'going off' – you might notice a change in the smell or colour, for example – it's time to stop using it and make a new batch. Typically products will last longer and remain fresher if kept in the fridge. Those with water should always be in the fridge; those without can be stored in the butter compartment of the fridge until you are ready to use it. Many products can be frozen if your batch is too large to use swiftly. You're using natural ingredients so your skincare is akin to the food you make, meaning it will have a shelf life and is best made and used fresh.

Look after your spare ingredients well too. Keep fresh herbs in the fridge and dried ones in a cool, dark place. Keep bottles of natural oils cool and dark. Don't pour unused oil back into the bottle and be careful to avoid cross-contamination when using several oils at once. Buy ingredients in the smallest practical quantities, as they all have a shelf life and are best used as fresh as possible.

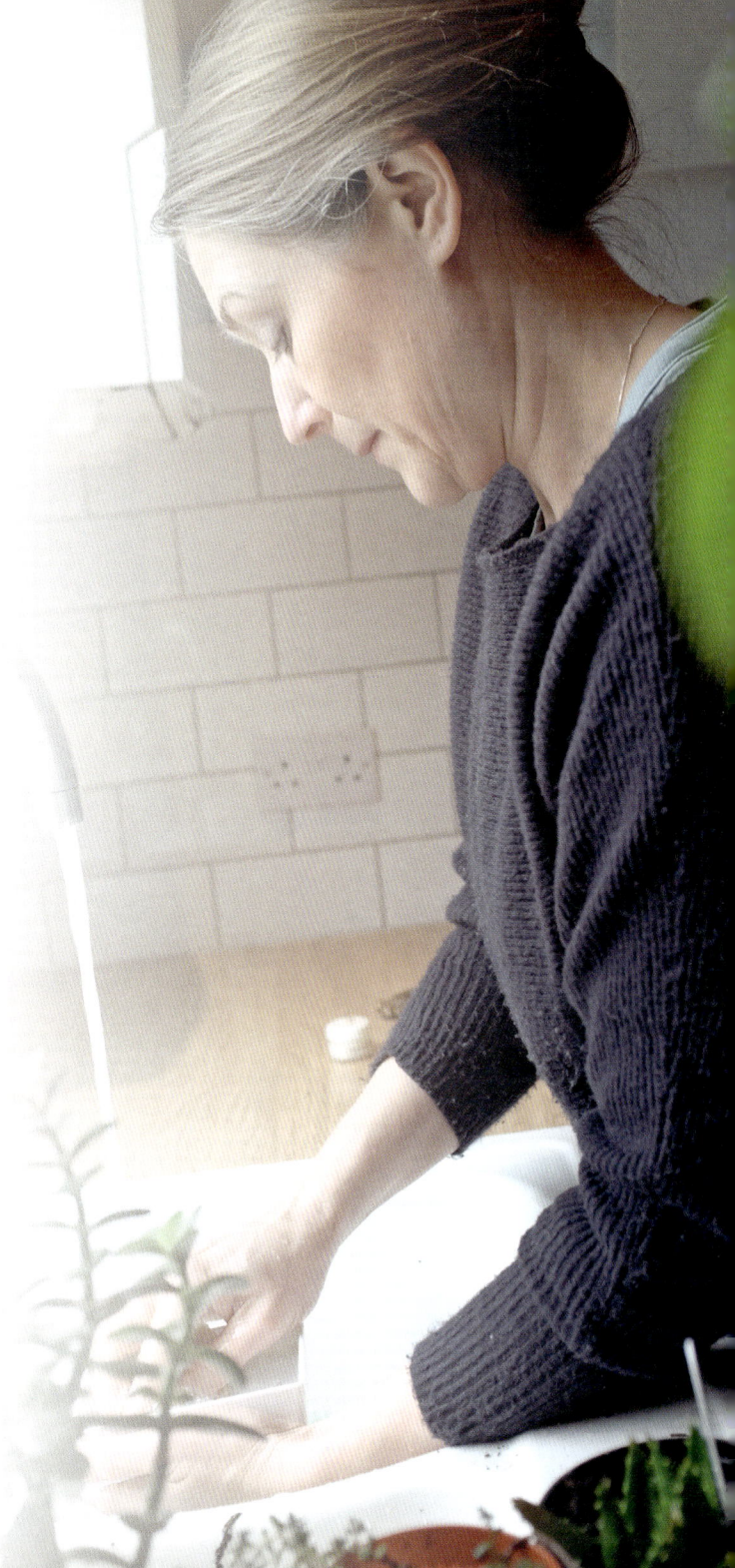

2. Equipment

❋ Measuring equipment

You need to accurately measure out your ingredients when making skincare. In the recipes in this book I've given teaspoon or tablespoon equivalents where possible so you can quickly use simple kitchen equipment to measure. Kit yourself with standard spoons and a small measuring jug to get started. When you need to weigh ingredients it can be quite tiny amounts (a few grams or parts of a gram) so you'll need micro scales and/or a syringe for accurate measuring.

Little battery-operated scales can be bought inexpensively online and are well worth investing in.

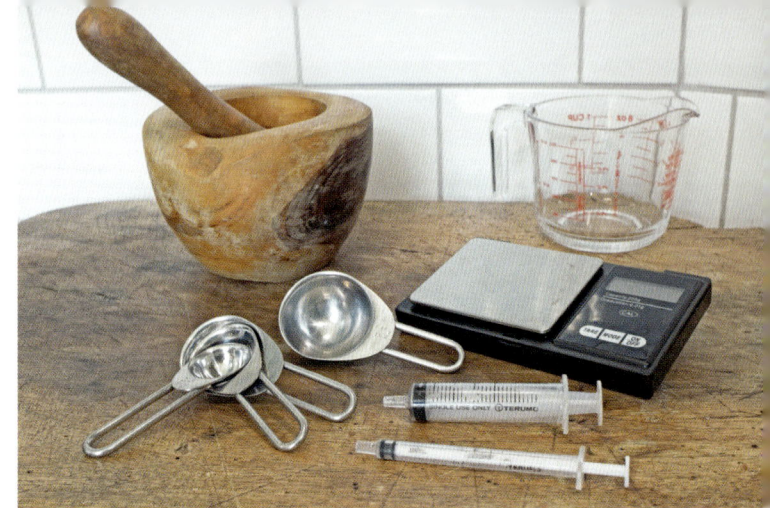

Conversion data for skincare makers

Imperial	Metric (ml)	ml/g (approx.)	Imperial (oz)	Metric (g)	Essential oils (approximations)*
		0.03-0.04			1 drop
1/10 teaspoon	0.49	0.5			12-15 drops
1/5 teaspoon	0.98	1			
1/4 teaspoon	1.23				
1/2 teaspoon	2.46				
3/4 teaspoon	3.69				
1 teaspoon	4.93	5			120-150 drops
1 tablespoon	14.79	15			
2 tablespoons	29.58	30	1	28	720-900 drops
1/4 cup	59	60	2	55	
1/3 cup	78		3	85	
1/2 cup	118		4	115	
2/3 cup	158				
3/4 cup	177				
1 cup	237		8	225	
1 pint (US)	473		16	455	
1 pint (UK)	568		20		
1 quart (US)	590				
1 quart (UK)	1140				

* Essential oils have different viscosities and are supplied in bottles with varying dropper types and flow rates, so use these figures as rule-of-thumb guidance only to help estimate ingredient requirements for recipes.

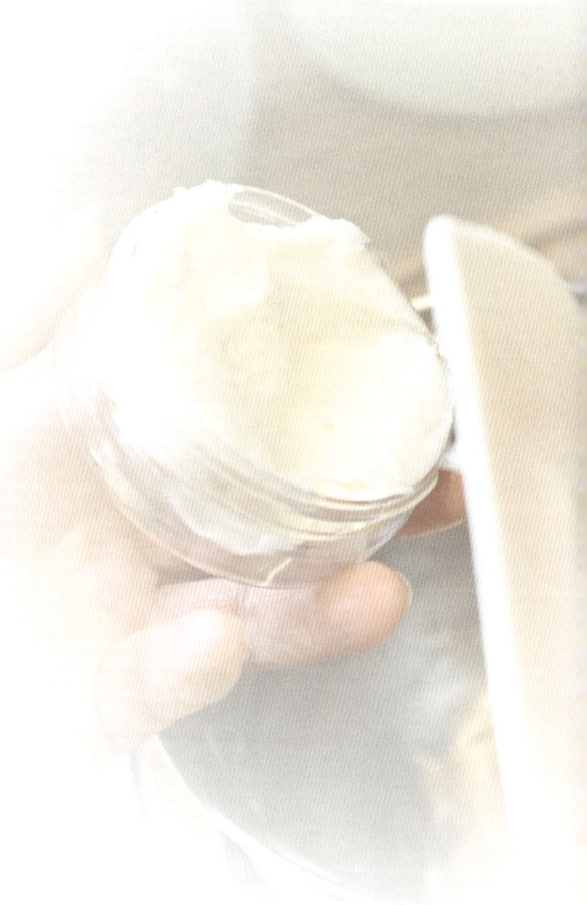

❋ Stirring equipment

There's a lot of stirring involved in making skincare. Ideally use a wooden spoon or stick for this, a chopstick works well. I also favour a simple looped whisk sold as an 'egg whisk' as an efficient way to get the oil and water molecules colliding rapidly when making an emulsion. A silicone spatula is ideal for scraping your creams into the containers, and a teaspoon to help tidy it up once in the pot.

❋ Double boiler

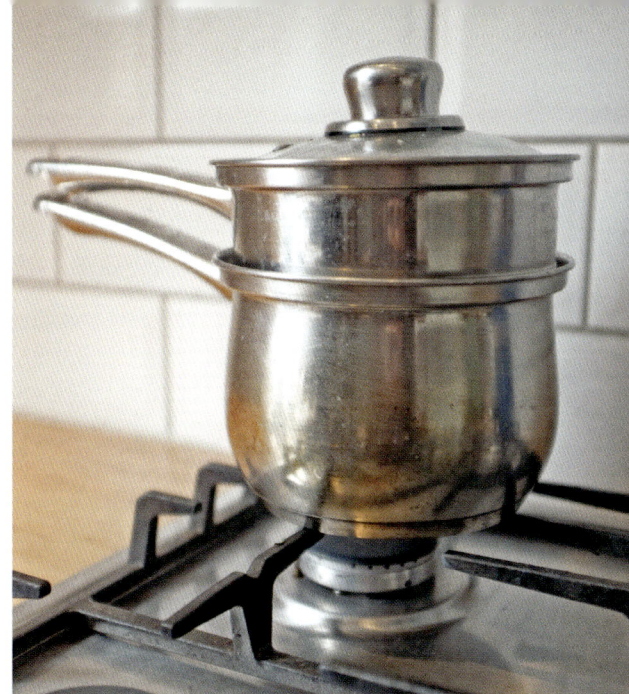

Infusions can be made in a normal saucepan but when working with oils it's best to use the gentle heat achieved by placing a bowl over boiling water, so it cooks in the steam, not directly on the flame. That way you can be sure not to burn your product as it will not get hotter than 100°C (212°F).

You can create your own double boiler by using a heat proof bowl over a saucepan, or you can buy a double boiler saucepan, sometimes sold as a porringer or bain marie. These are great pieces of kitchen equipment, but quite an investment. An alternative for making small quantities of skincare is a melting pan that sits over the top of your ordinary saucepan and still has the advantage of a handle and a pouring lip.

If you are using an improvised bowl-over-water option, make sure there's a good match in size between bowl and pan (it shouldn't wobble), and minimise gaps that let the steam seep out to avoid burns. Know how you'll pick up and pour from the pan once it's hot.

It's useful to have a second heatproof bowl with cold water in it to transfer your product over when you get to the cool stage of the recipe.

❋ Other useful equipment

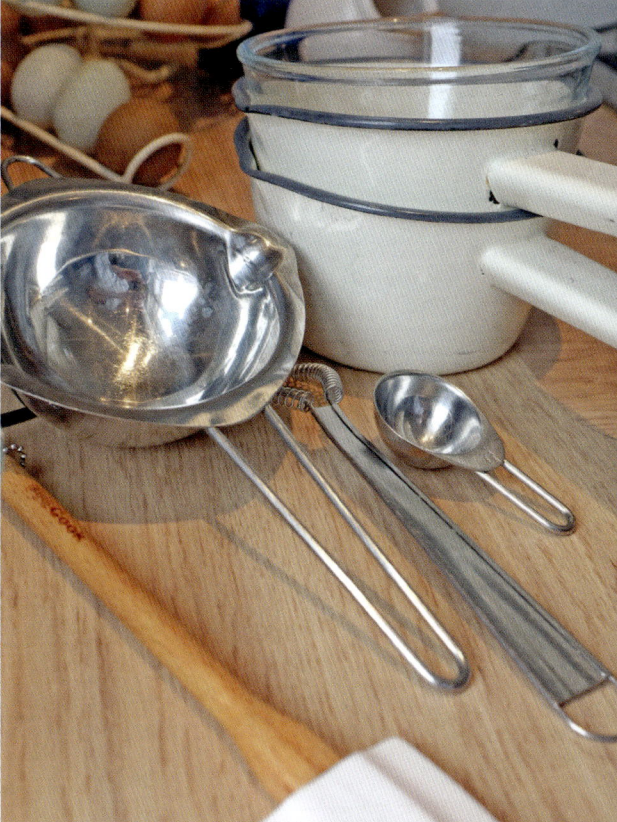

Depending on the recipe, you may need fine sieves or muslin for straining off herbs. You may want to use a pestle and mortar for preparing herbs, and scissors, chopping board and knife. Jugs and funnels are also a great help for transferring products into the container.

3. Storage

You'll need clean bottles and jars to store your products. Glass is ideal as it can be more easily cleaned and sterilised for repeated use. Dark colours are good to protect your product from sunlight. The wider the neck on your bottle or jar, the easier to fill with product, but the greater chance of contamination from dirt on your fingers during use, so choose and use your jars wisely.

Tot up the total weight of all ingredients in your recipe (not forgetting any added water) to know roughly how much you will be making and need to store. Decide whether this is best kept in one or several jars. Smaller jars mean you can have some product in use and some stored untouched (potentially frozen) or to give away.

Around 50g of face cream will usually last in daily use for two to three months; the same quantity of body cream may be good for five to ten applications. More specialist products like eye creams, serums or balms may typically be purchased in quantities of 10-30g and a lip balm stick is usually less than 5g of product and will last six to eight weeks with frequent use.

For some products it's good to use spray-top bottles, pump-action bottles or tube or stick dispensers. All these can be bought easily online in various types and sizes.

While making, you may also need to deploy ice cube trays or small moulds. You can buy specific trays or soap moulds, or use containers you find. There are so many things that can be cleaned and put to use rather than discarded: trays that fruit come in, bottle and jar tops, chocolate and biscuit box inners. Be creative.

4. Labelling

Whatever you're making, label it in detail. It's amazing how quickly you can forget when you made something, or what went into it. Take pride in your creation and let the label tell its story.

- Say when and where it was made, and who by
- Give a suggested use by date (taking into account the ingredients' shelf lives and whether you have added preservative or not)
- Note storage requirements
- List ingredients saying why they're included and where they came from

Make notes for yourself about how you made it, exact ingredient quantities and methods and any changes you'd make in the future. Note why you chose particular ingredients and any alternatives you considered.

Personalise it and have fun.
Whether it's functional or beautiful, it's up to you, it's your creation.

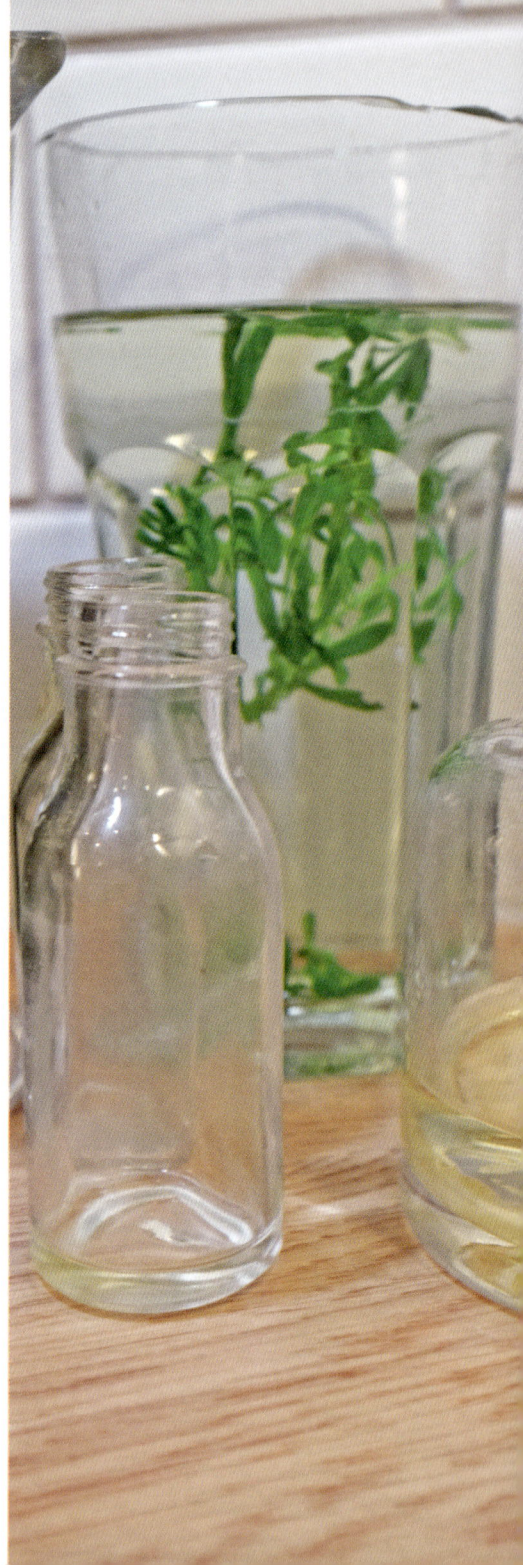

Blend Like a Pro

Blending your own skincare is really simple, but there are a few tips and techniques that are worth knowing to make you feel like a professional as you're working, and to prevent disappointment in your final product.

✦ *Some general tips to always remember are:*

- Work cleanly and accurately (see the details above)
- Minimise air getting into your product (think 'Stirred, not shaken')
- Use gentle heat (hence the double boiler technique)
- Keep stirring your product, especially as it's cooling down. Patience (and a bowl of cold water) are wonderful things to the skincare maker
- Remember, most things can be 'saved', often with more stirring

✦ *Special advice for creating an emulsion*

Many skincare products require combining oil and water to create a stable product. As oil and water won't combine on their own, an emulsifier is needed to bring them together successfully. It does this by breaking the surface tension of the ingredients to be emulsified. It is able to do this because it contains both oil and water (it's lipophilic and hydrophilic) and so can attract both oil and water to it.

There are a number of emulsifiers available to skincare makers. Some are 'water-in-oil' (W/O) emulsifiers which work best if you add the water to the oils; others are 'oil-in-water' (O/W) which you typically use when you plan to add the oils into the water. The emulsifier you use will depend on the oil:water ratio of the product you want to create. As a general rule, choose the emulsifier you can add to the larger component.

Theoretically, the emulsified ingredient can hold its own weight again in water (i.e. a 50:50 oil:water blend) but limiting the addition to 30% or less gives more guarantee of a good result.

The amount of emulsifier you require will depend on your choice of emulsifier, the amount of water, oils, waxes and butters you are using in the product and the consistency of the product you are looking to create. So it's difficult to give a useful rule of thumb. At a maximum, your emulsifier would be equivalent to 20% of the ingredient you add it to (e.g. with 100g of oil, combine 20g of emulsifier) but it can be as low as 0.5% for lotions, especially if also adding 'help emulsifiers'.

Recipes often include emulsifying wax (or E-wax). E-wax is a generic term encompassing many products with varying blends of raw ingredients that have been specifically developed to make emulsification simple (e.g. combinations of cetearyl alcohol, glyceryl stearate and Polysorbate 60). The results you will get depend on the particular brand of E-wax you use.

In the recipes in this book, where an emulsifier is needed, I use either cetyl alcohol (that also adds body and velvetiness to the product) or a specific branded emulsifier: Emulsifier L, which is particularly good for lotions. Do make your own substitutions as you choose. Some people avoid cetyl alcohol and cetearyl alcohol (a slightly milder blend of cetyl alcohol and stearic acid) because they can be made from palm oil (which may not have been farmed sustainably). However, there are now palm-oil-free versions available (e.g. made from rapeseed), and as E-wax typically contains cetearyl alcohol it's still important to know that it has been sourced sustainably.

Other emulsifiers you may come across include: stearic acid (a wax derived from coconut or palm oil), glyceryl monostearate (a blend of stearic acid and palmitic acid), vegetal, sucragel (glycerine, sweet almond oil, sweet orange water, sucrose laurate) or easymuls plus (a liquid natural emulsifier), among others. Each emulsifier will have its own requirements with regard to pH, temperature and whether to add the oil to the water (O/W) or the water to the oil (W/O). Check these things when you are trying new methods and make notes as you experiment.

Some emulsifying waxes are made from petroleum-derived ingredients and are therefore typically avoided by producers of natural skincare, so check the source ingredients and use what you are comfortable with. Also check for whether the wax contains Polyethylene Glycol (PEG); these are designed to enhance penetration and so can increase sensitivity to ingredients, especially when used on damaged skin.

You can also include 'help emulsifiers'. These aren't capable of emulsifying on their own, but do help create good conditions for a successful emulsion. Ones that are often included in skincare recipes include: lecithin (naturally found in egg yolk and also soya, sunflower and thistle, so the oils of these in your blends can help the emulsion), lanolin, beeswax and cocoa butter. Lanolin is the fat from sheep's wool, their equivalent of our sebum. Lanolin has got a bad press for causing skin reactions. Typically however, it is the chemicals in the lanolin from the treatment given to the sheep that cause reactions. Untreated lanolin does not cause adverse reactions.

Techniques for achieving a good emulsion:

- Ensure the oil and water components that you want to blend are at the same temperature when you bring them together
- Add the water to the oil (or oil to the water) gradually, stirring all the time; you want to give maximum opportunity for every water molecule to collide with an oil molecule, so keep stirring
- Use a stick blender or whisk to maximise agitation between the molecules
- Keep your blender or whisk in contact with the base of your pan or bowl to ensure minimising the air getting into the blend
- Take the combined oils and water up to over 75°C (167°F) to secure the chemical bond
- Keep stirring as your mixture cools, and allow it to cool gradually
- Include a 'help emulsifier' in your blend to strengthen the bond

It is truly satisfying to see your ingredients come together and the creamy consistency that results.

Once the emulsion is made there is a small capacity to add further ingredients, but these will be held in suspension within the emulsion and not chemically bonded. You will need to create a strong emulsion to be able to hold ingredients in suspension within it. Typically, you will not be able to add more than 10 percent of the emulsion's volume as suspension.

✲ Special advice for preserving products

One of the reasons people turn to making their own products is to avoid the need to use preservatives. Products without water (e.g. blends of oils, butters and waxes) can last quite well without preservatives. They may be good to use for six to twelve months. However, once you add water to a product, it will go off very quickly, typically lasting a couple of days to a week at most.

This is not a problem if you're making just what you need for immediate use. But if you are making a product with water and want it to last, you will need to include some form of preservative. The good news is that, because you only need it to last from the time you make it until it is used up, you don't need the levels of preservative that are needed for products that need to be able to sit on a shop shelf for weeks or months. The golden rule with preservatives is to use as much as you need, but no more than you need.

There are ingredients that have a preservative quality that you may choose to include in your products, but it is not possible to get the full spectrum of preservative qualities required this way. Either they are not effective enough against all the moulds and bacteria, or to include enough would be far too skin sensitising. To protect against all the fungal material, bacteria and moulds that could attack, you will need a proprietary preservative within your blend. As you're putting effort into creating something great, it's worth learning how to make it last.

Tips for maximising your product with safety and integrity:

- Work cleanly and accurately
- Use the freshest ingredients available to you, always be aware of their 'best before' dates
- Use appropriate containers with good lids and seals
- Keep products containing water in the fridge
- When including botanical material as infusions, make them on the day you intend to incorporate them into the product so they're as fresh as possible
- Minimise in-use contamination by only handling your product with clean hands, and by using a suitable container or dispenser (small-necked jars and bottles, pump action, tubes and sprays mean much less contact with the product)
- Incorporate a preservative as soon as possible into your blend so it can start taking effect
- Minimise the number of active ingredients: the more there are, the more complex to preserve

✲ Preservatives

The main function of a preservative is to extend the life of your product. The amount of preservative you need will depend on how long you want your product to last.

As their role is to create hostile conditions for moulds and bacteria, it is inevitable that they may also be challenging to some of the natural, beneficial bacteria in our skin. This is why it is not possible to have a completely benign preservative, and why we look to use just the amount required, and no more.

Conventional preservatives tend to be strong and effective, but this can be associated with more allergic potential. Natural preservatives may be milder but often need to be used in combination to be fully effective.

A simple way to start is by using an off-the-shelf natural full-spectrum preservative. These are specially formulated to provide protection against moulds and bacteria. Be careful which you choose as some are designed to work at specific pHs. Always follow the manufacturer's guidance on the maximum percentage to include in your product. A good starting point is Preservative Eco (INCI: benzyl alcohol, salicylic acid, glycerine, sorbic acid), this can be incorporated at a maximum of 1.15% (just over 1g per 100g of product).

Without preservative you can estimate that a product with water will only last a few days. One without water (just oils, butters and waxes) will last a few months. The lifespan of the final product often depends on how fresh the ingredients are going into it. As a rule of thumb, plant seed oils may be good for two years before they start to go rancid, but this is by no means true for all oils, and it will depend for many on the way they have been processed and whether any antioxidants (such as rosemary essential oil) have been added. By using the freshest ingredients, your products will have the longest shelf life; use oils that you've had in the cupboard for a while and you can't expect your product to feel fresh for so long.

The recipes in this book deliberately try to keep the ingredients list short and use the simplest, most accessible ingredients to support the vital herbs. They've been curated to enable you to make a full range of products without the need too purchase too many supplies. There are lots of wonderful skincare ingredients beyond the ones used in these recipes. As you become familiar with the structure of skincare formulas and blending techniques you will develop confidence to try different ingredients and have fun experimenting, but it will still be possible to meet most of your skincare needs using the simplest approaches.

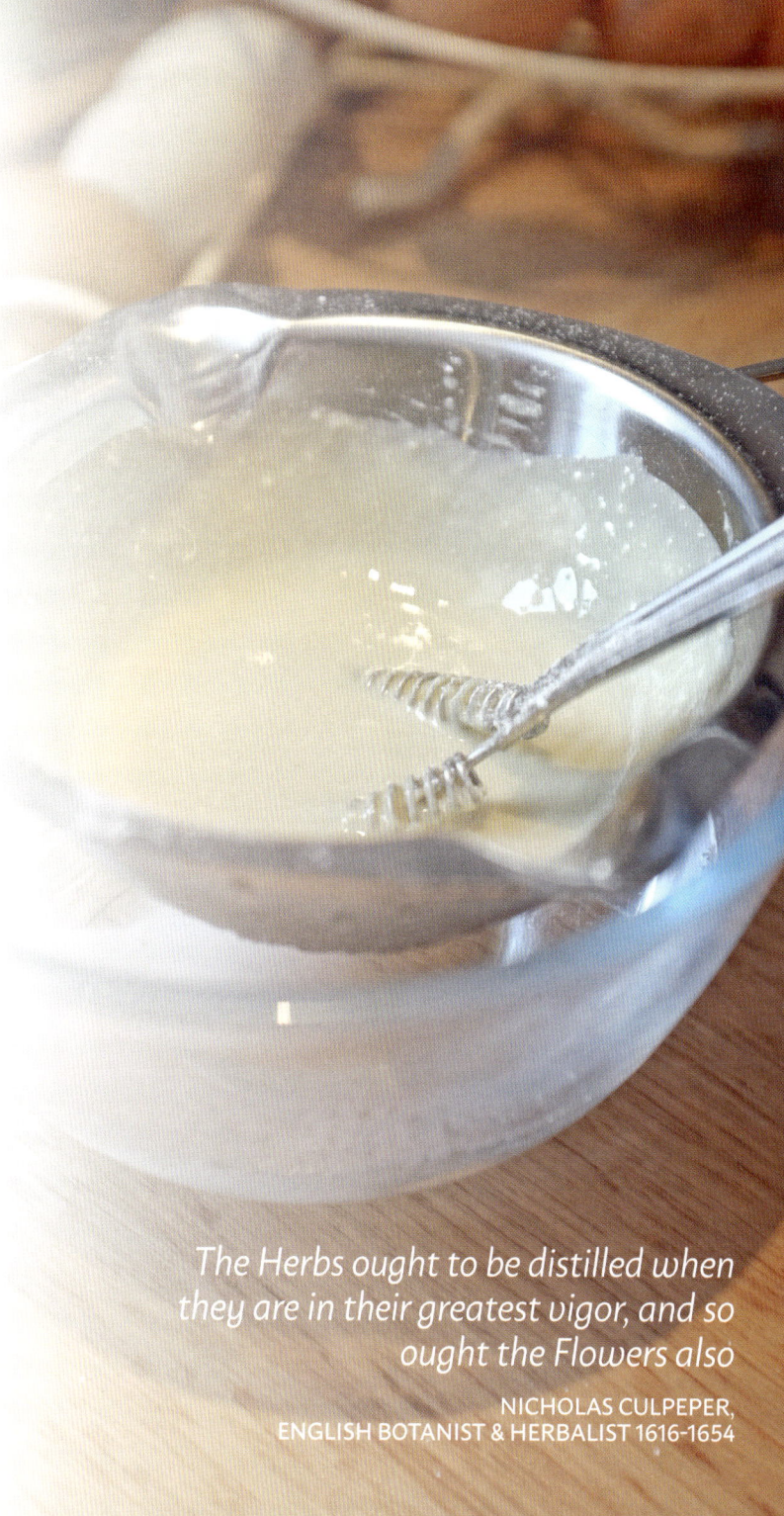

The Herbs ought to be distilled when they are in their greatest vigor, and so ought the Flowers also

NICHOLAS CULPEPER,
ENGLISH BOTANIST & HERBALIST 1616-1654

Part 5
Vitality

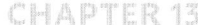

powerhouse seed oils – bringing vitality to your skincare with plant seed oils

Seeds hold the potential for life. Inside each seed is a store of oil (triglyceride) that will be the energy for the seed as it germinates. They are potent packs of vitality.

Pressing plant seeds and nuts expresses their oil. We have been doing this for thousands of years, and using plant oils on, and in, our bodies. They are gentle and work in sympathy with our skin's own oils, so are easily absorbed.

To increase that affinity, I choose to use oils derived from plants that thrive in the same climate and conditions as me, so I focus on temperate plants from which a wealth of different seed oils are derived. Historically people would always have used the plants growing closest to them.

My top ten favourites are:

Borage oil (Starflower oil)
Broccoli seed oil
Camelina oil (Gold of Pleasure or Wild Flax oil)
Hazelnut oil
Hemp seed oil
Pumpkin seed oil
Rosehip oil
Sunflower oil
Thistle oil (Safflower oil)
Walnut oil

Plant oils can have high levels of fatty acids, vitamins and minerals and have antioxidant, anti-inflammatory and moisturising properties. Together they can heal, protect, nourish, soothe, pamper and revitalise skin. They vitally provide the essential fatty acids our bodies need but cannot produce for itself. We often use them in combination to bring an array of synergistic properties to skincare products.

As plant oils are from living sources, they do have a lifespan. This varies with each oil but, typically, we can expect plant oils to last for about two years. This contrasts with petroleum-based oils that are from dead sources and last indefinitely. Petroleum oils do not have the same affinity with skin as they can't be absorbed and don't contain essential fatty acids or nutrients.

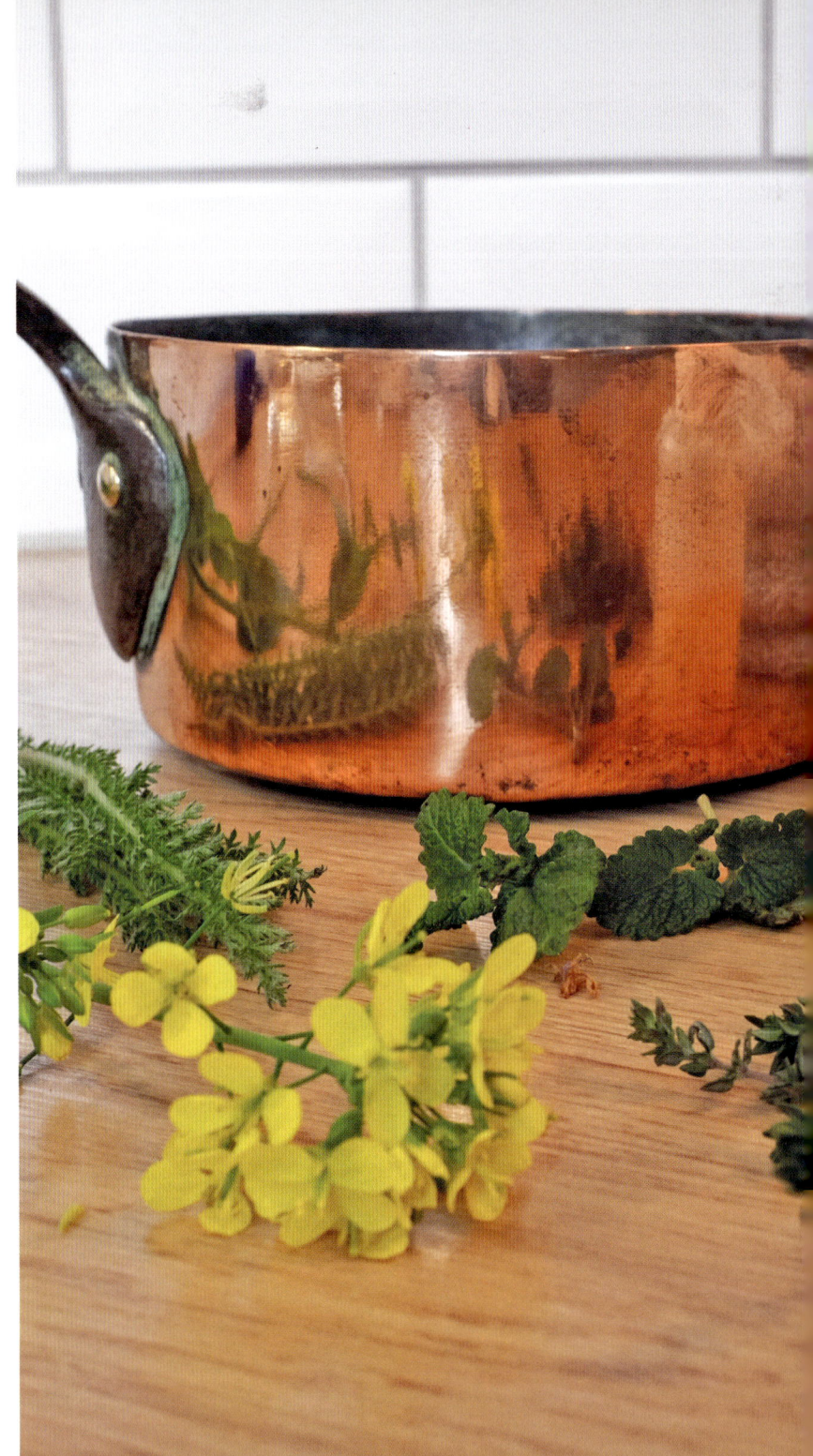

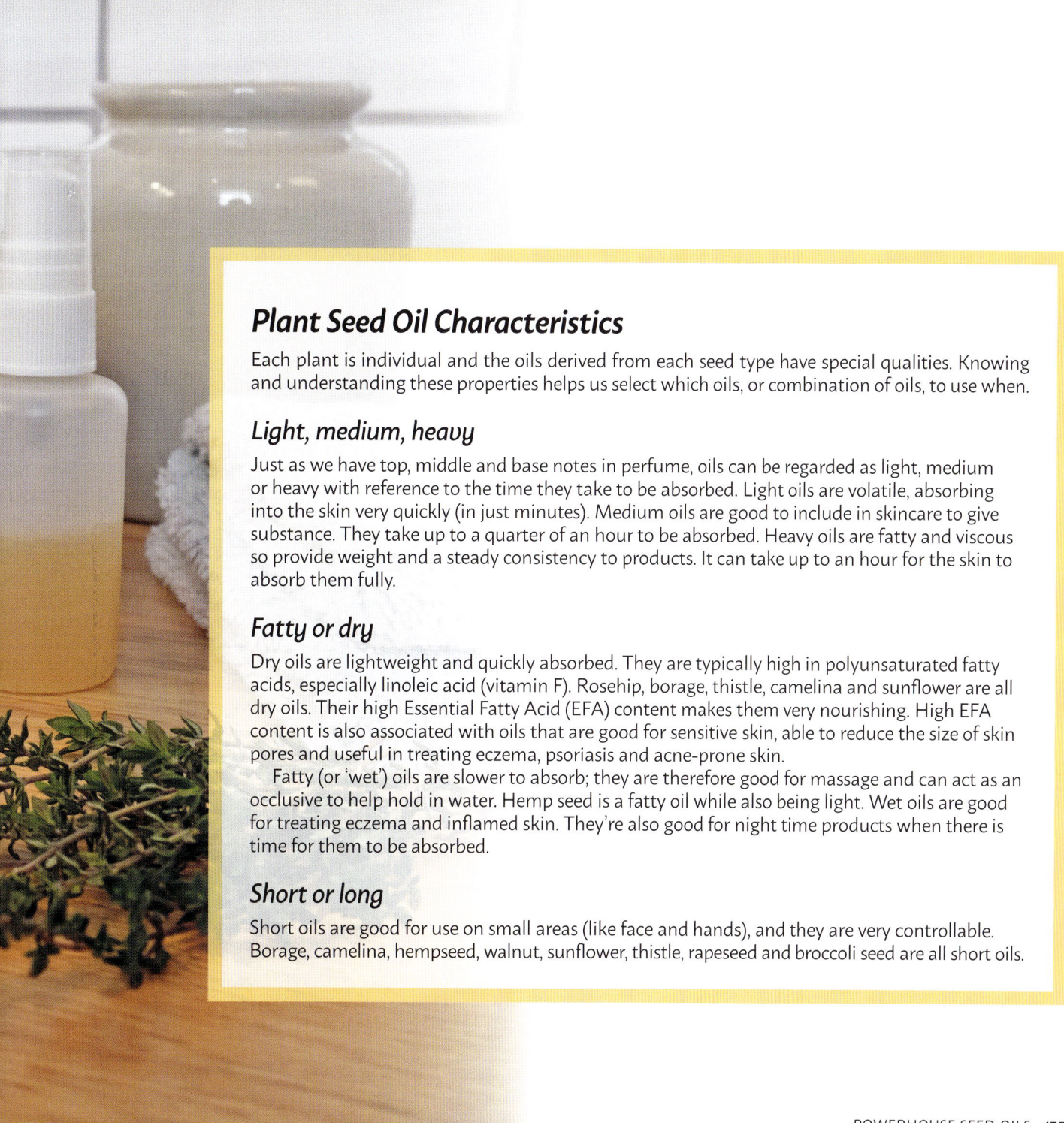

Plant Seed Oil Characteristics

Each plant is individual and the oils derived from each seed type have special qualities. Knowing and understanding these properties helps us select which oils, or combination of oils, to use when.

Light, medium, heavy

Just as we have top, middle and base notes in perfume, oils can be regarded as light, medium or heavy with reference to the time they take to be absorbed. Light oils are volatile, absorbing into the skin very quickly (in just minutes). Medium oils are good to include in skincare to give substance. They take up to a quarter of an hour to be absorbed. Heavy oils are fatty and viscous so provide weight and a steady consistency to products. It can take up to an hour for the skin to absorb them fully.

Fatty or dry

Dry oils are lightweight and quickly absorbed. They are typically high in polyunsaturated fatty acids, especially linoleic acid (vitamin F). Rosehip, borage, thistle, camelina and sunflower are all dry oils. Their high Essential Fatty Acid (EFA) content makes them very nourishing. High EFA content is also associated with oils that are good for sensitive skin, able to reduce the size of skin pores and useful in treating eczema, psoriasis and acne-prone skin.

Fatty (or 'wet') oils are slower to absorb; they are therefore good for massage and can act as an occlusive to help hold in water. Hemp seed is a fatty oil while also being light. Wet oils are good for treating eczema and inflamed skin. They're also good for night time products when there is time for them to be absorbed.

Short or long

Short oils are good for use on small areas (like face and hands), and they are very controllable. Borage, camelina, hempseed, walnut, sunflower, thistle, rapeseed and broccoli seed are all short oils.

Gamma linolenic acid (GLA) helps maintain an optimal balance of prostaglandins. Prostaglandins cannot be stored by the body so we have to provide them regularly. Maintaining a regular supply keeps skin supple, more tolerant of sunlight and less susceptible to wrinkles. Good sources of GLA include borage oil, evening primrose oil, hemp seed oil and blackcurrant seed oil.

Borage oil

CHARACTERISTICS Dry, Rough, Short, Top, Emollient
GOOD FOR Most skin – normal, dry, oily, sensitive, mature

Borage oil is soothing, regenerating and revitalising. It is absorbed quickly without leaving an oily feeling on the skin. It penetrates well, helping to soften the skin making it less prone to eczema and acne. Particularly good for mature or dry, flaky skin, it helps retain moisture, absorb oxygen and withstand disease. Borage oil is especially valued for its high gamma linolenic acid (GLA). It also has a high oleic acid content making it good for oily and acne prone skin.

Broccoli seed oil

CHARACTERISTICS Emollient, Short
GOOD FOR All skin

Broccoli seed oil gives sheen and luminescence without greasiness. Penetrating easily, it is absorbed quickly and softens.

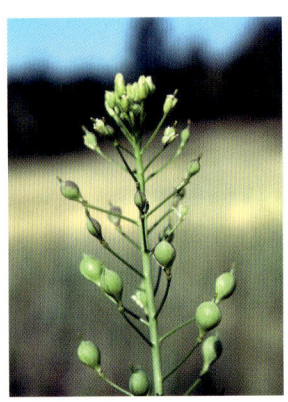

Camelina oil ('wild flax' or 'gold of pleasure')

CHARACTERISTICS: Dry, Rough, Short, Top, Emollient
GOOD FOR Oily, large-pores, mature and dry skin, avoid on sensitive skin

Camelina oil is very rapidly absorbed, penetrates well and is not oily. It has a high vitamin E content and has long been valued for skin rejuvenation. The high linoleic acid content improves skin elasticity, provides gloss and minimises wrinkles. Camelina oil is nourishing, good for damaged skin and can help strengthen the skin's barrier function, reducing transepidermal water loss (TEWL) and improving firmness. It has a high omega 3 content (like rosehip oil) and is great for face, neck and hands, and can help reduce skin redness.

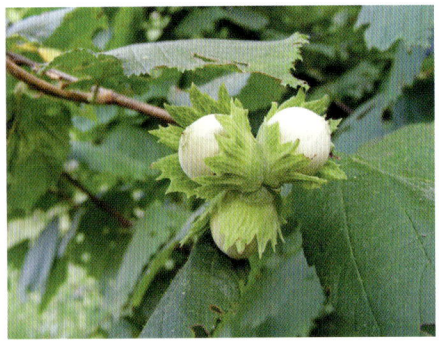

Hazelnut oil

CHARACTERISTICS Long, Emollient
GOOD FOR All skin including acne-prone, rough, tired and damaged skin plus dry, sensitive, oily and mature skin

Hazelnut oil is easily absorbed without a greasy residue. It is a good, temperate grown substitute for sweet almond oil. Immediately softening and moisturising, it is also toning and firming and encourages cell regeneration. Its slight astringency makes it good in defending against acne.

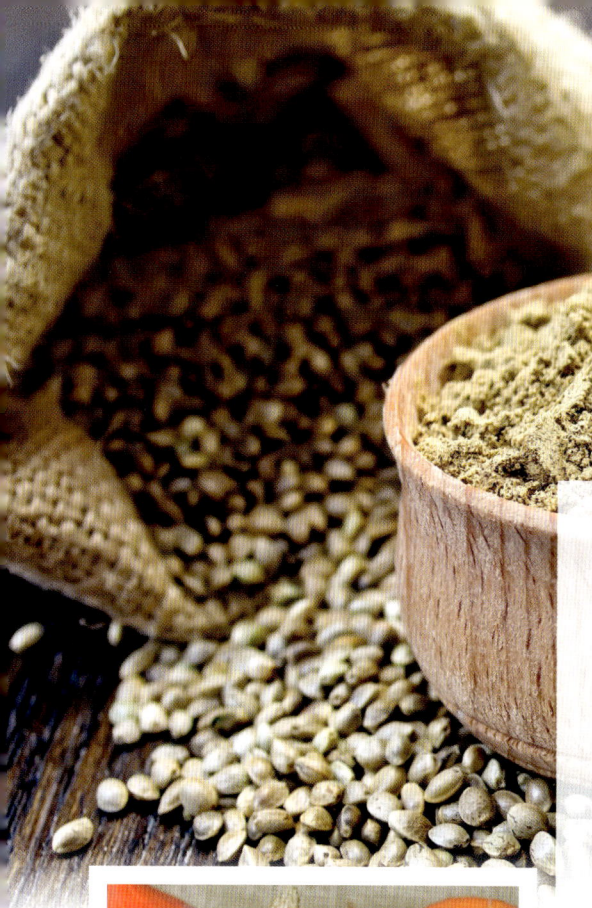

Hemp seed oil

CHARACTERISTICS Dry, Rough, Top, Light, Fat, Occlusive, Short
GOOD FOR All skin – especially oily, large-pores, dry, mature

Hemp seed oil is reputed to help slow down the signs of ageing as it smoothes and softens. Penetrating deeply, it is helpful for those suffering from eczema, psoriasis and acne. With a high vitamin E content, it is good for balance and tone, and it has one of the highest essential fatty acid contents for plant oils. It is great for dry skin. Hemp seed oil leaves little residue and helps skin absorb other active ingredients. It's also great for face serums.

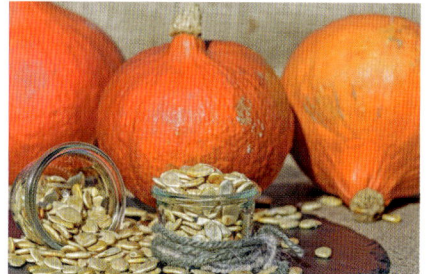

Pumpkin seed oil

CHARACTERISTICS Long, Fatty
GOOD FOR All skin, including dry, mature or damaged skin

Pumpkin seed oil has lots of zinc, so can be uplifting and good for mature, dry or damaged skin. It has compounds that give skin a bright and vibrant healthy glow, and vitamin A that helps cell regeneration. It moisturises deep down, is soothing and can help reduce redness. It smoothes skin and can help slow down signs of ageing.

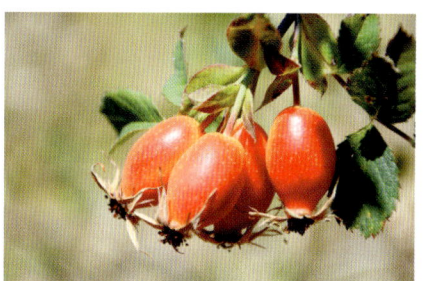

Rosehip oil

CHARACTERISTICS Dry, Smooth, Long, Top, Emollient
GOOD FOR Sensitive and delicate skin, dry, normal and ageing skin

Rosehip is a luxurious oil, known for its firming and anti-ageing properties. It helps reduce fine lines and supports skin cell regeneration. Absorbed quickly without leaving residue, it helps create a non-fatty blend. Rosehip oil is full of antioxidants and considered to be stimulating and toning.

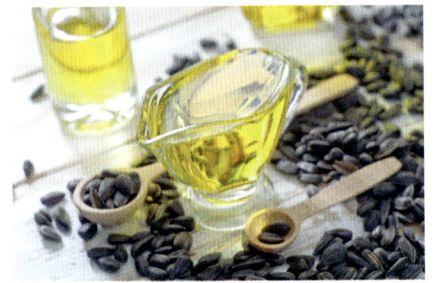

Sunflower oil

CHARACTERISTICS Dry, Light, Emollient, Short
GOOD FOR All skin – especially mature, dry, damaged, sensitive, large-pored

Sunflower oil is softening, nourishing and uplifting, with a high vitamin E content. It absorbs easily into the skin without feeling greasy, and helps other active ingredients absorb quicker. Its high lecithin content helps in emulsification.

Thistle oil (Safflower oil)

CHARACTERISTICS Dry, Rough, Thin, Light, Emollient, short
GOOD FOR Oily, large pores, mature, eczema-prone

Thistle oil is quickly absorbed without leaving a fatty residue. With high amounts of linoleic acid (vitamin F), among many other essential fatty acids, it is good for skin cell regeneration. It blends well with other oils and is rebalancing and nourishing. More likely grown in arid than temperate regions, thistle oil has been a vital skincare staple since Egyptian times.

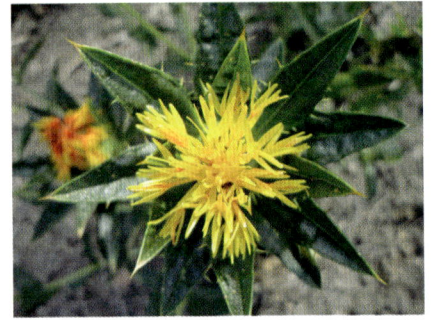

Walnut oil

CHARACTERISTICS Dry, short
GOOD FOR Oily, large pored, mature/ageing

Walnut oil helps with skin regeneration and is generally a good wrinkle-fighter. It increases circulation. It disperses well, leaving skin feeling soft and supple.

You can only perceive real beauty in a person as they get older

ANOUK AIMÉE,
FRENCH ACTRESS, 1932-

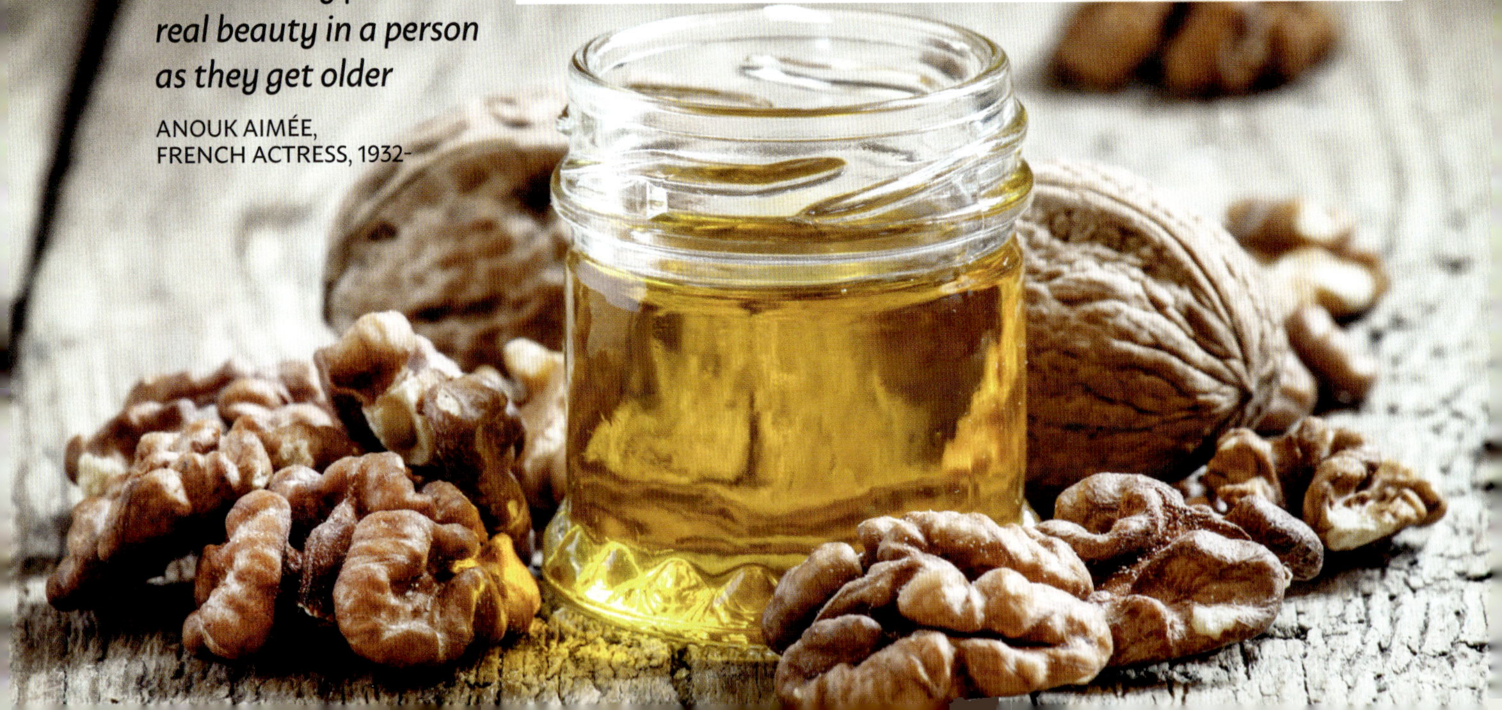

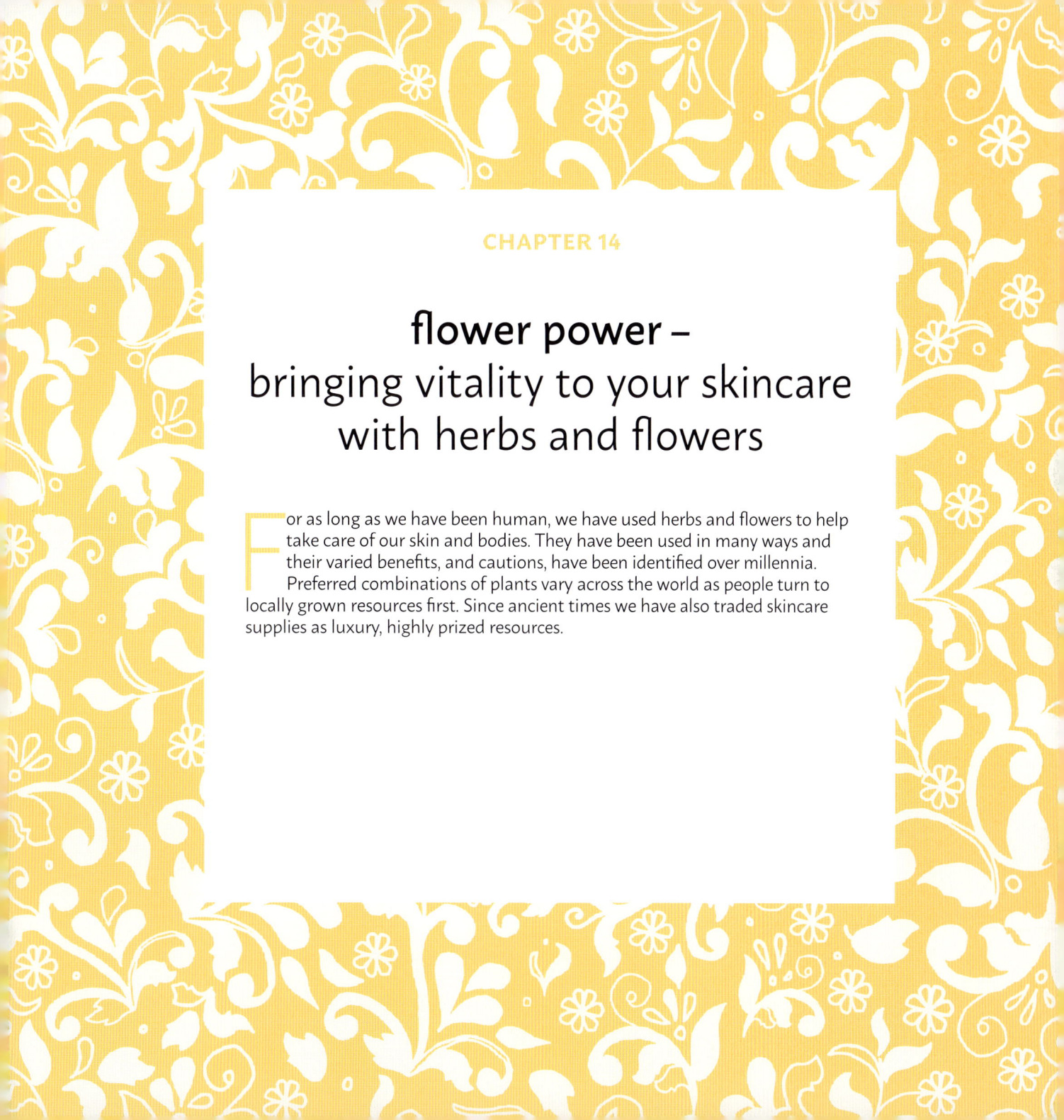

CHAPTER 14

flower power –
bringing vitality to your skincare with herbs and flowers

For as long as we have been human, we have used herbs and flowers to help take care of our skin and bodies. They have been used in many ways and their varied benefits, and cautions, have been identified over millennia. Preferred combinations of plants vary across the world as people turn to locally grown resources first. Since ancient times we have also traded skincare supplies as luxury, highly prized resources.

What is a herb? The range of plants studied and deployed by herbalists in medicinal, therapeutic and culinary ways can extend way beyond what we would typically find in a herb garden, or the herb section of the garden centre. It incorporates numerous trees, shrubs and flowers, as well as the classic array of herbs and hedgerow finds.

Studying herbalism involves embracing the accumulated knowledge of millennia, alongside learning from current scientific discoveries (many of which are confirming ancient traditions). Its skill often lies in understanding the whole plant in context – the climate and conditions it enjoys, how it cycles through the seasons, its reproductive techniques and how other plants and animals respond to it. It can mean a lifetime of learning, continually revealing new interests and pleasures.

To gain confidence in using herbs, it's good to hone in on just a few at first and really get to know them: where and how they grow, how to harvest and which parts to use and what they can help us with. Start by focusing on plants that grow around us, ones that we can commonly find in gardens or hedgerows. The wealth of goodness and properties they provide mean we have little need to go further afield.

It's good to vary the flowers and herbs you use in your skincare. Using the same one continuously may lead to irritation or a lessening of effectiveness over time. You're not looking for dramatic, immediate results, but a gentle, cumulative effect as your skin adjusts to the natural ingredients.

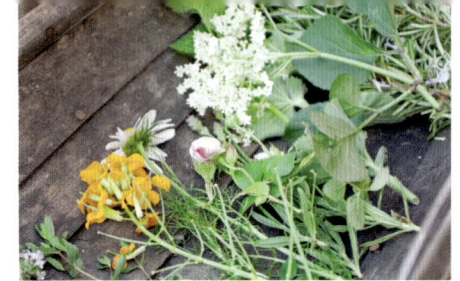

How to add Flower Power

Flowers and herbs can be incorporated pre, during or post making your product:

1. In preparation for making, you can use a variety of techniques to lace your component ingredients (especially the oils and water) with herbs
2. As you make your product, you can incorporate herbs into your blend
3. Post making you can embellish your products with herbs

1. Lacing Ingredients with Flower Power

❖ Adding flower power to oils: Maceration

In a maceration, the oil of your choice is steeped in herbs to extract their volatile oils. This can be done either fast or slow.

To achieve results fast, use the heat method; for a more gradual transformation, use the sun method suited to delicate flowers such as limeflower, St John's Wort or rose petals.

You can use fresh or dried herbs, but dried are preferable. With fresh herbs ensure every little bit of the herb is well covered in oil or it will go mouldy.

Macerations can also be made with vinegar, witch hazel or pure alcohol instead of oil.

Even if you've made your oil by the heat method, some herbalists recommend placing your bottle of herbal oil in sunlight and moonlight, for two to three weeks before using it.

Macerated oils can benefit from the addition of vitamin E, wheatgerm oil (up to 10% of the original oil volume) or a few drops of rosemary essential oil. This reduces oxidation so your carefully produced oil will last longer.

❖ Adding flower power to water: Infusion & decoction

The two different methods for steeping water with flower power are used according to the delicacy of the plant part you choose to use.

For delicate leaves and flowers, use the infusion method; for more robust twigs, bark, firmer leaves, roots and seeds, use the decoction method.

❖ Flower waters

Although very delicate, some flower petals can be made into waters using a method that is more similar to decoction than infusion. The petal to water ratio varies depending on the flower used.

Herbal waters, however they are made, have a much shorter shelf life than macerated oils, so are best made on the day you intend to use them. At best they will keep for a couple of weeks in the fridge. However, you can freeze your herbal water into ice cubes and defrost them when needed. Make sure you label your frozen herbal infusion clearly.

MACERATION – THE HEAT METHOD

60g herbs to 600ml oil

Place half your herbs in a bowl over hot water and cover with the oil. Using this bain marie method of a bowl over a pan of hot water will ensure the oil doesn't boil, but still be careful that it doesn't get too hot as that could destroy the properties of the plant, and it's a fire risk. Keep the oil at a constant low heat for an hour. Remove from the heat, strain the oil through a muslin, then put it back into the pan with the other half of herbs and repeat the process. The oil should darken with each batch of herbs added. Strain the macerated oil twice-over, through a muslin and then a coffee filter, and then put it into clean, dark bottles and label.

It can be difficult to keep the oil at a constant but low heat. If you have access to an oven that can maintain a steady, low temperature, you can use this to macerate oils overnight.

Try making macerations with: St John's Wort, calendula, comfrey and chamomile. Other herbs that macerate well include: birch leaves, dandelion, fennel seed, geranium, garlic, lavender, lemon balm, marjoram, mullein, peppermint, rosemary, sage, thyme and yarrow.

Try making decoctions with: burdock root, echinacea, fennel, marshmallow root or nettles.

MACERATION – THE SUN METHOD

Place your herbs in a clean, sterile jar with a tight-fitting lid. Add enough oil to cover the herbs and half as much again. Use a cold pressed oil for macerating using the sun method. Good oils to use are virgin olive oil, sweet almond oil, sunflower oil or rapeseed oil. Leave on a sunny windowsill for a minimum of two weeks, ideally six to eight weeks, shaking gently daily (just swirl it around, not too vigorously, you don't want to create air bubbles). Label the jar, or make a note elsewhere of exactly what and how much is in the jar and when you started the process, along with your target end date when the maceration will be ready. If your windowsill is in very bright light, you could put the jar into a paper bag to reduce the harshness. Check your jar each day and shake it, if there is any sign of moisture or condensation, carefully open the jar, wipe with a clean paper towel and reseal. Strain, bottle, label and record as per the heat method.

INFUSION

This is very similar to making a cup of tea and enables you to gently draw out the volatile properties of the herb.

Put your herb into a bowl or cup and pour on boiling water. Leave to steep for 10 minutes, preferably covered, before straining through a filter paper.

You can vary your infusion strength depending on the herb and the strength of the final product you require. A standard ratio is 1 tsp dried herb, or 1 tbsp fresh herb to 1 cup water.

Try making infusions with: borage, chamomile, cleavers, comfrey leaf, elderflower, lavender, lime-flower, lemon balm, calendula, marshmallow leaf and rose petals.

DECOCTION

This enables water-soluble active ingredients to be drawn out of the herbs, but is only suitable for plant parts that can withstand the heat. It's a good method to use if you are looking to draw out the vitamin and mineral components of a plant.

Use 30g of herb to 600ml of boiling water.

Chop up the herb and put it into a pan then cover with the water and a tight lid. If the herbs are too hard to chop, you can soak them first overnight in a cup or two of water to soften them. The next day, use this water as part of the fluid in the decoction. Slowly bring the water in the pan to the boil and simmer for 10 minutes. Strain as above. For a stronger decoction, you can leave the herb sitting in the water for 4-8 hours, or overnight, before straining.

FLOWER WATERS

Rosewater: use 150ml water with 220g petals, split into 2 batches
Calendula: use 400ml water with 50g petals, split into 2 batches
Elderflower: use 500ml water with 100g elderflower, split into 2 batches

Put half the petals into a pan and cover with the water. Bring to the boil, then simmer very gently for an hour. Strain and put the remaining petals into the pan, covering them with the strained flower water. Once again, bring to the boil, and then simmer gently for an hour. Leave to cool before straining first through muslin, then through a coffee filter to remove all the plant material. Store in clean bottles. It should keep for up to two weeks in the fridge.

❋ Tinctures and herbal vinegars

Some recipes ask for a herbal tincture. These are a stronger method of imparting flower power so are typically used in very small amounts. They can be made at home using a technique similar to the sun method maceration.

A tincture is made using alcohol. Anything from a 50/50 alcohol blend to pure alcohol can be used, 3 parts alcohol to 2 parts water is a good ratio for extracting most aromatics. Use the purest vodka available to you or, alternatively, heat cider vinegar in a pan and use this warm vinegar to pour over the herbs, instead of the alcohol.

Tinctures can have a distinctive smell so it's ideal to keep them as a small proportion of the overall recipe. They can also have a drying effect due to the alcohol.

Herbal vinegars are lovely to add to baths or use as skin toners, restoring pH balance. Lavender herbal vinegar added to a bath will relieve aching muscles and both rose and elderflower herbal vinegars can help relieve headaches and tension. Add about half a cupful to a warm bath.

When using herbal tinctures and vinegars directly on the skin, be sure to dilute them with water first. Tinctures should be diluted at least 1:4 and vinegars 1:6.

The classic Hungary Water is a tincture using multiple herbs. See page 162

TINCTURE

200g dried herbs or 400g fresh herbs to 1 litre liquid.

Pack your herbal material into a jar, then cover with the alcohol or warm vinegar, making sure all the herbage is submerged completely. Seal and store in a dark place, away from direct sunlight, for two to six weeks. Shake daily. Strain through muslin, and then through a coffee filter to ensure all the plant material is removed. Pour into a dark glass bottle, label and date. Store in a cool place away from sunlight. Tinctures will keep for a year or more.

● Try making a tincture with borage, cleavers, elderflower, lemon balm, calendula, lavender, nettles, rose petals, sage, thyme and yarrow.

2. Incorporating flower power into your blends

❋ Fresh or dried herbs

Both fresh and dried herbs are used in making skincare. Often it can be preferable to use dried to avoid adding water to the blend. Especially, for example, when blending dry ingredients that you want to keep for a while (such as a clay mask mixture) or when creating balms or other all-oil products.

It may be possible to substitute fresh herbs for dried in a recipe, but do so with care. Typically you'll need to double or triple the amount – so if the recipe calls for 5g of dried herbs, you'd add 10-15g of fresh herbs. This will change the overall weight of the product and proportion of the ingredients in relation to each other so it should be done with caution. When the herb is the main ingredient, you may need to substitute up to 10 times the weight of dried herbs. So, for example, 5g of dried herbs would be replaced with 50g of fresh.

When using fresh herbs, incorporate them as soon as they've been picked.

Some recipes use whole leaves and flowers, such as lady's mantle leaves in the sweet leaf mask (page 75) and lavender flowers in the sweet mud flower scrub (page 91). Sometimes you'll chop or shred the herb first before incorporating it. Often it is blitzed in a pestle and mortar or electric blender and pulverised before being incorporated into a cleanser, mask or cream.

Adding herbs (fresh or dried) to a steaming bowl of water, to a foot or hand bath, or to your main bath, are lovely ways to enjoy herbs directly. To minimise the mess of strewn herbs post-bath, fresh herbs can be tied into a bundle with string and dried ones can be gathered into a muslin cloth. For best results, hang the herbs so the water flows over and through them as the bath is drawn, then let the herbs float in the water. If you don't want the herbs themselves in the bath, get their benefit by making a herbal infusion and adding this to the bath.

for a bath use 5-10g of dried herbs or 50g of fresh herbs.

for a hand or footbath or facial steam, use 1.5-2g of dried herbs or 15-20g of fresh herbs.

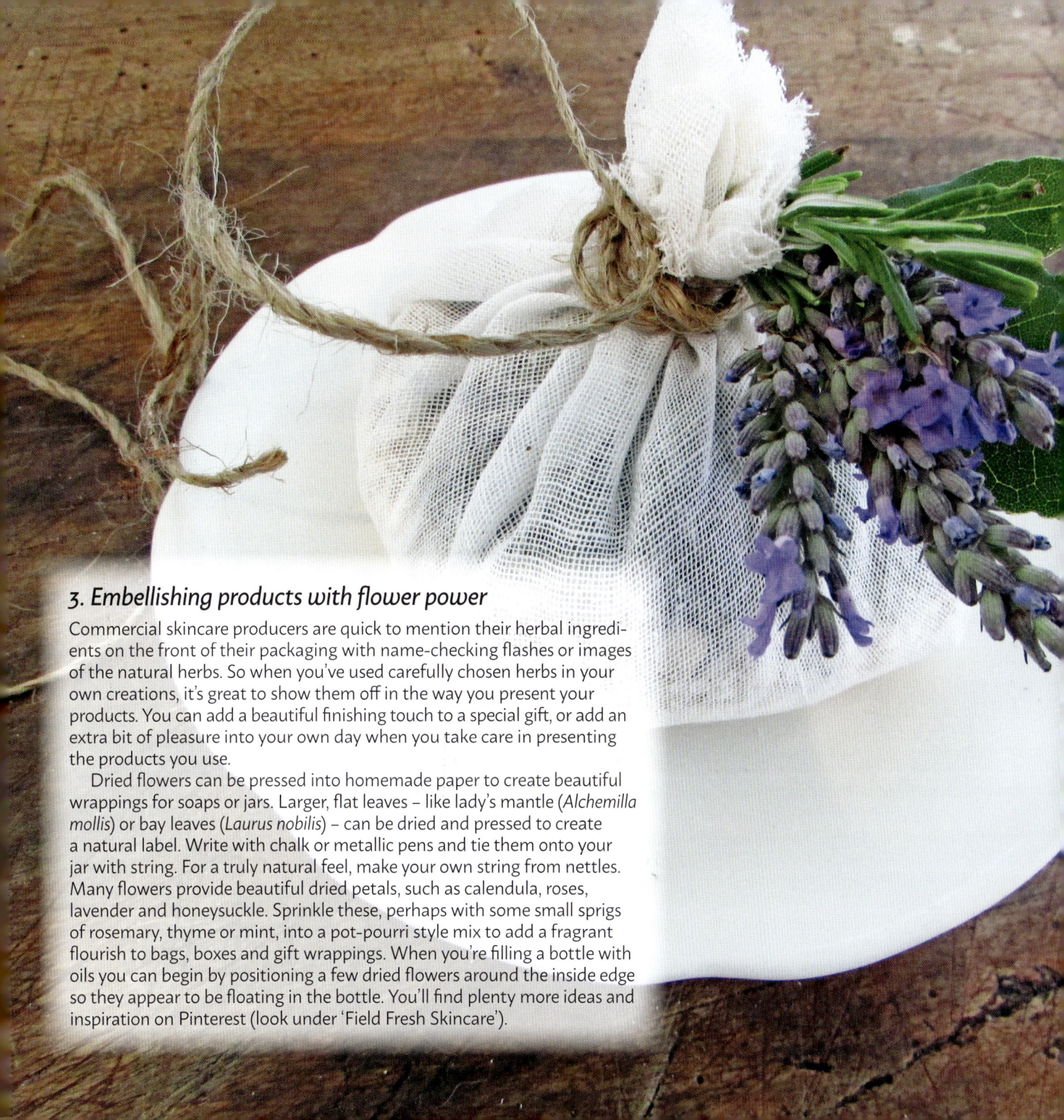

3. Embellishing products with flower power

Commercial skincare producers are quick to mention their herbal ingredients on the front of their packaging with name-checking flashes or images of the natural herbs. So when you've used carefully chosen herbs in your own creations, it's great to show them off in the way you present your products. You can add a beautiful finishing touch to a special gift, or add an extra bit of pleasure into your own day when you take care in presenting the products you use.

Dried flowers can be pressed into homemade paper to create beautiful wrappings for soaps or jars. Larger, flat leaves – like lady's mantle (*Alchemilla mollis*) or bay leaves (*Laurus nobilis*) – can be dried and pressed to create a natural label. Write with chalk or metallic pens and tie them onto your jar with string. For a truly natural feel, make your own string from nettles. Many flowers provide beautiful dried petals, such as calendula, roses, lavender and honeysuckle. Sprinkle these, perhaps with some small sprigs of rosemary, thyme or mint, into a pot-pourri style mix to add a fragrant flourish to bags, boxes and gift wrappings. When you're filling a bottle with oils you can begin by positioning a few dried flowers around the inside edge so they appear to be floating in the bottle. You'll find plenty more ideas and inspiration on Pinterest (look under 'Field Fresh Skincare').

Flower power for when your skin is feeling...

oily	dry or sensitive	overwhelmed	tired or old	normal
calendula	bay	comfrey	blackberry leaf	apple mint
comfrey	borage	chamomile	daisy	chamomile
fennel	chamomile	honeysuckle	dandelion	comfrey
geranium	chickweed	houseleek	elderflowers	jasmine
horsetail	cleavers	limeflower	lemon verbena	lavender
lavender	elderflower	marshmallow	liquorice root	lemon balm
nettles	honeysuckle		red clover	limeflower
peppermint	houseleek		St John's Wort	raspberry leaf
rosemary	lady's mantle		tansy	rose
sage	marshmallow			spearmint
yarrow	meadowsweet			thyme
	pansy			
	parsley			
	rose			
	salad burnet			
	sorrel			
	violets			

Gathering herbs

If you're new to herbs and plants, get to know them by growing a few things yourself. Grow in your own garden, offer to garden for a friend or get involved in a community garden. In a 'controllable' environment you can be more certain about what you've planted and what you expect it to look like. It's a good way to learn.

Only gather in the wild when you're absolutely sure what it is. The best way to learn what to look for is to go with other people. Look for a foraging group local to you – a quick search on Facebook or Meetup might find one.

When gathering, take the minimum you need, and certainly leave more than you take. Be sure the plant is healthy and will continue thriving. Don't lift roots in the wild or the plant will not grow again.

Be a bit picky and look for perfect leaves for use in your skincare. Avoid blemishes, bugs or signs of disease or animal presence.

Gather fresh ingredients as you need them, but if you're gathering to store for future use, know the best season to do so. This will vary with each plant. As a rule of thumb:

- Leaves are typically at their best just before the flowers open.
- Flowers are at their prime as they open
- Roots are at their best in autumn, when goodness has passed back into them from the leaves
- Bark is best in the spring when the sap is rising.

Use secateurs to make clean cuts, if necessary.

Don't ram your gathering bags full, better to make more foraging trips more frequently.

Remember that whatever time you spend gathering, you're likely to need twice that time preparing the gathered materials once they're back home. Don't gather what you won't have the opportunity to use.

Storing herbs

Most herbs can be stored for future use, but you'll need to prepare them for storage as quickly as possible after picking. There are several ways to store them.

Freezing

Many herbs take well to being frozen. As soon as they're gathered, make sure they are clean and transfer into airtight bags. Where appropriate, it's worth taking some time to strip leaves from stems and check for blemishes so you know you're only preserving the best. Label the bag clearly and make a record of what you're freezing in a notebook. For easy reference, include the date, where it was gathered and any notes about how you've prepared it or intend to use it.

Drying

Drying is the traditional way of preserving herbs and works well for most. There can be significant changes as dehydrated materials lose their colour and form. Although they look to have less vitality, reintroducing water when you're ready to use them (often in an infusion or bath) proves the flower power is still there as they scent the room.

There are various methods of drying; choose the mode most suited to the plant, the quantity you are drying and the space you have available.

- Tie small bunches together by the stalks and hang upside down. Ensure you can catch any falling parts, either by putting a tray underneath, or by loosely securing a paper bag around the leaves or flowers.
- Lay petals or leaves on a flat surface with plenty of air circulating (a muslin-covered rack is ideal). Leave them for a couple of days, and then turn them over and leave for another couple of days to ensure they are thoroughly dried.
- Speed up the rack drying process by laying your material on trays that can be sat in the oven on a very low heat for a few hours or instead put them into a solar drier if you're guaranteed a few days of warmth.
- Some herbs respond well to being layered in salt to dry and preserve them. Just keep layering plant material with salt until you've packed a jar full and seal it tightly. This is a traditional way of storing basil leaves.

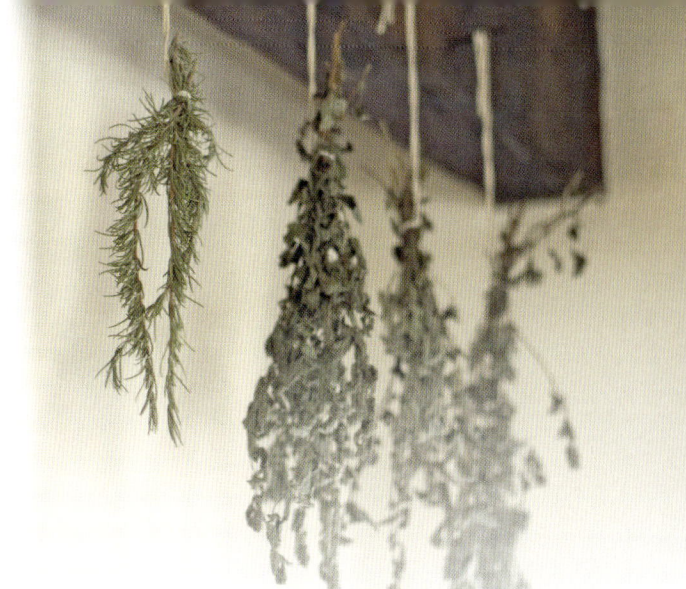

Do refresh and review your stocks of herbs on a regular basis, ideally replacing and replenishing stocks each growing season. Although dried herbs do keep for a few years, it's always best to use the newest material available to you.

Jars

You'll need a good number of wide-necked jars once you start collecting and drying your own herbs so you can store them cleanly and as airtight as possible. Ideally these should be dark glass jars. If necessary, you can use clean, sterile, dry jam jars (and larger catering sized jars for your more plentiful herbs) and keep them in a dark cupboard to minimise the impact of degrading UV light. Use a new jar for each gathering of herbs. Don't be tempted to pack fresh pickings on top of old. This means you can be sure you're rotating your stock properly (using the oldest first) and can trace your source for each batch. If you're short of space, dried herbs can also be kept in plastic bags with an airlock seal.

Labelling

Be meticulous about labelling. You can make it a joy by creating beautiful labels to either securely tie on or stick onto your jars. The label should clearly name the plant material in the jar, as well as giving details about where and when it was collected. It can also be helpful to weigh your material before it goes into the jar so you can make good estimates of stocks available when planning your product making.

Essential power

There is a third way of harnessing the power from plants to use in skincare. Alongside the powerhouse of plant seed oils and the flower power of using the plants themselves, we can also distil the essential oil of plants to bring their therapeutic qualities and scent into our products.

Magical and wonderful as they are, I have incorporated a very limited range of essential oils into the recipes in this book. There are a number of reasons for this:

- Essential oils are a very personal choice, and we often respond to them differently. While an aromatherapist will expertly be able to recommend specific oils for particular therapeutic qualities, the initial response for most people to an essential oil is based on whether we do or don't like the smell. A wonderful product can be rendered unappealing if the essential oil doesn't suit the individual. The base product with its herbs and seed oils can either be enjoyed in its simplicity, or you can add your own choice of essential oils, appropriate to your mood, need or the season.

- Essential oils are incredibly powerful and strong; just a few drops added to a pot of cream floods the product with their character and scent. I've therefore included them where I believe there is a benefit, but omitted them where it is preferable for the character of the plant seed oils and herbs to come through. Do make adjustments to the essential oils as you see fit, using your favourite blends or omitting them altogether.

- A large proportion of essential oils come from plants that grow in tropical climates. As I believe in the affinity of plants that have grown in the same conditions as us, when using essential oils I try to restrict myself to just those sourced from temperate grown plants, which creates limitations.

- Even though essential oils are highly concentrated, and therefore not hugely burdensome in terms of transport, by avoiding the use of those that come from afar I am minimising skincare miles and keeping products true to their local environment.

- It's important to consider sustainable sourcing when using essential oils. As they have become more popular, particularly in skincare but also for other uses, some have become scarce and we are beginning to encounter concerns about how to supply the world's demand for these precious ingredients.

However you choose to incorporate the vitality of plants into your products, be careful to scrutinise any recipe and know whether you are adding:

- A plant seed oil: expressed from the pressed seeds of the plant (some of these may be referred to as carrier oils, but I tend to avoid that term because I believe them to be more than a vehicle for delivering other ingredients).

- A macerated plant oil: created by steeping the plant material in a base oil.

- An essential oil: a quite different and highly concentrated distillation of the plant's vital oils.

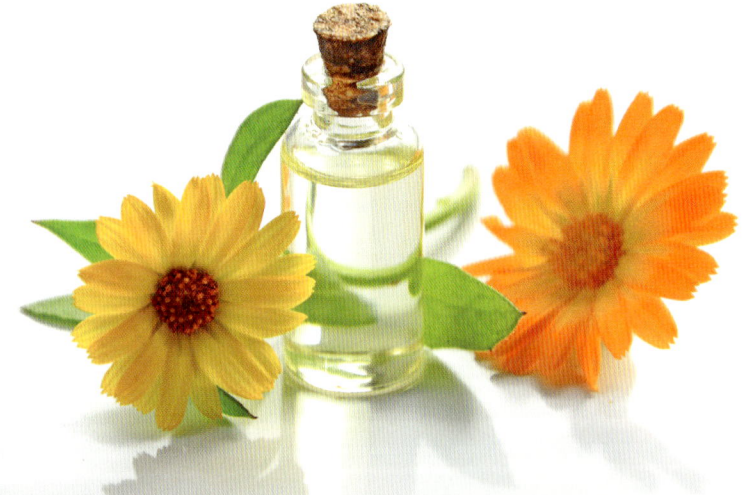

Beauty is truth, truth beauty – that is all ye know on earth, and all ye need to know

JOHN KEATS, ENGLISH POET, 1795-1821

CHAPTER 15

our closest herbs

As a starting point for using herbs and flowers in your skincare, here are suggestions for plants to look out for. I've selected easy-to-find examples in each of the main foraging and growing seasons: spring and summer. Getting to know just seven wild and seven cultivated plants in each season will give you a good repertoire of herbs and flowers to use in your skincare. From this you can continue to build, incorporating your own favourites or what grows locally to you.

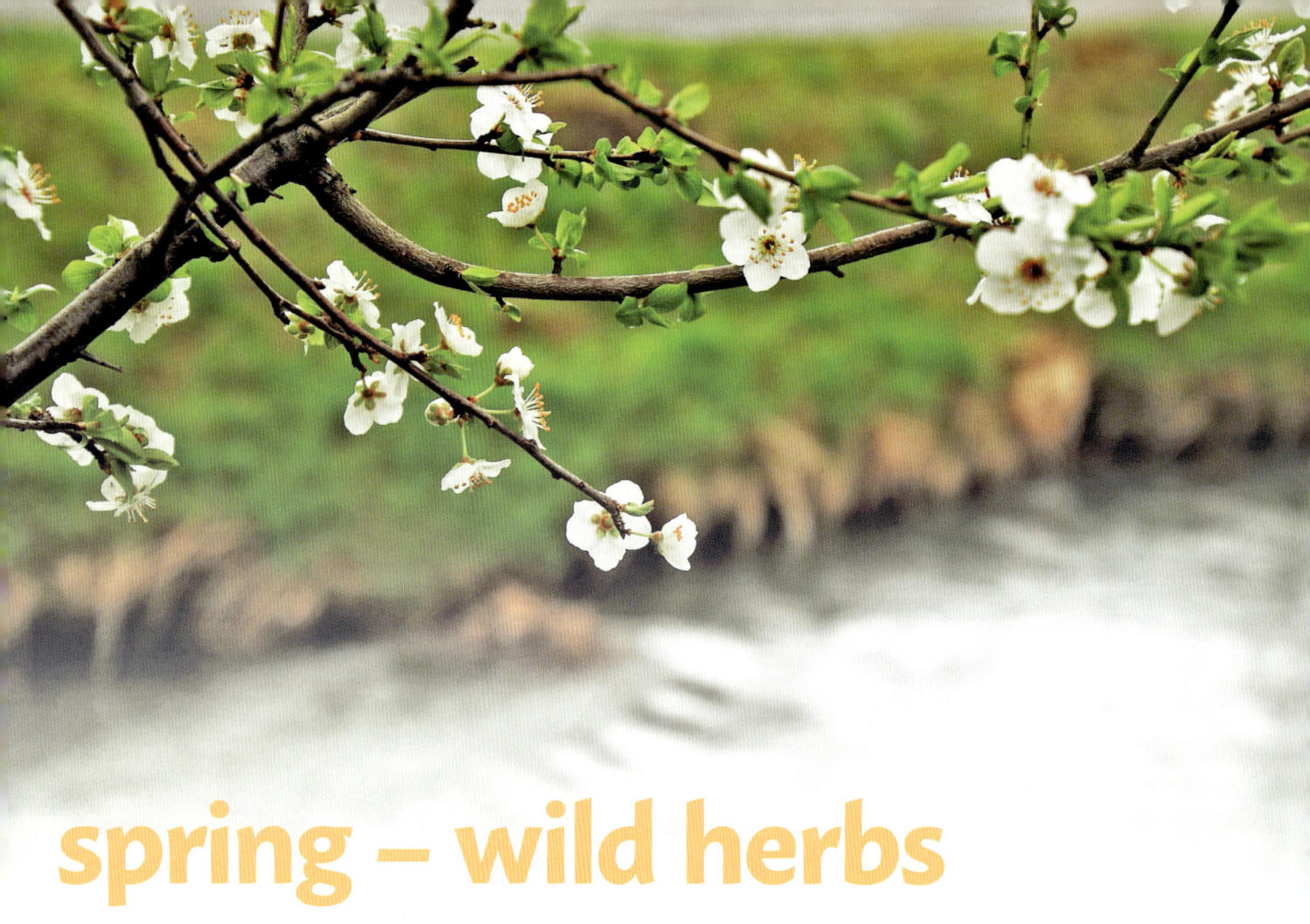

spring – wild herbs

Blackberry leaf
Chickweed
Cleavers
Comfrey
Dandelion
Horsetail
Nettles

Blackberry *Rubus fruticosus*

Think about the pace at which brambles can romp through the hedgerows (and gardens), with foot after foot of growth on a seemingly daily basis, and it's clear just what a powerhouse blackberry leaves must be – able to draw in the sun's energy and convert it into fuel for the bramble to grow and later produce succulent fruits. That is the little power pack of vitality that is offered up in a blackberry leaf. A constant, entanglement of hedgerows, superstition suggests it is possible to cure boils by passing through a loop of blackberry, formed when a shoot takes root.

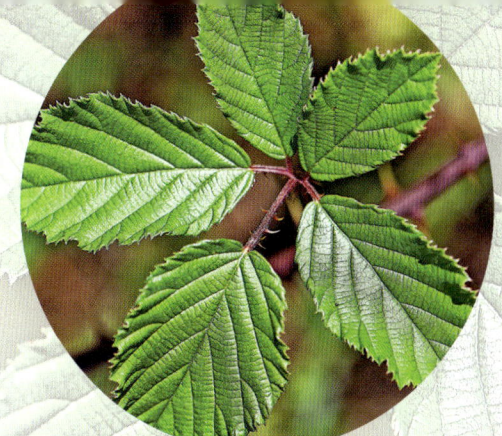

BLACKBERRY BATH SPLASH

Midway between a bath oil and a soap

A handful of blackberry leaves
1 litre rainwater
5 tbsp castile soap, grated

MAKE *Put the blackberry leaves into a pan and pour over 2 pints (1 litre) of water. Bring to the boil, cover and simmer for 15 minutes. Then remove from the heat and leave to infuse for 2 hours, before straining and discarding the leaves. Return the liquid to the pan, bring to the boil and whisk in the grated castile soap. Keep whisking until it has dissolved, then remove from the heat and set aside to cool. Pour into a bottle, seal and label.*

USE *Use in the bath or shower as liquid soap for the body.*

STORE *Keep in the refrigerator and use within one week.*

Benefits

Blackberry leaves are invigorating. They're a great addition to a bath to bring vitality back to your skin, refreshing and brightening it. Nicholas Culpeper, a 17th Century herbalist, tells us that the leaves make 'good lotions for sores in the mouth or secret parts'. So a good resource for help with itches and sores. An application of the leaves is said to help scalds and burns. For the hair, a blackberry leaf rinse will help deepen colour, especially good for greying hair.

Parts to use

Leaves

How to find, grow, harvest

Blackberries are plentiful in the countryside, making them easy to find. Gather leaves early in the year and dry and store for future use, or pick as you need them.

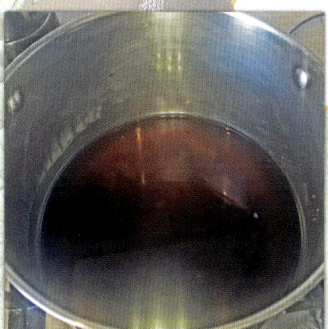
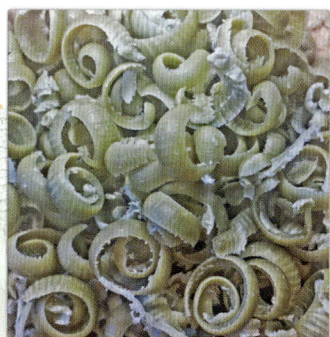
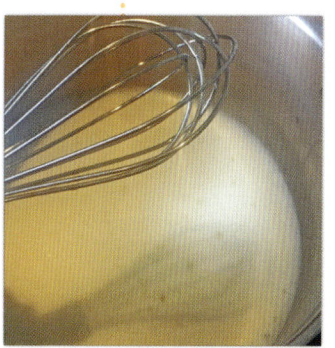

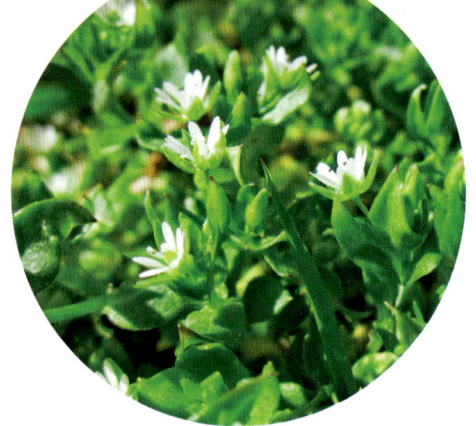

Chickweed *Stellaria media*

Chickweed's Latin name portrays it as a star of middle magnitude. It is an unobtrusive but fairly ubiquitous mini superstar of the herbal world. Lord Bacon, who carefully watched all changes in nature, said of chickweed: "When the flower expands bold and fully, no rain will happen for four hour or upwards; if it continues in that open state, no rain will disturb the summer's day; but if it entirely shuts up or veils the white flower with its green mantle, let the traveller put on his great-coat and the ploughman, with his beast of draught, expect rest from their labour." This closing of the leaves is known as the 'Sleep of Plants'.

CHICKWEED LOTION

A handful of chickweed

MAKE Put the chickweed into a bowl and pour over 2 cups (474ml) of boiling water. Cover and leave to infuse. When cool, strain and transfer to a screw-top bottle.

USE Apply morning and night to a cleansed face.

STORE Keep in the fridge and make a new batch every two or three days.

This can also be used as a body wash or added to the bath.

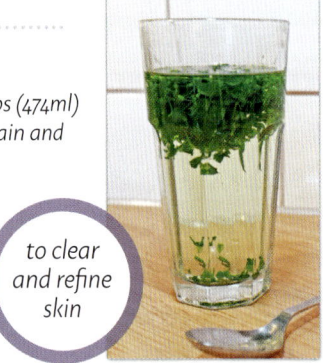

to clear and refine skin

Benefits

Chickweed has saponins (soap-like compounds) and mucilage (which makes it easy to combine into creams and lotions). It soothes and heals, so is helpful for irritated skin, inflammation, burns, scalds and soreness. Nicholas Culpeper advised its use to reduce redness in the face and Dr Fernie (Victorian herbalist) proposed it as a cure for scurvy. Chickweed juice can be used to ease insect stings and, incorporated into an ointment, it has been used to treat rheumatism. Other applications include helping with insomnia and soothing sore eyes. It's a great addition to a bath for aching pains and reducing skin irritations.

Parts to use Flowers, leaves, stems.

How to find, grow, harvest

Typically hardy, chickweed can be available all year-round, but take care in gathering as the stems can be fragile. It can also be dried to ensure a year-round supply. For drying, gather the most vibrant herbs in early summer but work with it quickly before it dries out. You'll find it in gardens, fields, along country lanes and in wastelands and watery places. Its spreading roots means it creeps over the ground, seeking out the richer soil. Low-growing, it has starry white flowers and soft, bright green leaves.

CHICKWEED OINTMENT

for irritated, sore or burnt skin

3 tbsp chickweed, chopped
1 tbsp (15ml) sunflower oil
1 tsp (5g) beeswax
1 tsp (5g) walnut butter

MAKE Macerate the chickweed in the sunflower oil using either the sun or the heat method (page 141) then strain. Melt the beeswax and walnut butter into the top of a double boiler and add the chickweed oil. Replace the water in the bottom of the double boiler with cold water and stir continually while the ointment cools. Put into a clean pot with a lid.

USE Rub the oil into the affected area as needed, repeating regularly until the condition heals.

STORE Keep sealed in a cool, dark place. Will keep for 12 months.

How to use

For sore skin, take a chickweed infused bath, and then apply chickweed ointment.

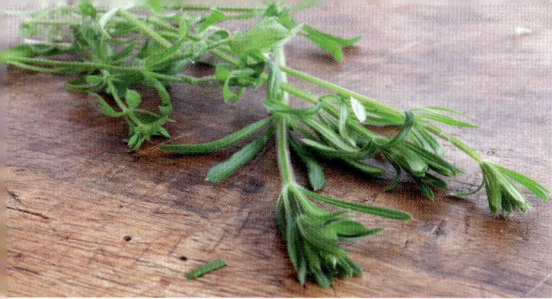

Cleavers *Galium aparine*

Commonly known as goosegrass, sticky weed, or 'organic sellotape'. Another name, 'Harriff' or 'Erriff' derives from the Anglo-Saxon 'hege-rife', a tax-gatherer or robber, because the plant plucks wool from the sheep as they pass through the hedge.

Benefits

Cleavers contain three distinct acids: tannic, citric and rubichloric. It's great for eczema and psoriasis and makes a good face wash to clear the complexion. It can also be used to treat sunburn and in an ointment for scalds and burns. In a hair tonic, it will improve texture and shine as well as treating dandruff. In addition, it is a good herb to use in making natural deodorants.

Parts to use

Leaves and stems.

How to find, grow, harvest

Cleavers grow in profusion around fields and wasteland, and sometimes too much in gardens. The bristly stems enable it to hook, climb and engulf. Whorls of leaves march up the stem, embellished with easily missable tiny white star-like flowers. These turn to little black balls of seed heads that cling and scatter everywhere. Gather the leaves and stems and extract their goodness through infusion or maceration. If you want to dry the plant for future use, gather in early summer.

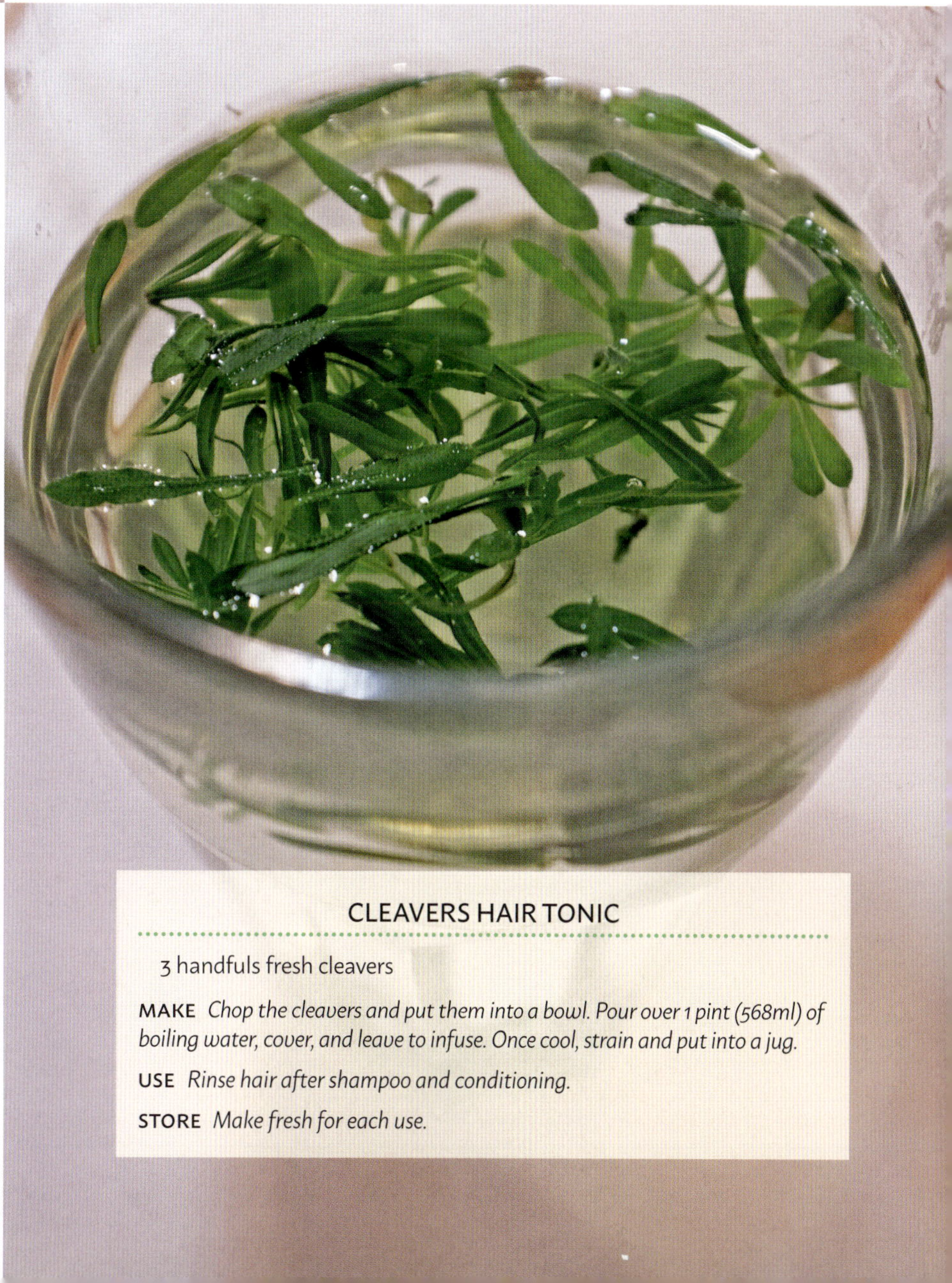

CLEAVERS HAIR TONIC

3 handfuls fresh cleavers

MAKE Chop the cleavers and put them into a bowl. Pour over 1 pint (568ml) of boiling water, cover, and leave to infuse. Once cool, strain and put into a jug.

USE Rinse hair after shampoo and conditioning.

STORE Make fresh for each use.

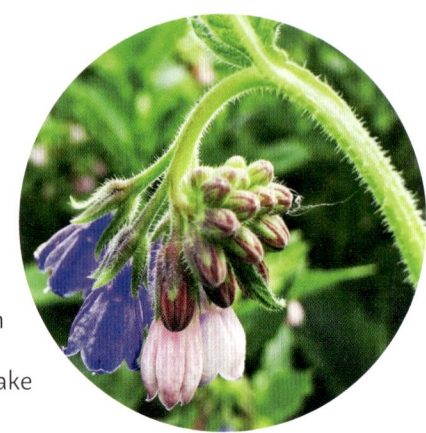

Comfrey
Symphytum officinale

In medieval times, comfrey was looked upon as a cure-all. The word *Symphytum* means 'to make whole' or 'heal'.

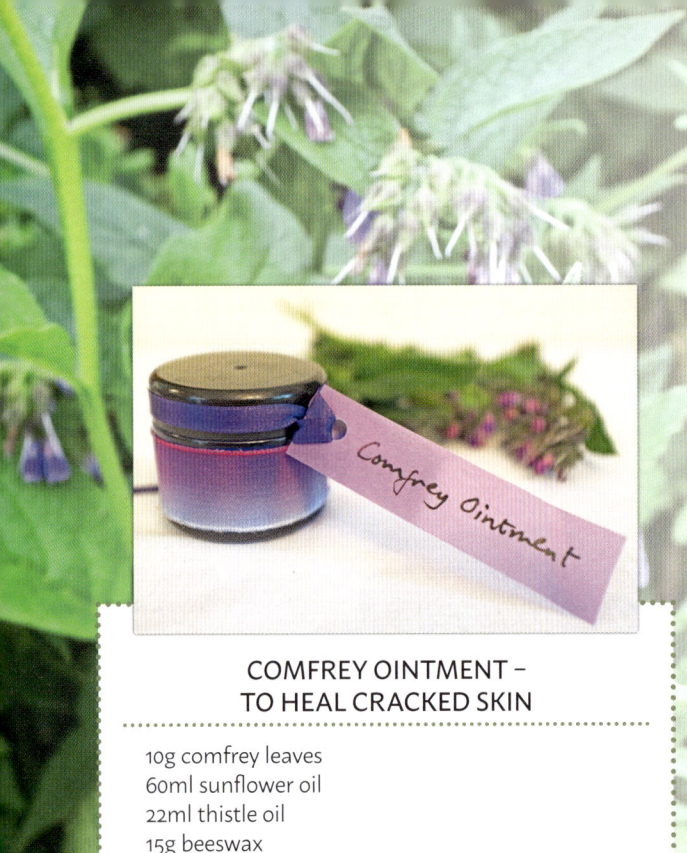

COMFREY OINTMENT – TO HEAL CRACKED SKIN

10g comfrey leaves
60ml sunflower oil
22ml thistle oil
15g beeswax
2ml vitamin E oil

MAKE First prepare by macerating the comfrey in the sunflower oil using either the heat or the sun method (see Chapter 14). When ready, put the macerated oil with the thistle oil and beeswax into the top of a double boiler and heat gently until it melts, stirring well to combine. Replace the water in the bottom of the double boiler with cold water and, as the ointment cools, add the vitamin E.

USE Rub into the affected area whenever required.

STORE Keep in a cool, dark place. Will keep for two years.

Benefits
Comfrey is a great skin conditioner and can be used in face packs, steams, creams and lotions, especially to help with eczema, acne, blemishes, rashes and dry skin. It softens skin and improves texture and youthfulness. On delicate skin it is gentle, while on oily skin it can be powerful. Including comfrey in a cream is good for cracked, dry skin. It contains allantoin, one of the most effective healing agents that speeds up the formation of new cells.

Parts to use
Use the leaves in infusion and the mucilaginous root in decoctions.

How to find, grow, harvest
Comfrey is rough and hairy so have gloves for harvesting. Its red, purple or cream flowers are bell shaped and held on long, thin stems above the large leaves in a curve said to resemble a scorpion's tail. Often found near water, ditches and moist fields and most recognisable in June and July when in flower.

Special care
There are concerns with comfrey root due to the presence of pyrrolizidine alkaloids (PAs) but these are much lower in the leaf. Comfrey leaf is considered safe to use externally but patch testing, as ever, is recommended (see how to do this in Chapter 7). In law, use of comfrey is restricted due to scares about liver toxicity.

How to use
- Use in creams and lotions to combat wrinkles
- Add infusions to baths and lotions to soften skin
- A decoction of the stems will help with scalp problems (rub it in during the final rinse when washing hair).

Dandelion *Taraxacum officinale*

In nearly all European languages the name for dandelion makes reference to the lion's teeth-like jagged edges of the leaf. In the Language of Flowers, dandelion is the Oracle, connecting the superstition that if you blow off all the seed heads in one puff, your wish will come true. There's also a tradition that the drifting seed heads carry your thoughts to a loved one. Dandelion is associated with faithfulness. We too readily dismiss dandelions these days as weeds; not so long ago they were a highly-regarded medicinal plant and livings were made digging the roots and sending them to London, a practice so common that a special 'green-herb' rate was charged by rail companies for transporting them.

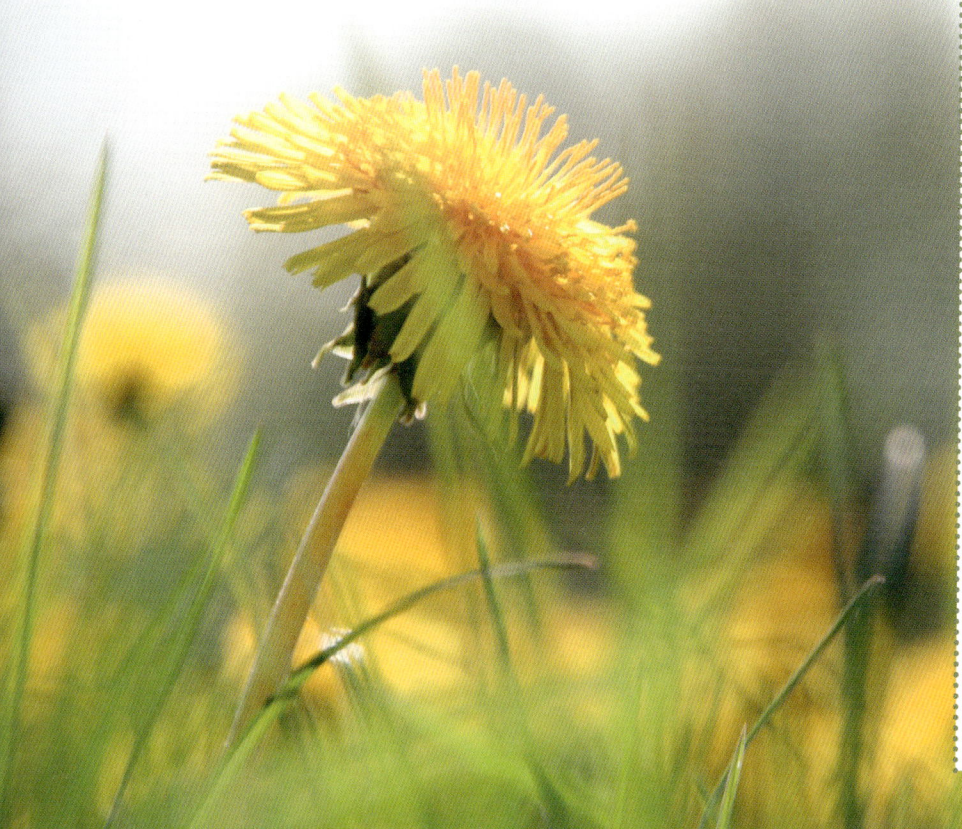

Benefits
Brightens dull skin.

Parts to use
Flowers, leaves, roots.

How to find, grow, harvest
Dandelions are ubiquitous, most noticeable in spring when in bright yellow flower. This is the best time to gather them, before they quickly give way to spherical fluffy seed heads.

How to use
Add an infusion of the leaves to the bath for cleansing.

DANDELION SKIN TONIC – A PICK-ME-UP FOR NORMAL SKIN

A generous handful of dandelion leaves
2 heaped tbsp of fresh thyme leaves
(or 1 tbsp of dried thyme leaves)
1 tsp (5ml) witch hazel

MAKE *Put the herbs in a bowl and pour over 300ml of boiling water. Leave to infuse for 20 minutes then strain through a sieve. Add the witch hazel. Bottle and shake well.*

USE *Apply to face in the morning as a refreshing wake up for the skin or in the evening to sweep away the last traces of cleanser.*

STORE *Keep in the fridge and use within 2-3 days. Freeze supplies in ice cubes and bring out to defrost when needed.*

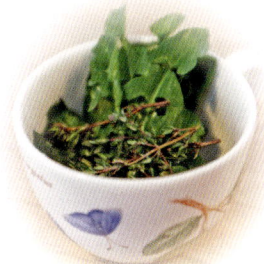

Horsetail *Equisetum arvense*

Horsetail has abrasive properties that were used from the Middle Ages until the 18th century for scouring pots and pans, especially pewter. Its massive tap root means it pulls minerals up from deep in the soil. Playing with horsetail, you'll find it breaks neatly at the stem nodes and stems can be stacked together, giving it the name 'Lego plant'.

Benefits

Horsetail contains alkaloids (including nicotine) and various minerals. Its unusual chemistry makes it a unique plant to use in skincare. Rich in silica it helps to keep skin, hair, nails and teeth healthy, preserving the natural elasticity in skin and restoring skin tone (especially after illness). It's the go-to herb for broken nails and lifeless hair. Horsetail is sometimes known as the 'hair gloss herb', such are its conditioning properties.

Parts to use

Use the stems either fresh or dried (though it's more effective fresh).

How to find, grow, harvest

Horsetail looks like a throw-back to Jurassic times, the basic structure of the plant has changed little since dinosaurs roamed the land. Horsetail is often found in wastelands or along canals or railways, especially on sandy soils where it spreads easily. It is a curious looking plant with segmented stems, from which pine-needle-like leaves radiate. Do not plant in your garden as it's incredibly invasive. Avoid gathering plants with brown spots as this is a fungal disease. Dry carefully without damaging the stems. When dry it becomes very difficult to cut, so you may prefer to chop your stems when freshly picked to have pre-prepared dried herb ready to use.

Special care

An irritant, best combined with demulcent herbs, and restricted to short-term use.

How to use

Add a strong decoction to the bath to soothe skin irritations and help heal minor abrasions. It's good combined with dandelion, fennel and seaweed.

HORSETAIL SHAMPOO

7 tbsp (105g) grated, dried soapwort
7 tbsp (105g) snipped horsetail stems

MAKE Prepare by putting the soapwort to soak overnight and then drain ready for use. Put the herbs into a pan and pour on 2 pints (1.2 litres) of water. Bring to the boil, cover and keep boiling for 15 minutes, then remove from the heat and leave to infuse for about an hour. When cool, strain into bottles, seal and label.

USE You'll need about a cup (250ml) of the shampoo each time you wash your hair.

STORE This will keep for about a week in the fridge, but you can make batches of 300ml to freeze in pots or freezer bags.

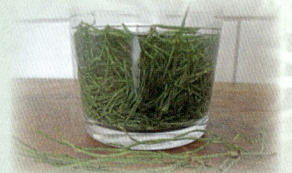

HORSETAIL SKIN TONIC

2 tsp freshly cut horsetail

MAKE Put the horsetail into a small pan and pour over ½ cup (118ml) of water. Leave to soak for several hours before bringing to the boil. Simmer for 10 minutes, then cover and leave for a further 10 minutes before straining and putting into a screw-top jar.

USE Apply morning and night after cleansing using cotton wool pads. Smooth it all over the skin and allow to dry.

STORE Keep in the fridge and make a fresh batch every two to three days.

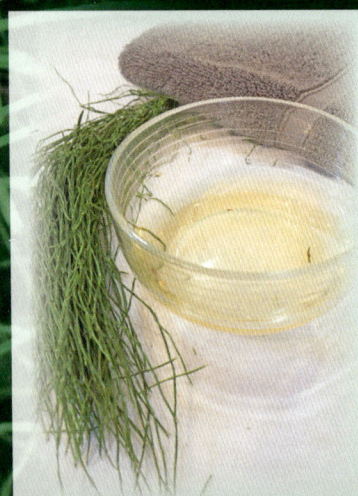

HORSETAIL NAIL BATH

3 tsp chopped horsetail
150ml boiling water

MAKE Put the horsetail into a bowl or cup and pour over ⅔ cup (158ml) of boiling water. Cover and leave to infuse.

USE While still warm, put the infusion into a bowl and soak your nails for 10 minutes. Repeat every other day. It is good to alternate this with soaking your nails in warm oil for 5 minutes every other day. (There is an example of an oil nail soak as part of the Hand Spa recipes in Chapter 11.)

STORE Make up a fresh batch for each use.

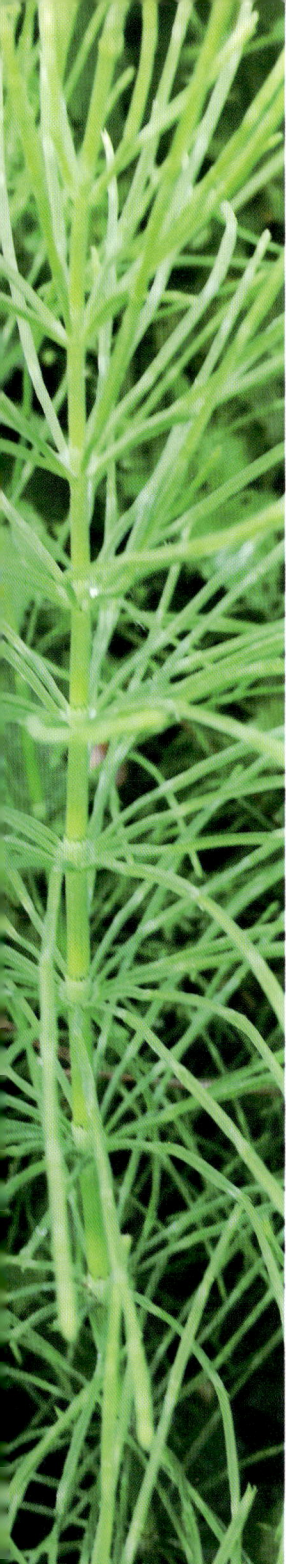

Nettles *Urtica dioica*

Nettles are said to have been introduced to Britain by the Romans. In our cold climate they could be stuffed inside garments or used to thrash limbs and stimulate circulation to help keep warm (each to their own). 'Uritication' or flogging with nettles was an old remedy for rheumatism or loss of muscle power. The name nettle either came from a derivation of 'needle', possibly referencing its sharp sting; or from 'net' meaning spin or sew, referencing the fibres (similar to hemp or flax) that were valued in cloth making. Nettle could be made into cloth reputedly as fine as linen.

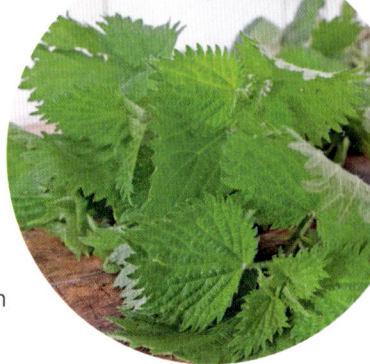

Benefits
Helps with arthritic pain, gout, sciatica and neuralgia, burns and insect bites. Also good for the scalp and as a stimulating, astringent tonic for the hair. Nettle infused oil is good for inflamed psoriasis. It has mucilage, like mallow and comfrey, which makes it easy to combine into creams and lotions.

Parts to use
The leaves are high in nutrients such as vitamins A, C and D, iron, potassium, manganese, calcium and nitrogen. They also contain minerals, formic acid, beta-Carotene and phosphates.

How to find, grow, harvest
Nicholas Culpeper wrote, stinging nettles "need no description: they may be found by feeling, in the darkest night". They should be collected in May and June, before flowering. Although the whole plant can be used, gathering just the fresh tips is recommended.

Special care
Take care when harvesting not to touch the bristly hairs that contain histamine and formic acid, which sting. If stung, rubbing with a dock leaf is the well-known antidote, but rosemary, sage and mint leaves will perform the same function and, remarkably, the nettle's own juice is an antidote to its sting. Once prepared in a recipe, all sting will go from the leaves.

How to use
Use an infusion of the leaves or decoction of the roots as a hair conditioner (rub in well).

NETTLE AND DANDELION BATH

refreshing and good for the skin

4 handfuls of nettles
4 handfuls of dandelion leaves
5-6 cups of boiling water

MAKE Put the herbs in a bowl and pour over 5-6 cups of boiling water. Cover and infuse for 15-20 minutes then strain into a jug.

USE Add directly to the bath water

NETTLE HAIR TONIC

to help prevent hair loss and make hair soft and glossy

A handful of nettles

MAKE Put the nettles into a pan and cover with 1 litre of water. Bring to the boil and then simmer for 2 hours. Leave to cool, then strain and bottle.

USE Saturate the scalp with the lotion every other night, leaving for half an hour before shampooing.

STORE Keep in the fridge. It will last for a week.

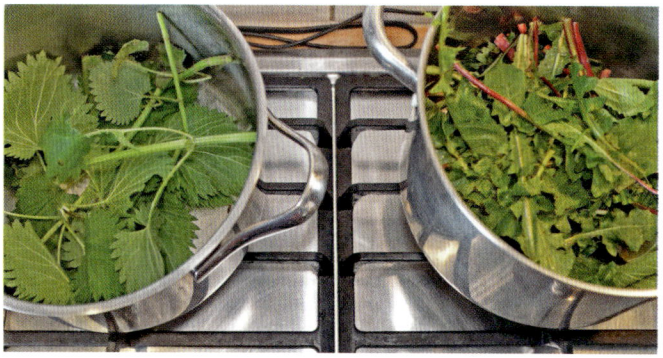

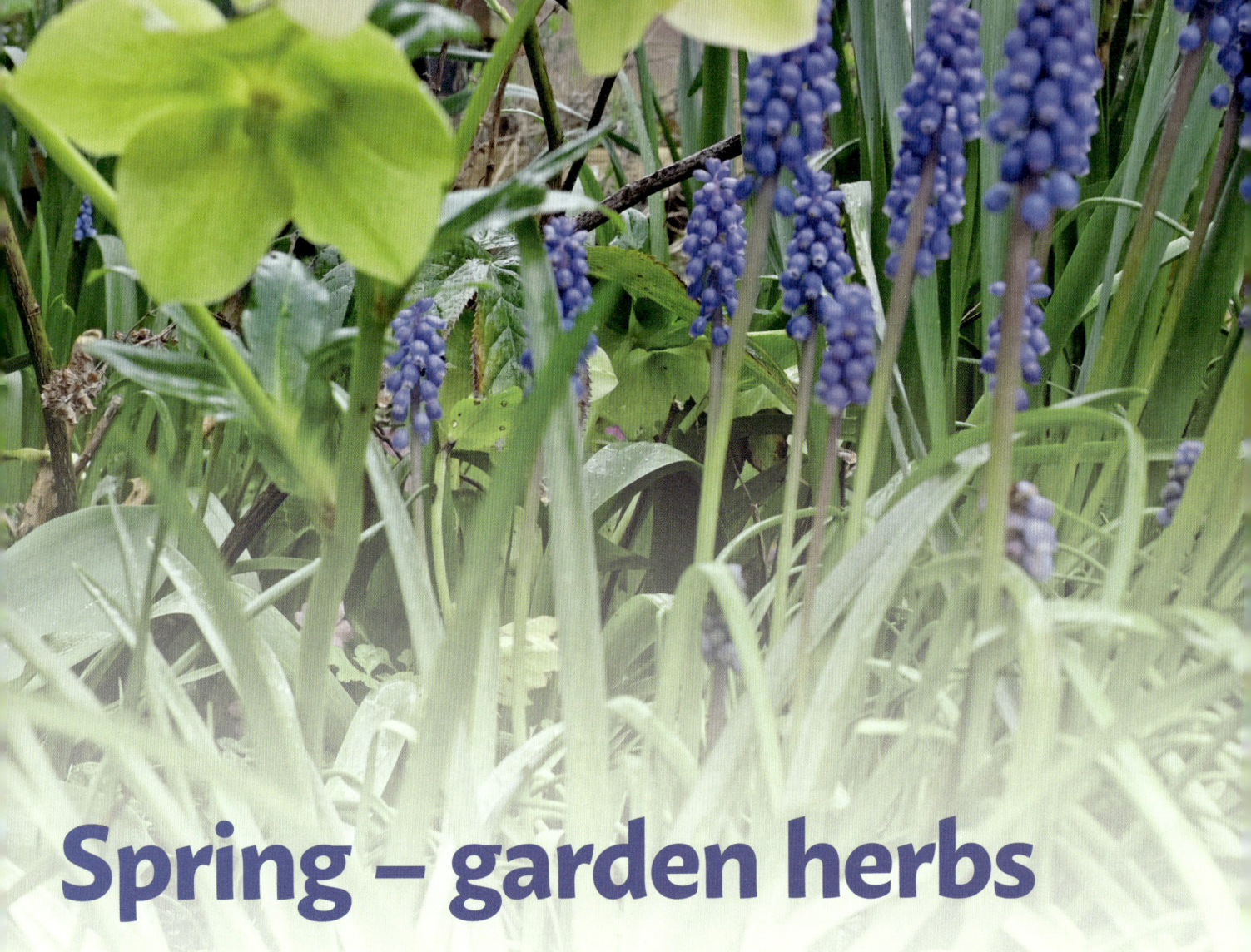

Spring – garden herbs

Bay
Houseleek
Lady's mantle
Lemon balm
Parsley
Raspberry leaf
Rosemary

Bay *Laurus nobilis*

Laurus is from the Latin *laus* meaning 'praise' and refers to the crown of bay leaves worn by the victorious Romans. This draws on an association with Apollo, the Greek god of philosophy, poetry and healing, making bay a symbol of wisdom and glory. Bay leaves were consumed by the priestess at Delphi; they may even have induced her prophetic trances (being slightly narcotic in large doses). Nicholas Culpeper assures us of the ancient wisdom that 'neither a witch, nor devil, thunder nor lightning, will hurt a man in the place where a Bay tree is'.

Benefits
Bay relieves aching limbs, so it's good added to a bath with a tablespoon of vinegar to relax muscles. Oil infused with bay is good for weary travellers and can help with scars and bruising, itches, scabs and wheals. Bay can help with dandruff when used as an oil for pre-shampooing scalp conditioner.

Parts to use Leaves

How to find, grow, harvest
Bay is often grown as an ornamental tree, clipped in shapes and positioned by doorways and entrances. Left unchecked it can grow into a large, bush-like tree. The leaves can be picked at any time of year.

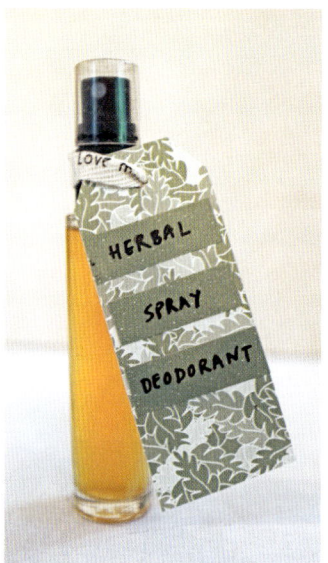

HERBAL SPRAY DEODORANT

Rind of 2 lemons, finely chopped
Rind of 2 oranges, finely chopped
10 fresh bay leaves, finely chopped
3 tbsp fresh pine needles, finely chopped
3 tbsp fresh thyme leaves
2 tbsp (30ml) glycerine
250ml vodka (or just enough to cover the ingredients)
100ml orange blossom water

MAKE Place the rinds, bay leaves, pine needles and thyme in a Kilner jar and cover with vodka, then seal and leave in a dark place for 2-4 weeks to macerate. Strain into a jug, then stir in the glycerine and orange blossom water and pour into a bottle with a spray nozzle.

USE Do a 24-hour test on a small patch of skin before using. Allow to dry fully to avoid staining.

STORE Keeps for up to 1 year if stored in a cool, dry place.

HERBAL CREAM DEODORANT

There are quite a lot of ingredients in this recipe. However, I have restricted it to things you can find at the supermarket or in fairly basic skincare making supplies. Deodorants are one of the most sensitising products to create and very much a personal thing. It may take a couple of days to get used to, if you have irritation after this point, try making another batch eliminating or reducing any ingredients you may be sensitive to. Bicarbonate of soda, salt and lemon are the first ones to try isolating. You can alter the quantities of other ingredients to keep the oil/dry ingredient ratio the same. Or change the essential oils, perhaps relying more on lavender than the more citrusy oils.

Once you get the combination you like, it's good to make up a larger batch of the macerated oil, as this will keep for six months, and will then be ready for you to easily blend your fresh batch of deodorant each time your pot needs refilling.

Try to change your standard products every so often. The two options here mean you can alternate between the spray and cream deodorant.

See overleaf for ingredients and method.

HERBAL CREAM DEODORANT

1 tbsp calendula
1 tbsp sage leaves
1 tbsp bay leaves
1 tbsp lemon peel
3 tbsp (45ml) hazelnut oil (absorbs quickly into the skin so it's not greasy)
2 tsp (10g) walnut butter
3g beeswax (protective and soothing, it's good to have some wax to give substance but minimise this to reduce greasiness)
1 tsp (5ml) witch hazel (astringent, anti-inflammatory, antibacterial, soothing, prevents razor burn)
1 tsp (5ml) glycerine
Juice from 10 houseleek leaves (you can substitute this with 5g of aloe vera gel)
2 tsp (10g) kaolin or bentonite clay (detoxing and absorbs moisture)
1 tsp (5g) bicarbonate of soda (neutralises pH and helps with body odour; eliminate this if it is irritating)
1 tsp (5g) arrowroot (absorbs excess moisture; too much arrowroot makes it firm)
1 tsp (5g) cream of tartar
1 tsp (5g) icing sugar
1 tsp (5g) salt (antibacterial, inhibits growth of odour-causing bacteria)
0.5g lemon juice (helps deodorise and the acidity reacts with the baking soda alkalinity to enable the powders and oils to say mixed together; otherwise the powders would sink to the bottom)
2 drops lavender essential oil
2 drops rosemary essential oil
2 drops lemon essential oil
2 drops grapefruit essential oil
2 drops clary sage essential oil
(the first 4 essential oils are all antibacterial, and clary sage is astringent, helping you to stay dry)

MAKE First macerate the herbs and lemon in the hazelnut oil using either the heat or sun method. When ready, melt the butter and wax into the top of a double boiler, then add 1 tablespoon (15ml) of the macerated oil. Add the witch hazel, glycerine and houseleek juice (or aloe vera gel), followed by the dry ingredients and then the essential oils and lemon juice. Transfer to a jar.

USE Apply with your fingers onto clean armpits and allow to dry for a few moments before getting dressed.

STORE Keep in a cool, dark place. It will keep for 1 month.

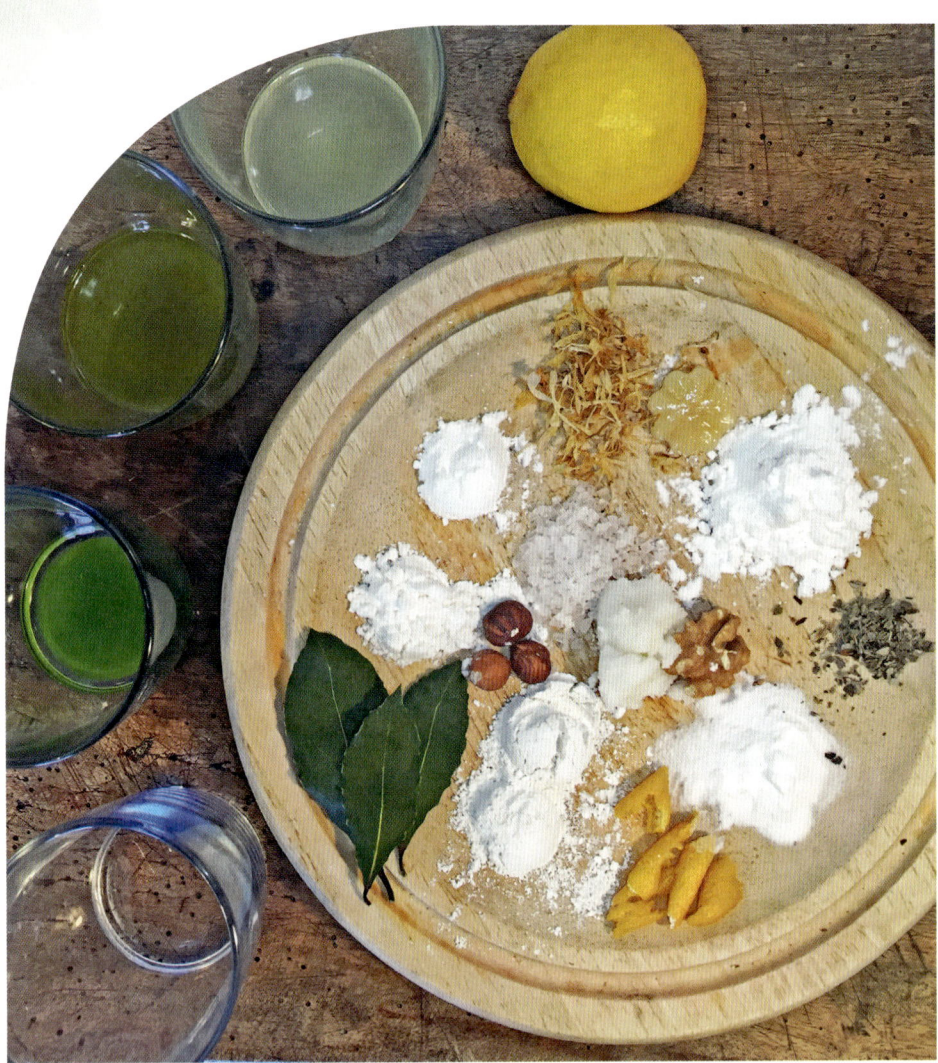

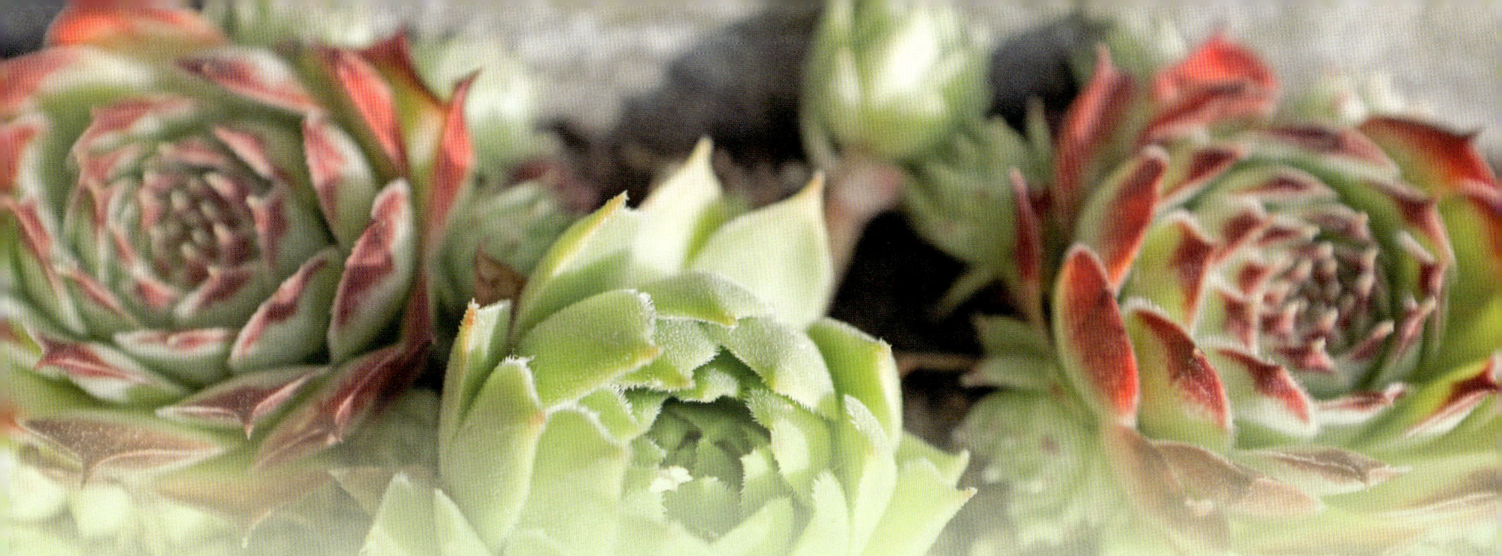

Houseleek *Sempervivum*

Houseleek's common name comes from the Anglo-Saxon leac, meaning 'a plant' (so you could say these are the original houseplant). Romans grew them in containers at their front doors, believing them both a protector and an aphrodisiac. The Latin name, *semper* means 'always' and *vivus* 'alive', as these are drought-tolerant plants. The Emperor Charlemagne decreed that his subjects should grow houseleeks on their roofs to ward off lightning; they are still traditionally planted for this purpose. In the language of flowers, houseleek symbolises vivacity and industry.

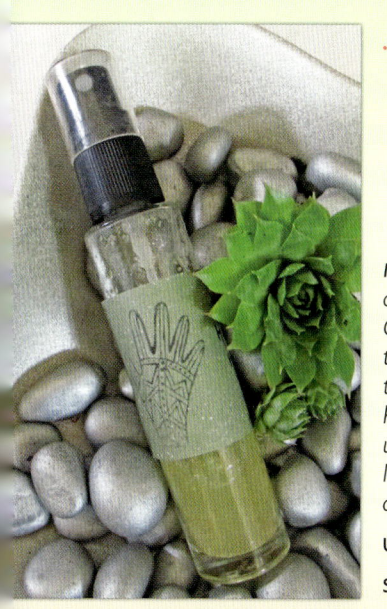

HOUSELEEK HAND SANITISER

- 1g lavender flowers
- 2 tsp (10ml) sunflower oil
- 10 houseleek leaves
- 1 tsp (5ml) thyme tincture
- 10 drops lavender essential oil
- 10 drops eucalyptus essential oil

MAKE Prepare by macerating the lavender in the sunflower oil. With small amounts it's best to use the sun method (see Chapter 14). When your lavender macerated oil is ready, blitz the houseleek leaves and sieve to extract the juice. Put this into the top of a double boiler to heat gently and slowly add the herbal infused oil, whisking thoroughly together. Replace the water in the bottom of the double boiler with cold water and keep stirring as it cools. Add the thyme tincture and essential oils. Pour into a pump or squeezy bottle, seal, label and date.

USE Spray on hands whenever there is a need.

STORE Keep in a cool, dark place for up to a year.

Benefits

The gelatinous leaf is a good alternative to aloe vera. Use it for stings, bites, warts, burns, sunburn and inflamed or itchy skin. It contains tannins and mucilage that soothes and heals damaged tissues.

Parts to use

Leaves – these can be blitzed whole for use in a recipe, or halved and the gelatinous parts scraped out. Traditionally they were halved and applied directly to the affected skin.

How to find, grow, harvest

Do as the Romans and keep a planter with houseleeks by your door, or in your house. Give them space to spread and they will form little plantlets (known as 'mother-and-chicks') and multiply.

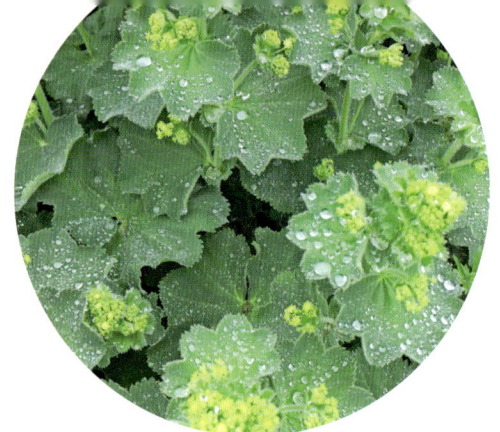

Lady's mantle *Alchemilla vulgaris*

Alchemilla means 'little magical one', from the Arabic for alchemy, because the way in which the leaves hold water was thought to be magical. In the Middle Ages *Alchemilla* was reputed to preserve youth and was prescribed for female complaints. The pleated leaves are like a cloak and became associated with the Virgin Mary, hence the name 'Our Lady's Mantle'. Although *Alchemilla mollis* is the more commonly found variety, *Alchemilla vulgaris* is the plant used in skincare and *Alchemilla alpina* is considered to be the most effective variety.

Benefits
Lady's mantle soothes inflamed skin and can help with minor infections, windburn and sore eyes. It is used to defend against fine lines and large pores as well as helping with acne. Useful as a toner and for cleansing. The leaves are astringent, so good for oily skin.

Parts to use
Leaves. Use in an infusion, or use the leaves directly by soaking them in warm water or blitzing them to a paste.

How to find, grow, harvest
Fuzzy greeny-yellow flowers and pleated leaves are held aloft on thin stems; a delight post rain or in the early morning dew, when sprinkled with charming, clinging waterdrops. They will be in flower from early summer to early autumn. However, the best flowers are in late June and early July so pick then for drying. It will often self-seed and spread itself, but you can also propagate it by division or collect seeds for sharing with friends.

How to use
- Use an infusion as a toning facial wash (add a little witch hazel for toning oily skin).
- Soak pads of cotton wool in an infusion from the flowers and leaves to create a cold compress for eyes.
- Soak the leaves in warm water and lay them directly on the face to manage fine lines, or on the breasts to ease soreness.

LADY'S MANTLE AND BUTTERMILK LOTION

10g lady's mantle leaves
¼ cup (60ml) buttermilk (to make buttermilk, see page 66)

MAKE *Put the leaves into a bowl and pour over ¼ cup (60ml) boiling water. Cover and leave to infuse. When cool, strain off the liquid and add the buttermilk.*

USE *Wipe over your face to cleanse and wash off with warm water.*

STORE *Keep in the fridge. Make new supplies every other day.*

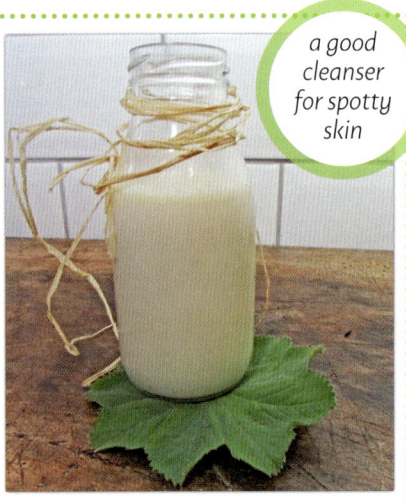

a good cleanser for spotty skin

LADY'S MANTLE JUICE FOR ACNE

A handful of young lady's mantle leaves and flowers.

MAKE *Put the leaves into a juicer or blender. If blending, add sufficient water to make a pulp and then squeeze through a muslin.*

USE *Dip cotton wool pads in the juice and swab the affected area, leaving on the skin to dry.*

STORE *Make a fresh batch each time.*

SKIN FRESHENER – A TONIC FOR WAN SKIN

30g lady's mantle leaves

MAKE *Put the leaves into a bowl and pour over 1 cup (237ml) of boiling water. Cover and leave to infuse for 10 minutes.*

USE *Soak a face cloth in the infusion, wring it out and then place over your face and lie down for 10 minutes. If your skin is particularly dry, you can apply some oil before using the cloth.*

STORE *Keep in the fridge; lasts for 2 days.*

Lemon balm *Melissa officinalis*

It's easy to go barmy for lemon balm – the bees certainly do. Melissa is the Greek word for 'honey bee'. It used to be said that a swarm of bees would never desert a hive where lemon balm was planted close. Traditionally lemon balm is said to help heal a broken heart. Paracelsus (1493-1541) called lemon balm "the elixir of life" and John Evelyn (1620-1706) described it as "sovereign for the brain, strengthening the memory and powerfully chasing away melancholy…"

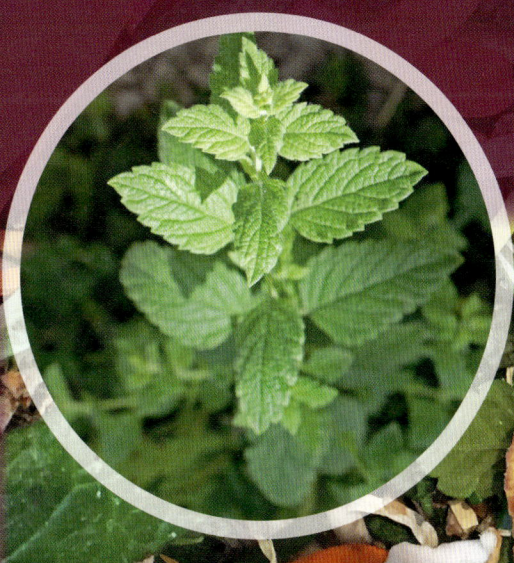

"…a herbe greatly to be esteemed of Studentes. For that by a special propertie, it driveth away heavinesse of minde, sharpneth the understanding and the wit, and encreaseth memorie"

Benefits
Lemon balm is a soothing astringent. An infusion of it therefore makes a good cleanser and a useful rinse for greasy hair. It will add a cheering scent to your bath and is considered to help with depression, nerves, memory, headaches, insomnia, colds and fevers, as well as treating insect bites and cold sores. An ingredient in 17th century Carmelite water ('Eau de Carmes'). It was originally taken to ease nervous headaches and neuralgia.

Parts to use
Use the leaves in infusion or maceration.

How to find, grow, harvest
Identify it by the lemon scented leaves (which look a little like mint leaves) and delicate white flowers that cluster up the stem. If you can't find it, watch the bees and they'll show you where it is. It will grow in most soils but will be stronger scented and more effective in moist, fertile soils.

How to use
- Add an infusion to the bath for relaxation
- Use the leaves in perfume and colognes
- Infuse as a facial steam or as a rinse for greasy hair

HUNGARY WATER

25g fresh lemon balm leaves or 1 tbsp dried lemon balm
50g fresh rosemary leaves
1 fresh mint sprig (use only fresh; omit if you don't have any)
Thinly pared rind of ½ lemon
300ml vodka
125ml orange flower water
125ml rosewater

MAKE Chop the lemon balm and put all the herbs and the lemon rind into the bottom of a glass jar. Add the vodka, cover tightly and shake well. Leave in a warm place – or on a windowsill – for three weeks, remembering to shake it every day. Then strain and, as a last step, add the orange flower and rosewater. Decant into a sterilised bottle.

USE Splash and spritz all over for instant freshness and fragrance.

STORE Keep in a dark, cool place and use within six months.

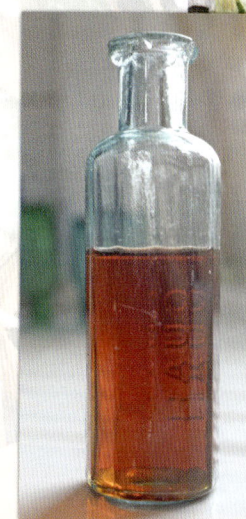

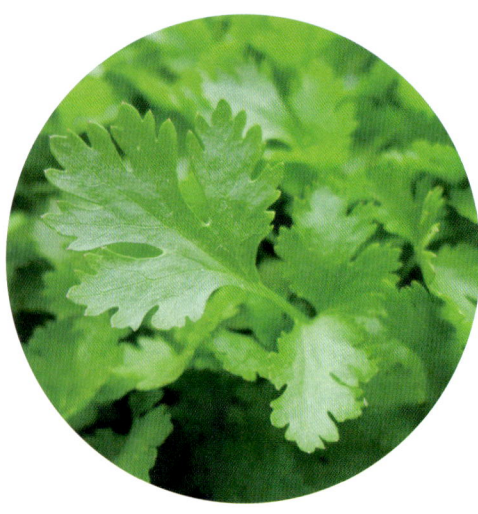

Parsley *Petroselinum crispum*

Parsley has a reputation as a health herb. It was originally used as a medicinal plant before people started including it in food. Important in Greek and Roman culture and noted by Pliny the Elder (1st century AD) as consumed by people from all walks of life. Folklore tells us that parsley grows well in a household where 'the woman wears the trousers'.

Benefits

Parsley is good for cleansing and conditioning, but beware of its skin-lightening properties. It can be included in face packs, lotions, creams and cleansers and is especially good for those with oily skin or thread veins. A tonic will help improve sallow or blotched complexions and help dilated veins and bruises. A compress of parsley can help with swollen breasts, insect bites, painful swellings and sore eyes. As an astringent, parsley will help with enlarged pores.

Parsley also makes a great hair tonic and conditioner with anti-dandruff and deodorising properties.

Parts to use

Use the leaves and stems in an infusion, or crush the leaves and extract the juice. Parsley can be especially good combined with other strong green herbs such as mint, dandelion or comfrey.

How to find, grow, harvest

Parsley is best gathered and used before it flowers. It grows well in warm, moist ground and, if sown successively, you should be able to keep fresh supplies going all year round, especially if you can use cloches to protect it at the coldest times. Alternatively, gather supplies for drying at the end of summer, or keep it in the freezer. You can use the flat or curly-leaved variety of parsley in your skincare, whichever is more readily available to you.

How to use

Expressed parsley juice with egg white is a good tightening and boosting mask.

GREEN HEALING FACE PACK – A TONIC FOR SKIN

1 handful parsley
1 handful spinach
2 tbsp (30g) fine ground oatmeal

MAKE *Chop the greens and put them into a pan and pour over 1 cup (237ml) of water. Bring to the boil and hold for 5 minutes, then cover and leave to cool. Press through a fine sieve to fully extract the juices. Mix with enough oatmeal to make a smooth paste. If your skin is oily but also sensitive, add natural yoghurt to the mixture.*

USE *Apply to face, avoiding eyes, and lie back for 10 minutes before rinsing off with warm water and finishing with a soothing oil.*

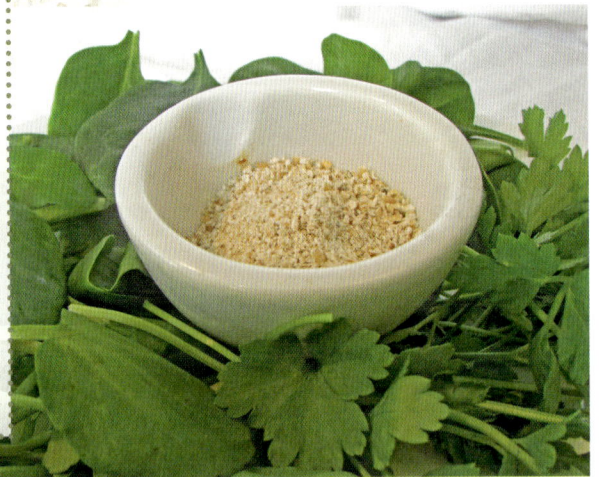

Raspberry leaf *Rubus idaeus*

Raspberry does grow wild in Britain, especially in damp woodland, but is more commonly found cultivated in gardens, typically grown in a fruit cage to protect from raiding birds. Another name for it is 'hindberry' meaning 'berry eaten by deer in the woods'. Dreaming of raspberries is said to be a good omen for a love affair.

Benefits
A raspberry leaf tea can be good for cleansing, treating wounds and as an eyewash or compress for inflamed eyes.

Parts to use
Leaves

How to find, grow, harvest
A shrubby and long-stemmed plant with succulent red fruit. The leaves have a characteristic coating of dense, white hairs.

Special care
Raspberry has long been associated with pregnancy and is very helpful in strengthening uterine muscles in the later stage of pregnancy, but should be avoided in the early stages.

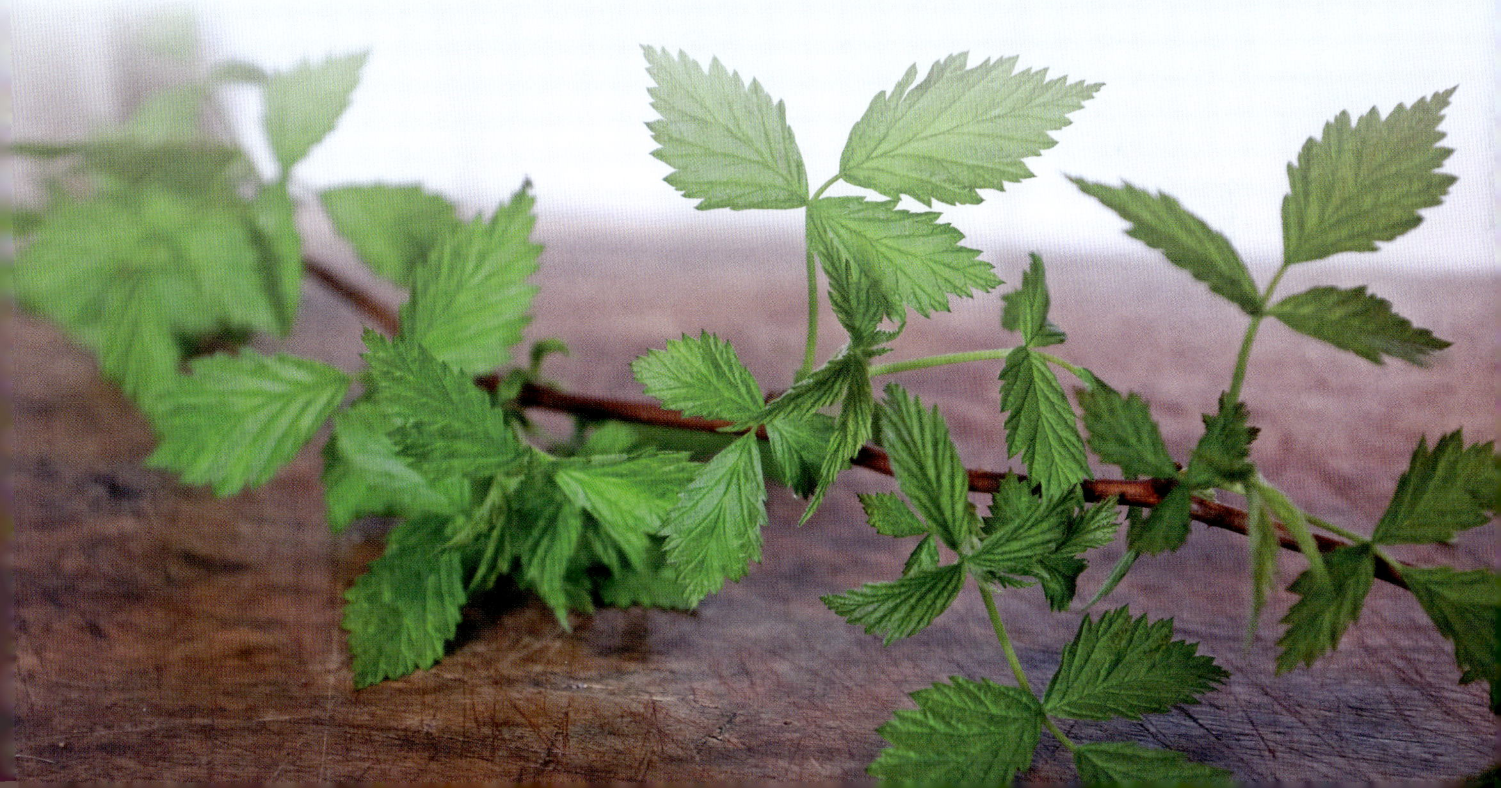

RASPBERRY LEAF SKIN CLEANSER

1 handful raspberry leaves

MAKE Put the raspberry leaves into a bowl and pour over 1 pint (568ml) of boiling water. Leave to infuse for 10 minutes before straining and bottling.

USE Use daily as a wipe-on, wipe-off cleanser.

STORE Keep in the fridge and make fresh supplies every few days.

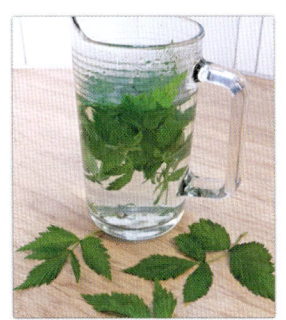

Rosemary *Rosmarinus officinalis*

The name rosemary means dew (ros) of the sea (marinus). It is a classic plant of the Mediterranean. Rosemary is associated with remembrance; during some funerals today we hand out sprigs of rosemary as we remember the departed loved one. In the Middle Ages sprigs of rosemary were dipped in gold and tied with ribbon as a keepsake for wedding guests. The sprigs were also given on New Year's Day as the year changed from old to new. Rosemary activates the brain so it is good to have present when studying. Follow on by taking a sprig of rosemary into an exam to help recollect your study time.

Benefits
Rosemary is one of the great cosmetic herbs, used traditionally in toilet waters, such as Hungary Water. It has a practical use as an antioxidant, often used to prolong the life of herbal macerations. The active antioxidant components are carnosic acid and carnosol. Great for the hair, rosemary stimulates circulation to improve the scalp and it is also used for rheumatism, arthritis, neuralgia, muscular injuries and wounds. It is included in herbal body oils to relieve muscle pain, boost body circulation and stimulate brain activity.

Parts to use Leaves and flower

How to find, grow, harvest
The small grey-green leaves will release their aromatic oils as you brush against them. Rosemary has small, pale blue or white flowers that may appear at any time in the year, although spring is their main flowering season. True to its Mediterranean origins, it likes dry soil and good light.

Special care
The high concentration of phenol derivatives can make rosemary an irritant for skin and eyes.

How to use
- Add rosemary oil to create a stimulating bath
- Use rosemary leaves in an infusion for steaming the face
- Steep rosemary leaves to make a hair rinse

Some traditional advice for using rosemary

The Physicians of Myddfai, 13th century:
'By washing each morning with the decoction and allowing it to dry naturally, the aged will retain a youthful look as long as they live.'

Bancke's Herbal, 1525:
'Boyle the leaves in white wine and wash the face therewith and thy browes and thow shalt have a faire face'

'Also put the leaves under the bedde and thou shalt be delivered of all evil dreames'

'Smell of it oft and it shall keep thee youngly'.

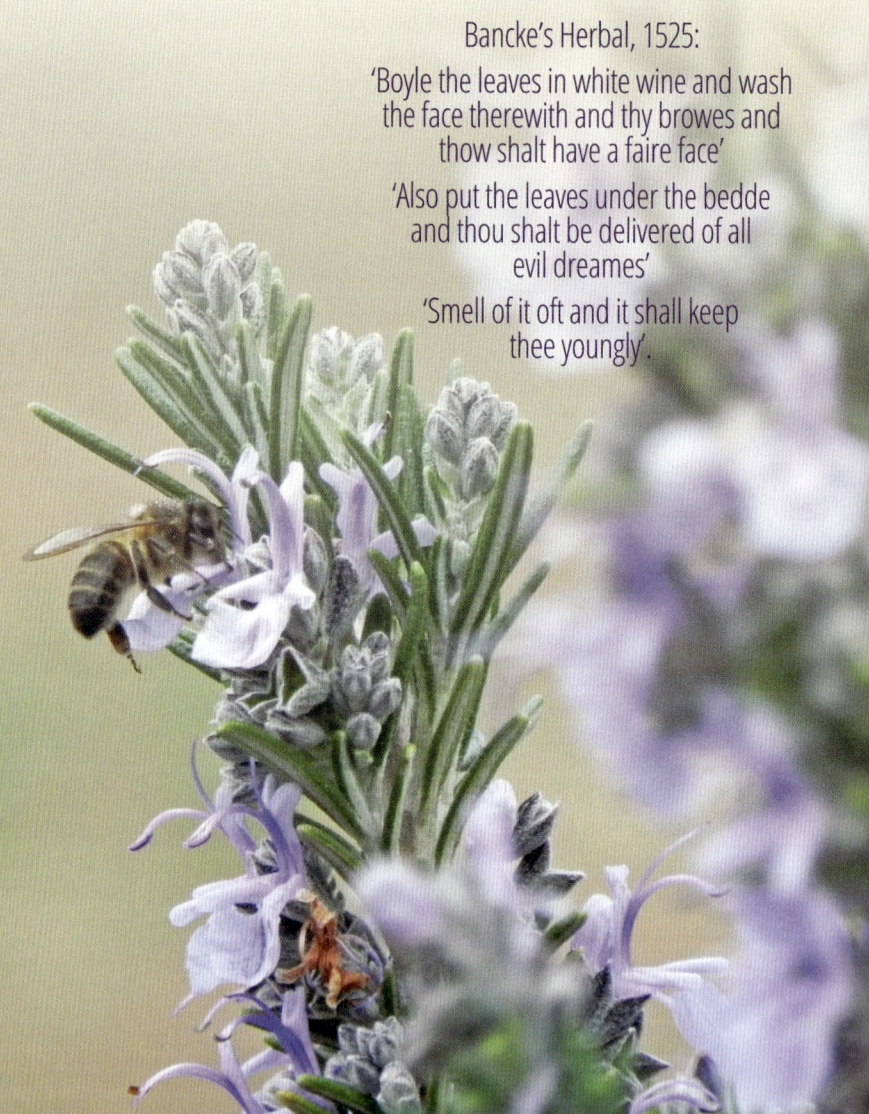

ROSEMARY FACE RINSE

2-3 handfuls (30g) of fresh rosemary

MAKE Put the rosemary leaves into a pan and pour over ½ pint (284ml) water. Bring to the boil and keep hot for 5 minutes before covering and leaving to cool. Strain and bottle.

USE Wipe over your face as a refresher and to hydrate before applying moisturiser.

STORE Keep in the fridge and make fresh supplies every few days.

ROSEMARY HAIR CARE – FOR GREASY HAIR

2-3 handfuls (30g) of fresh rosemary
300ml apple cider vinegar

MAKE Put the rosemary into a jar and cover with the cider vinegar. Leave it to stand for 10 days and then strain.

USE Add ½ cup of the rosemary vinegar to your final rinsing water when washing hair.

STORE Keep in the fridge. Will keep for 4-6 weeks.

ROSEMARY HAIR CARE – FOR DRY HAIR

2-3 handfuls (30g) of fresh rosemary
300ml sunflower oil

MAKE Infuse the rosemary in the oil using the sun or heat method (see Chapter 14).

USE Rub the rosemary infused oil into your scalp and wrap with a hot towel. Leave for 30 minutes before washing off with a gentle shampoo.

STORE Will keep for 12 months in a dark bottle.

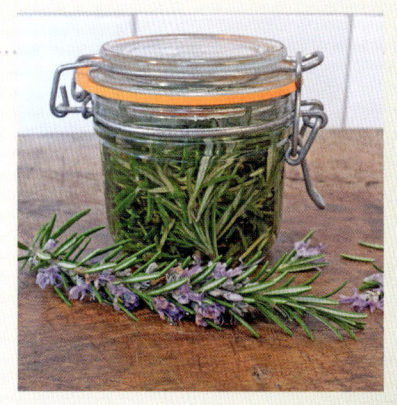

ROSEMARY AND MINT MOUTHWASH

25g fresh rosemary (or 10g dried rosemary)
25g fresh mint (or 10g dried mint)
2 tbsp (30ml) vegetable glycerine
10-12 drops peppermint essential oil
5-10 drops myrrh essential oil

MAKE Put the herbs into a bowl and pour over 2 pints (1 litre) of boiling water, then leave to infuse. When cool, stir in the glycerine and add the essential oils. Pour into a sterilised bottle.

USE Shake before use. Rinse around mouth morning and night after brushing teeth. Don't swallow it, though if you do it won't do you any harm.

STORE Keep in the fridge. Keeps for two weeks.

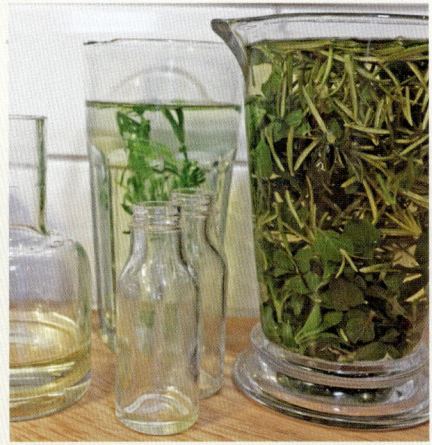

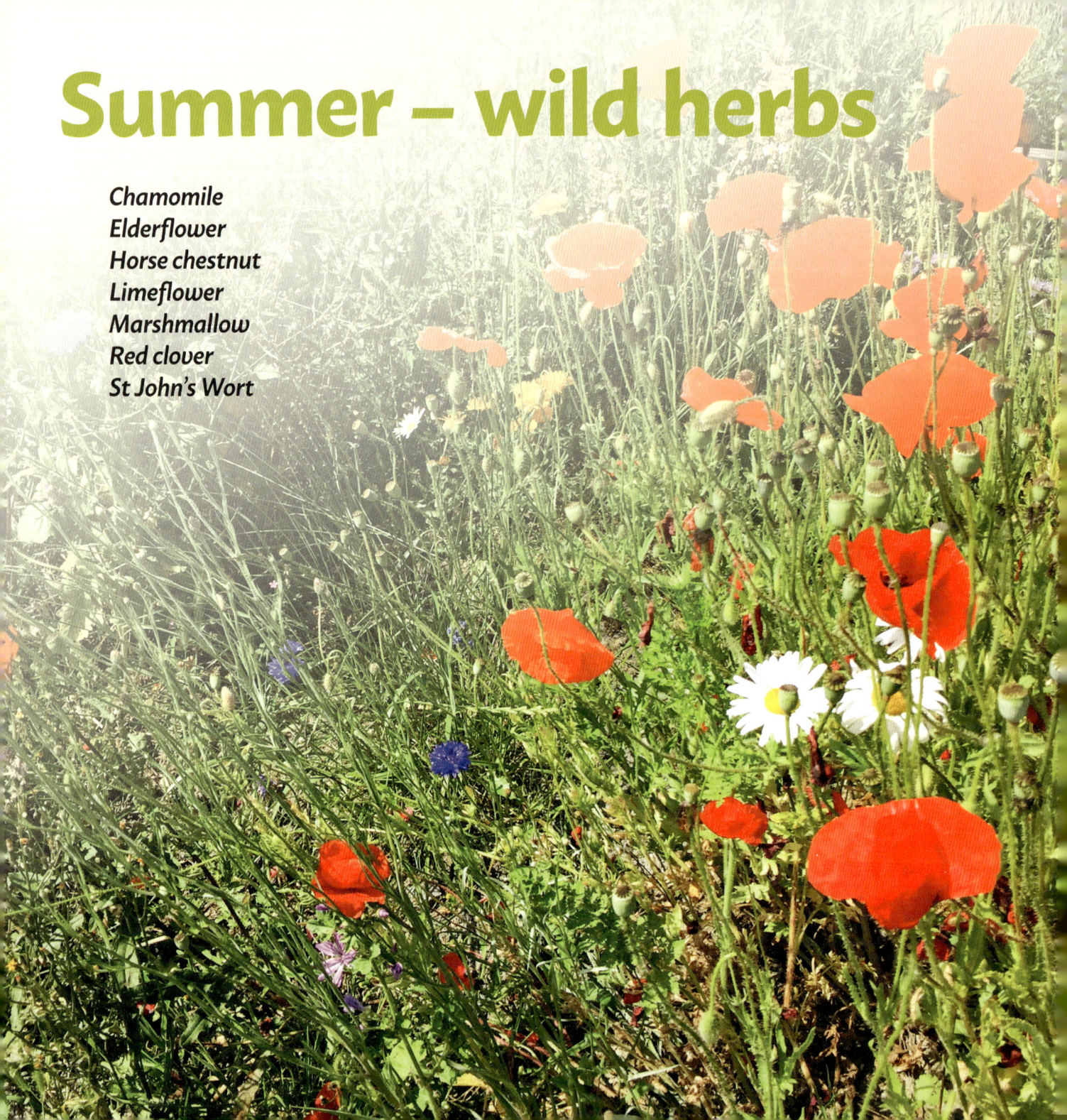

Summer – wild herbs

Chamomile
Elderflower
Horse chestnut
Limeflower
Marshmallow
Red clover
St John's Wort

Chamomile Matricaria recutita
(German chamomile, scented mayweed)

Chamomile is one of the nine sacred herbs from Anglo-Saxon times, and it was revered above all other herbs by the Egyptians who dedicated it to the sun. German chamomile is closely related to Roman chamomile (*Chamaemelum nobile*) and both are used in skincare, and can be blended together. German chamomile has similar chemistry to Roman chamomile but a less pronounced aroma. It's the flower we drink in chamomile tea. The name comes from the Greek *chamaimēlon* meaning 'apple on the ground'. There's a strong scent of apple when it is trodden upon. It was commonly used as a strewing herb, and seems to thrive being trodden on, as Shakespeare appreciated.

> 'Harry, I do not only marvel where thou spendest thy time, but also how thou art accompanied. For though the chamomile, the more it is trodden on, the faster it grows, yet youth, the more it is wasted, the sooner it wears' Henry IV, Part I, Act II, Scene 4

Roman chamomile is considered 'the plant's physician', as ailing garden plants are supposedly cured by planting chamomile beside them, and cut flowers revive and last longer with the addition of chamomile tea to the water.

Benefits
Chamomile is great for dry and normal skin and can be helpful to problem skin of all types and ages, and a comfort to irritated skin. It is gentle, calming, soothing and softening as well as being healing and anti-inflammatory. It's an astringent, good for cleansers, conditioners, face packs and steams. Often used in hair products and rinses to lighten and condition, it's also a soothing and healing addition to bath oils and lotions.

Parts to use
Flowers

How to find, grow, harvest
You'll find chamomile at field edges, often in gateways. Patches of chamomile will shift around cultivated fields from year to year with human disturbance. All traces disappear over winter necessitating an early summer search to discover where they'll emerge this year. Starting as a feathery cluster of leaves, it can grow to knee or thigh high. The white flowers have a bright yellow centre and smell of apples. When you can, use the flowers fresh; otherwise preserve their goodness in macerations. You can also freeze them for later use to make the most of their volatile oils which can be lost a little in the dried flowers.

Special care
Significant terpene content means this is a skin sensitiser and skin and eye irritant.

How to use
- Add an infusion for a relaxing bath
- Use as a cleanser in facial steams or lotions
- Add to oatmeal face packs
- Use an infusion to rinse hair
- Add to creams for dry skin

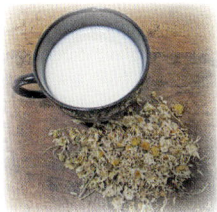

SUNBURN LOTION

1 handful of chamomile flowers
1 cup (237ml) milk

MAKE *Put the flowers in a small pan and pour the milk over. Bring to the boil then simmer gently for a minute. Cover and allow to infuse for 5-10 minutes before straining.*

USE *Bathe the affected skin.*

STORE *Keep in the fridge for two days.*

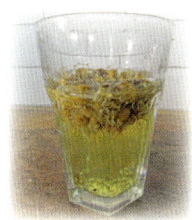

GOLDEN HAIR RINSE

2 handfuls of chamomile

MAKE *Put the chamomile into a bowl and pour over 2 cups (474ml) of boiling water. Leave to infuse for 30 minutes, then strain.*

USE *Ideally use the infusion as a rinse after shampooing. Catch the infusion as you rinse and pour it through your hair 2-3 times.*

Elderflower *Sambucus nigra*

Elderflower is an essential summer scent, a classic element in the hedgerow medicine chest and has been used since Roman times. As one of the white-flowered queens of the hedgerow, elder was a reminder of the White Goddess and therefore revered. The name sambucus is from the Greek 'sambuke', a musical pipe. New shoots of elder bushes were traditionally used to make tuneful pipes. Show respect to an elder by tipping your hat. An elder tree in your garden is very lucky, especially if it is self-sown. Elder wood and bark is believed to be physically warmer than that of other trees because they bloom at the peak of the sun's strength, at midsummer.

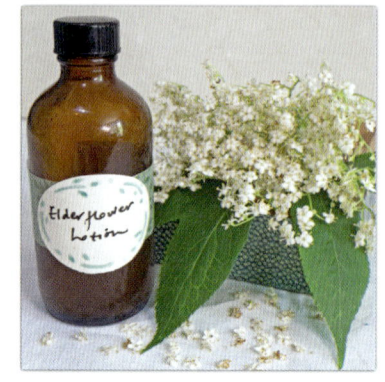

ELDERFLOWER LOTION FOR ROUGH, CHAPPED HANDS

3 tbsp elderflowers
1 tbsp (15ml) glycerine

MAKE Put the elderflowers into a cup or bowl and pour on 4 tablespoons (60ml) of boiling water. Leave to infuse and, when cool, add the glycerine, mix well and transfer to a bottle.

USE Smooth into the hands to keep them soft and supple.

STORE Keep in the fridge for up to a week.

SOME TRADITIONAL ELDERFLOWER USES:

ELDERFLOWER OINTMENT

450g elder leaves
225g plantain leaves
100g wormwood
50g ground ivy
1kg lard

for swellings & wounds

MAKE *Cut the herbs very small. Boil the lard, stirring continually until the leaves become crisp. Then press out the ointment for use.*

OIL OF SWALLOWS

Also known as
Oil of Elder Leaves or Green Oil

1 part bruised fresh elder leaves
3 parts linseed oil

MAKE *Macerate the leaves in the oil.*

When sold commercially this is often coloured with Verdigris.

a traditional treatment for piles

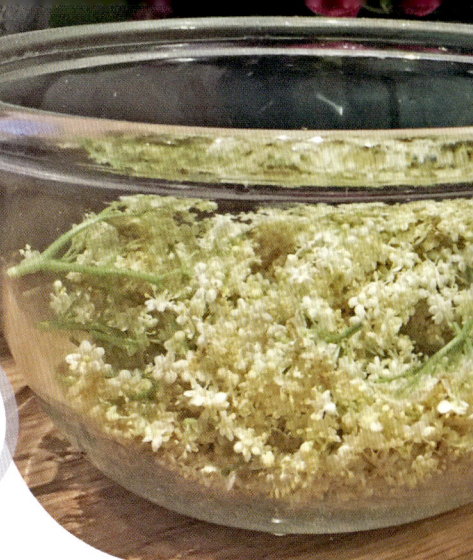

Benefits

Elderflower was the go-to complexion enhancer on every dressing table in the past. It is widely used in skincare for its conditioning and skin lightening properties that can be handy for reducing freckles and sunburn and for treating greying hair. Elderflower water (Aqua Sambuci or Eau de Sureau) is an infusion of elderflowers popularly used for softening cleansers, toners and conditioners for hands, face and body (for details on how to make it see 'Flower Waters' in Chapter 14). It is soothing for irritated and inflamed skin and can be used against skin infections, chilblains and chapped hands. Nicholas Culpeper recommends washing hands with a distillation of elderflower morning and night. It's also good for sore feet.

Elder leaves are good for blemished, sun or wind-burned skin and are also a traditional insect repellent (traditionally bruised and tucked into a hatband, or rubbed on the face). The elder leaf is also a useful addition to ointments for bruises, sprains and chilblains and to emollient creams and cooling ointments.

Elderberries improve the colour of greying and dark hair.

Parts to use   Flowers, leaves and berries.

How to find, grow, harvest

Collect the flowers when first in bloom and gleaming white (ignore any that are yellowed or starting to smell 'catty'). Traditionally this is in the three weeks that straddle midsummer, although I find you have to get out earlier to find the best blooms. Shake them down from the boughs onto a sheet or pick blossoms and throw them into a heap where they will become warm. The corollas will loosen and can be easily gathered by sifting. Infuse the flowers or decoct the leaves. Elderflowers used to be salted (at a ratio of 10:1 flower:salt) to preserve them for future use in distillation – these would be referred to as 'pickled' elderflowers. These pickled flowers take on a gentler fragrance than the fresh flowers and are preferred for making elderflower water. For future use in infusions, elderflowers need to be dried. This is best done in an oven, sooner rather than later. Traditionally elder leaves would be gathered on the last day of April.

How to use

- Elderflower water is mildly astringent and a gentle stimulant. It is good to use after bathing in salt water or in creating lotions for skin and eyes.
- For its insect repellent properties, make an elder leaf infusion. Use it neat, combine in a cream or add to a bath.
- Use an elderflower infusion to rinse blonde hair that is greying; use an elderberry infusion to rinse greying dark hair.

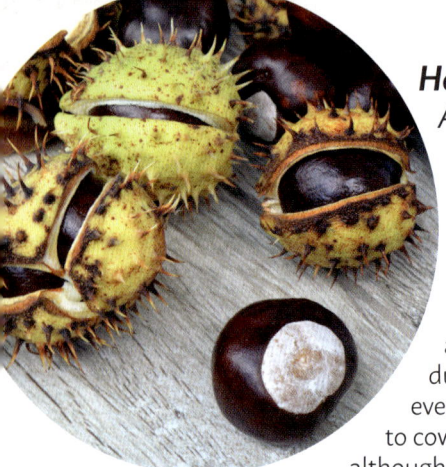

Horse chestnut
Aesculus hippocastanum

The horsechestnut tree got its name from the observation that eating the seeds (conkers) cured horses of chest complaints. Though wrongly classified as a chestnut, the name has stuck.

Horse chestnuts are not edible by humans and not recommended for livestock, but, during World War I, it was estimated that for every ton of horse chestnuts harvested and fed to cows and sheep (made palatable by soaking first, although pigs would still refuse them), half a ton of grain could be saved for human consumption so, indirectly, increasing the national food supply.

Benefits
Conkers are used to treat chest pain in humans, as well as circulation issues such as frostbite, swelling, cold feet, rheumatism, varicose veins and sprains or other injuries. It's the aescin within them that helps as this promotes circulation and reduces swelling.

Parts to use
Use the white flesh of the seed, taken out of its spiky case and shiny outer.

How to find, grow, harvest
The horse chestnut tree is distinctive in spring with its white or pink 'candles', a great attraction for bees. By autumn these have given way to spiky round cases which often split open as they drop to the ground, revealing shiny brown conkers. This coincides with the start of the new school year in September. Passing a horse chestnut tree on the school walk often includes a little treasure-hunting to collect conkers for fun, festooning or fights.

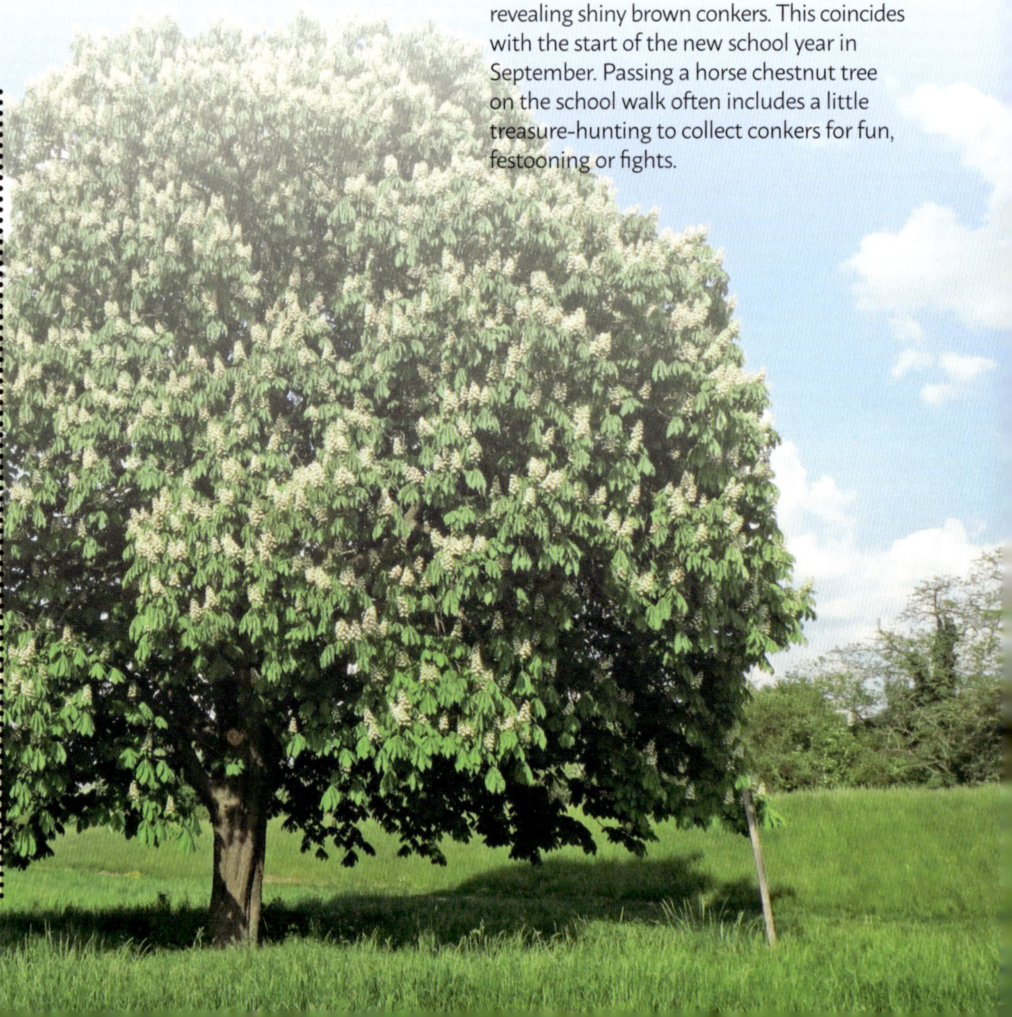

HORSE CHESTNUT OIL

30g conkers, peeled and chopped into the smallest pieces you can
100ml sunflower oil

MAKE Place the conkers into the top of a double boiler and pour over the oil. Keep on a low, gentle heat for three hours, stirring occasionally. Leave to cool, then strain the conker pieces from the oil by passing it through a coffee filter and collecting the oil in a clean, sterilised bottle.

USE Apply to varicose veins, spider veins, swelling, tired legs or in a sports massage. Do not use if you're pregnant or breastfeeding.

STORE Keep in a cool, dark place. Will keep for 12 months.

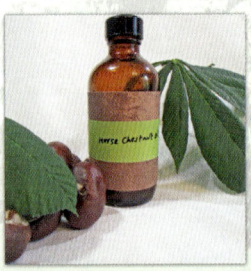

Limeflower
Tilia cordata (small-leaved lime), Linden tree

The lime tree grows all over Europe. Despite its size, the lime tree remains relatively inconspicuous until July, when they come into their own. Their flowers open, and a sweet fragrance fills the air as bees buzz in among their branches. The honey made from lime pollen is especially good, so do try some if you get a chance. You may be surprised to find it has a slightly minty flavour, which is absolutely delicious. Also known as the linden tree, limes are said to date back 70 million years.

A simple way to try tasting limeflower yourself is by steeping a few sprigs in boiling water to make a tea. In France this is a traditional bedtime drink, enjoyed from childhood onward. It's likely that the calming effects of limeflower tea have aided healthy hearts more than red wine. It's a good drink to have if you're suffering from a cold or flu, as it promotes perspiration.

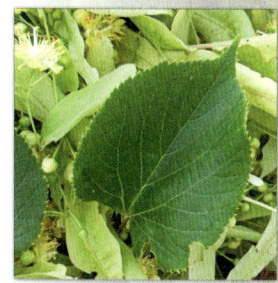

Benefits
Limeflower is one of the most helpful of skincare plants. It's skin-conditioning, helps soothe skin and smooth out tiny wrinkles, helps fade freckles and improves circulation. Using limeflowers brings the heart of summer into every day. Known as 'tilleul' in perfumery, it is used in many classic scents, helping recall a bright summer's day.

Parts to use
Flowers and bracts.

How to find, grow, harvest
Limeflowers bloom and can be gathered for just a few short weeks in July, so do head out and find your local trees while you can. Collect the flowers and the bracts; they're best when just open and the stamens are full of pollen.

Special care
Avoid old flowers when making preparations as they may produce symptoms of mild intoxication.

How to use
- Limeflower footbath for aching feet and ankles
- Lime water hair rinse to keep hair soft and in good condition.

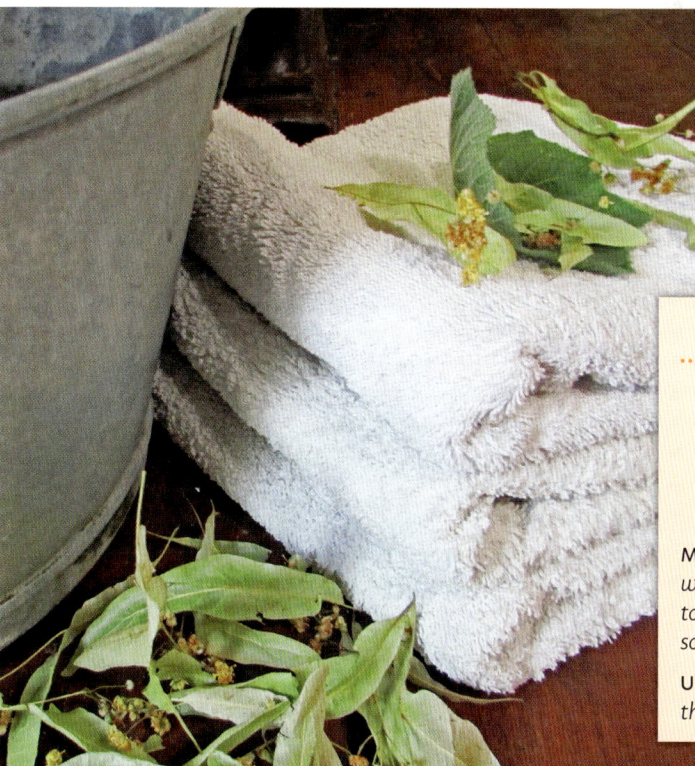

SOOTHING FOOT BATH

4g limeflowers
2g marshmallow leaves
2g comfrey
1 tbsp (15ml) apple cider vinegar
2 tbsp (30g) arrowroot

MAKE Put the herbs in a pan and pour over 3½ pints (2 litres) of water. Bring to the boil, simmer for 5 minutes then cover and allow to cool to a comfortable temperature. Transfer to a suitable bowl for soaking your feet and add the cider vinegar.

USE Soak your feet while relaxing for half an hour and then dry them meticulously and powder with arrowroot.

OUR CLOSEST HERBS

Marshmallow *Althaea officinalis*

Mallow has been grown as a medicinal plant since Roman times and was considered a 'cure-all'. Its name *Althaea* comes from the Greek *altha* 'to cure'. It is the plant from which our sticky sweets get their name, which were originally made using the mucilage from the stems of this plant, an ingredient also used to make Middle Eastern halva. The name 'mallow' derives from the Old English 'malwe' meaning 'soft' and refers to the abundant mucilage, which is the useful skin-softening component. You'll notice a similarity between the marshmallow plant and hollyhocks, they are related: 'hoc' was the Old English word for 'mallow'.

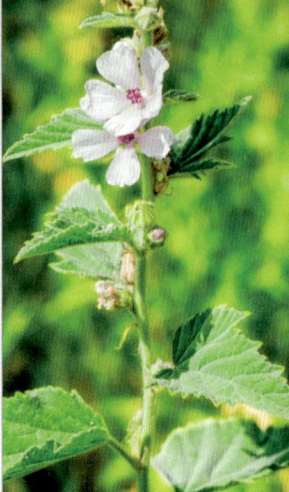

MARSHMALLOW HAND CREAM

5g marshmallow root
2 tbsp (30g) ground almonds
1 tsp (5ml) milk
1 tsp (5ml) cider vinegar

MAKE First make a decoction of marshmallow root by placing it in a bowl and pouring over 150ml water, then leave overnight. Strain the next day and use 2 tablespoons (30ml) of the decoction. Mix this with the almonds, milk and cider vinegar, beating them together until well blended. Put into a screw-top jar.

USE Apply whenever hands feel dry.

STORE Keep in the fridge. Will keep for one week.

CARROT AND MARSHMALLOW MASK

for dry and sensitive skin

1 large carrot
2 marshmallow leaves
1 egg yolk, beaten
1 tbsp (15ml) double cream

MAKE Grate the carrot and pound the marshmallow leaves, then mix them together with the egg yolk and add just enough double cream to make a firm slush.

USE Use your fingers or a brush to apply to your face, sit back and relax for 10-15 minutes. Then wash off with warm water and pat dry.

Benefits
Great for softening skin and conditioning and long used traditionally for this purpose, along with many other applications including treating irritations, boils, burns, sores, ulcers, wounds and inflammations. Marshmallow is gentle enough to use on babies' skin or sensitive skin, while also being rejuvenating for older skins on the face or body. It's anti-inflammatory, antimicrobial and moisturising (helping to maintain levels of hyaluronic acid in the skin). In hair products it can help nourish, detangle, condition and may counteract hair loss.

Parts to use
Leaves and roots. Make an infusion or maceration from the leaves and a decoction or maceration from the roots.

How to find, grow, harvest
On making my first attempts to find marshmallow growing wild I was disappointed to find Nicholas Culpeper's description: 'Common mallows are generally so well known they need no description'. So discovery has been something of a labour of love, and I prize my sightings of marshmallow, even though now I recognise it can be quite common when driving along country roads. It is typically found in damp conditions, so near streams, rivers and marshes. You'll recognise it easiest when in bloom; pale flowers appear in late summer, with no fragrance, and all die down in autumn. It has five-lobed roundish, soft leaves that are densely covered in hairs. There is a saying that marshmallow grows only near a happy home.

How to use
Use an infusion in a rinse for dry hair.

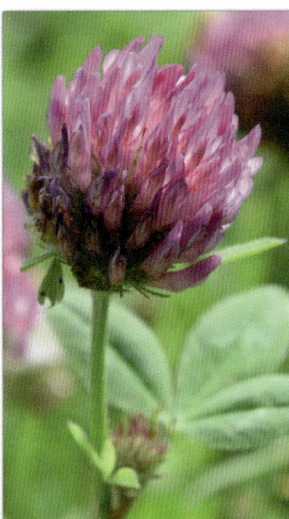

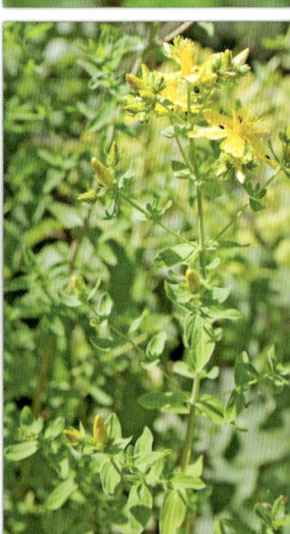

Red clover Trifolium pratense

Clover has been important since the Middle Ages as a forage crop, containing more nutrient for cattle than any other fodder. It is sensitive to weather, as Pliny the Elder observed: 'Its leaves do start up as if afraid of assault when tempestuous weather is at hand'.

DUCHESS AND DAIRYMAID SKIN SOFTENING BATH

- 1 tsp lavender
- 1 tsp thyme
- 1 tsp grated orange peel
- 1 tsp chickweed
- 1 tsp cowslip
- 1 tsp marshmallow leaf
- 1 tsp elderflower
- 1 tsp red clover
- 1 tsp comfrey leaf
- 2 tbsp (30g) oats
- 1 tbsp (15g) dried milk powder

In the 18th century, the romantic, pastoral ideals led aristocracy to play-act as farm labourers. This bath remedy recalls that whimsy by using cultivated herbs and imported citrus in a rich and elegant infusion, worthy of a duchess, along with meadow herbs tied together with oats in a muslin scrubbing bag.

MAKE Put the lavender, thyme and orange peel into a bowl and pour over 1 litre of boiling water. Leave for an hour to infuse. Meanwhile, mix together all the other herbs with the oats and dried milk powder and tie this in a muslin.

USE Hang the muslin over the taps as you draw the bath. Strain the infusion and add this to the bath. While bathing, you can use the muslin herb sack as a washcloth.

Benefits
Clover tea can calm the mind and promote sleep, and the tea can be applied as a very gentle soother to any part of the skin.

Parts to use
Flowers and leaves

How to find, grow, harvest
Find clover in open meadows, often the ones with the happiest cattle. The phrase 'living in clover', references how happy cattle are in its presence. It is more prevalent on sandy ground. Look for the distinctive egg-shaped heads of purple-red flowers and broad, oval leaflets. They're often given away by their sweet smell; in fact sailors returning home to the Scottish island of Papa Stour in the Shetlands are said to have been guided by the fragrance.

St John's Wort Hypericum perforatum

Known as the 'happy flower' or 'sunshine flower' because it contains hypericin which is an antidepressant. This has a fluorescent red pigment that can ooze like blood from the crushed flowers, leading to an association with wounds. It was used by the Crusaders to heal wounds. St John's Day is the 24th June, and on that day the flower was traditionally placed on religious pictures to keep off Midsummer evils. Its Greek name, hypericum, means 'over an apparition', possibly referring to its attributed power to dispel evil spirits. If gathered with dew on it, it is believed to help you find a husband or conceive.

ST JOHN'S WORT OIL

A handful of St John's Wort flowers
½ cup (118ml) sunflower oil

MAKE Put the flowers into a jar and gently bruise them using a wooden spoon. Pour over the sunflower oil and put the lid on the jar. Gently swirl the flowers in the oil and place on a windowsill. Swirl and turn the jar each day for two weeks, or until you see the oil turn a deep red. Then strain, bottle, label and date.

USE Rub the oil into the affected area as needed, repeating regularly until the condition heals.

STORE Keep sealed in cool, dark place. Will keep for 12 months.

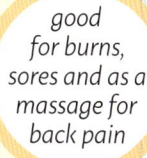
good for burns, sores and as a massage for back pain

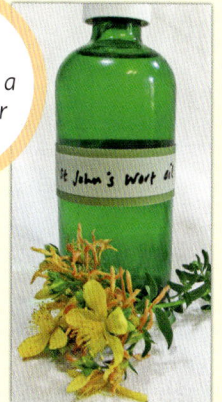

Benefits
Helps with burns, bruises and injuries, sores, cramps and sprains. Good for creams and lotions and helps keep skin soft and supple. Rub over hands to reduce age spots and keep skin smooth.

Parts to use
The whole plant – there is oil in the leaves and in the star-like, bright yellow flowers.

How to find, grow, harvest
Find St John's Wort in woods and hedgerows, along country lanes, dry banks and wasteland. Nicholas Culpeper considered it 'a great ornament to our meadows'. About 30-60cm high, its square, branching stems are reddish in colour and its small, thin leaves have tiny perforations. These are the oil glands, which you can see these the leaf up to the light. Pick it in full flower, being careful not to let the oil seep out and stain your fingers.

Special care
Can have photosensitivity issues so best used in nighttime products.

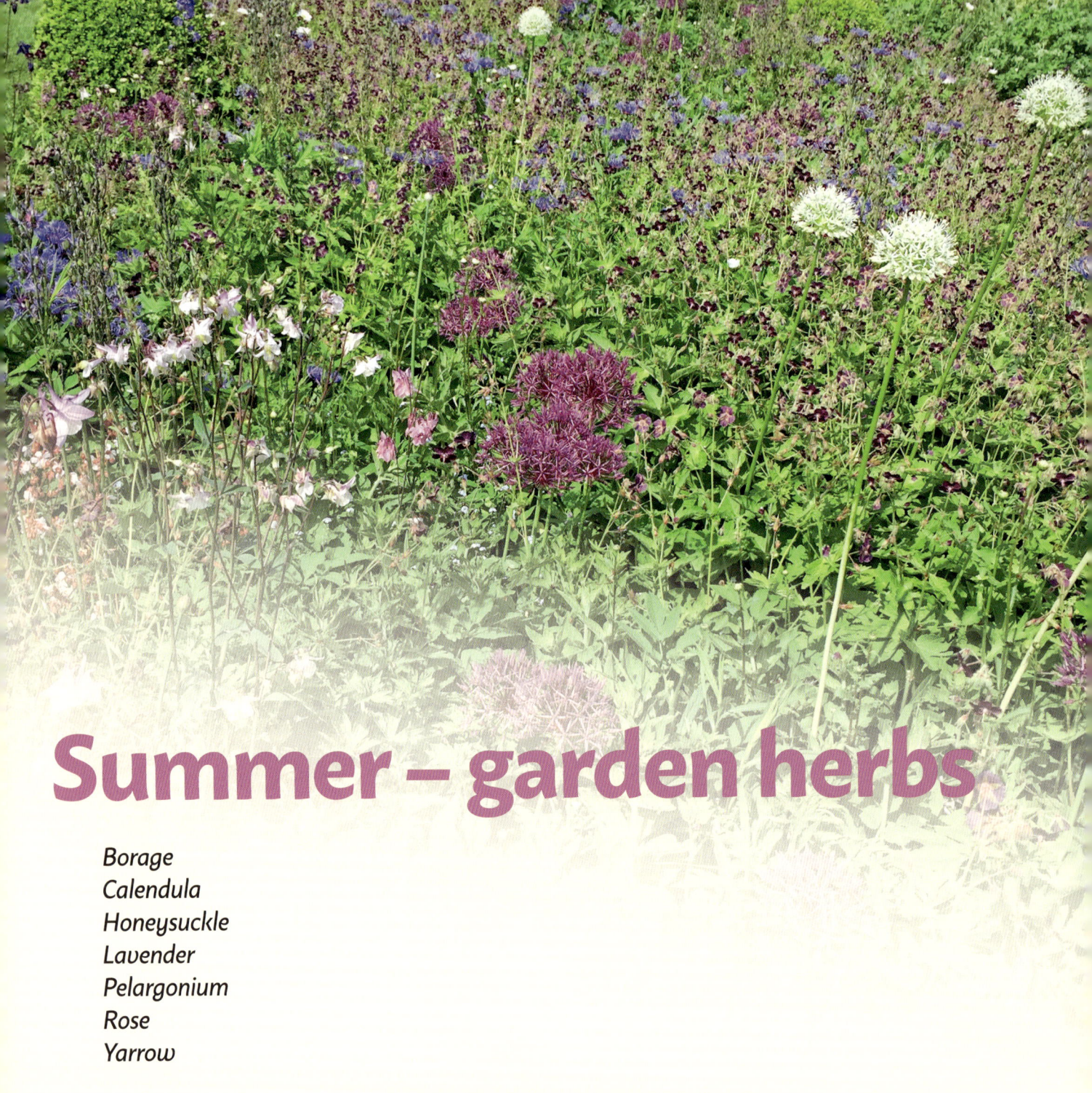

Summer – garden herbs

Borage
Calendula
Honeysuckle
Lavender
Pelargonium
Rose
Yarrow

Borage Borago officinalis

Pliny the Elder called borage Euphrosimum because of its euphoric effect. It has a reputation for lifting the spirits, enhanced by John Gerard's description of it (in his 1597 herbal, Generall Historie of Plantes):

> "Those of our time do use the floures in sallads to exhilarate and make the minde glad. There be also many things made of them, used for the comfort of the heart, to drive away sorrow, and increase the joy of the minde. The leaves and floures of Borrage put into wine make men and women glad and merry, driving away all sadnesse, dulnesse and melancholy, as Dioscorides and Pliny affirme. Syrrup made of the floures of Borrage comforteth the heart, purgeth melancholy and quieteth the phrenticke or lunaticke person."

The cheerful blue flowers, scattered over salads, floated in drinks or frozen into ice cubes or ice bowls, certainly raise a smile. They were floated in the stirrup cups given to Crusaders to offer them courage. The Celtic name *borrach* meant 'courage' and the Welsh name *Llanwenlys* means 'herb of gladness'. Research suggests borage works on the adrenal gland, where courage begins.

Benefits

Borage is good for dry skin, and soothes damaged or irritated tissues. It is considered a mild sedative with antidepressant effects. The seeds are a rich source of gamma-linoleic acid and their oil can help regulate hormonal functions.

Parts to use

Leaf, seeds, flowers

How to find, grow, harvest

Borage's bright blue, pinkish or occasionally white star-shaped flowers hang over a cluster of black anthers, sometimes described as their 'beauty spot'. Gather the leaves in spring and summer as the plant starts to flower. The stems, leaves and flower buds are covered in silvery hairs that, while very pretty in sunlight, can make harvesting a little rough, so wear gloves. Use them fresh or dry them. These will deteriorate quickly so process them with haste and replenish dried herbs each year. Extract their benefit through infusions and macerations. Borage has a long, fleshy taproot so it doesn't transplant well. Instead let it grow where it pleases, or gather seed and sow where you please. It will disappear completely over winter (with new plants emerging in spring) but you can keep supplies going by sowing a few seeds for a pot on a windowsill or greenhouse.

Special care

All parts of the herb, except the seed oil, are subject to legal restrictions in some countries.

The plant (but not the oil) contains small amounts of pyrrolizidine alkaloids that may cause liver damage. It has the potential to be a skin irritant and possible allergen, so do a patch test.

SPOT TREATMENT LOTION

1 handful dandelion leaves
1 handful watercress
1 handful borage leaf

MAKE Blitz all the herbs together in a blender and then pass through a sieve.

USE Clean your face and then smooth the extracted juice over the affected areas. Allow to dry completely before washing the face again.

STORE Always prepare a fresh juice mixture for each application.

Calendula *Calendula officinalis*

Calendula is also known as marigold, but I prefer to use its lilting Latin name to distinguish it from the African marigold (*Tagetes*), a much more blousy, pungent plant that should not be used in skincare. Calendula's gentle presence is, as its name suggests, almost year round. The Latin *calendulae* means 'first day of the month', and once established, they always seem to be in flower then (and every day). Its habit of opening and closing its petals with the sun is so reliable, Victorian gardeners would jest that they could set their clocks by it. In *The Winter's Tale*, Shakespeare described the calendula's habit of closing up when there is no sunshine 'Te Marigold that goes to bed wi'the sun, and with him rises weeping'. This mourning of the sun is why calendula is associated with grief.

Benefits
Calendula is very versatile and can be blended into oils, creams, lotions, face packs or steams and massage oils. It's great for dry or sensitive skin, is often used after sunburn and is especially good for cracked skin and chapped lips. Antiseptic, soothing, anti-inflammatory, cleansing, healing, softening and conditioning, calendula is also effective at reducing scars. It's been used for dyeing and medicinal purposes since Ancient Greek times.

Parts to use
Leaves and flowers. The petals are particularly lovely to harvest and use. Incorporate these directly into recipes; you can macerate to make calendula oil or create an infusion.

How to find, grow, harvest
Grow a patch of calendula in your garden or a window box and harvest regularly as the flowers appear. Lay the petals out on a fine drying rack or a piece of kitchen paper and allow them to dry for a couple of days, gently turning them occasionally. The plants will keep flowering right through to the first frosts. Flowers left on will form seed heads. You can gather these and scatter elsewhere, or else leave them to fall and reseed naturally.

How to use
- Add an infusion of the petals to the bath for their cleansing and astringent properties
- Use in creams and oils for dry skin
- Use in lotions for oily skin
- Use an infusion in a toning face wash.

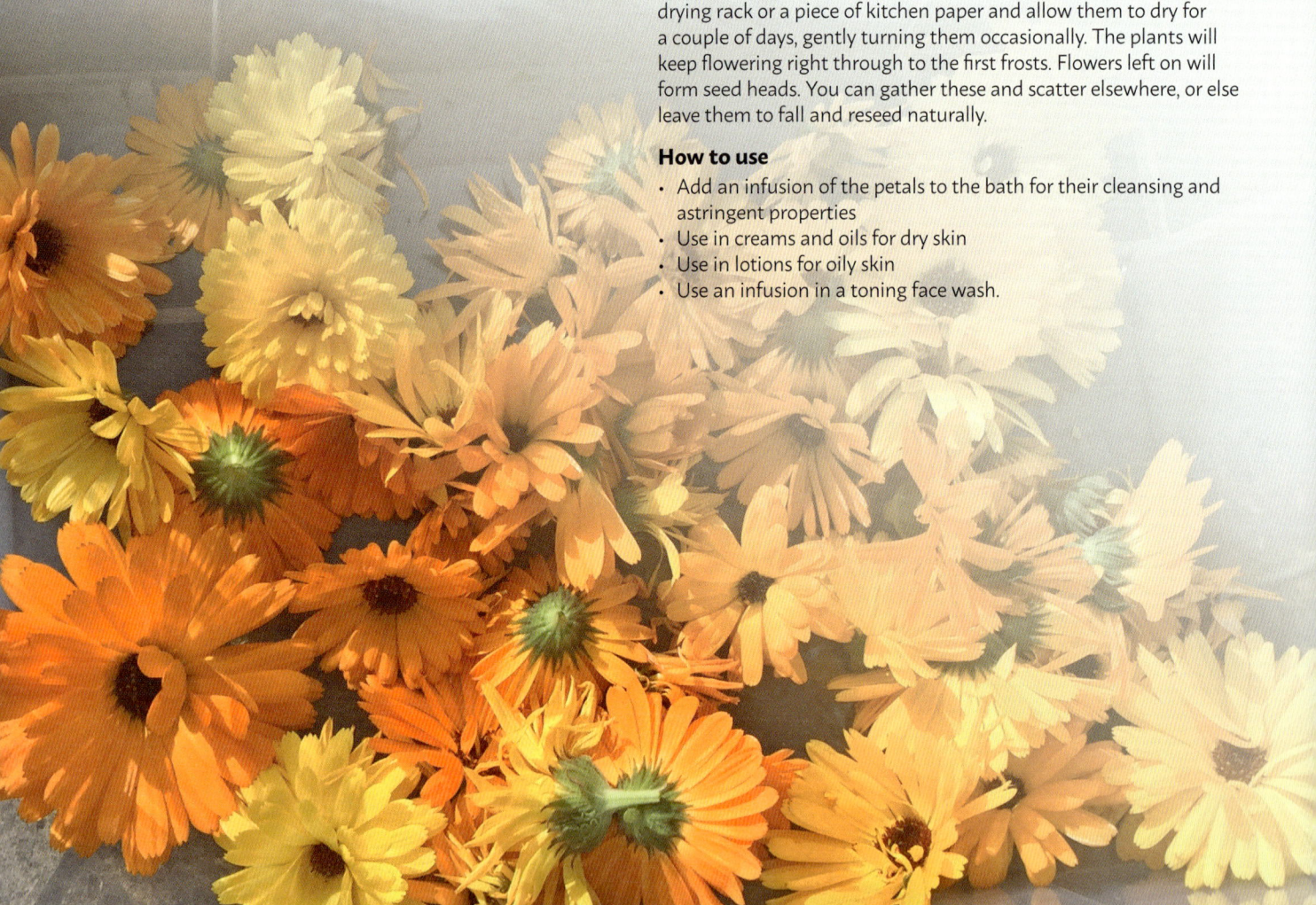

CALENDULA OIL

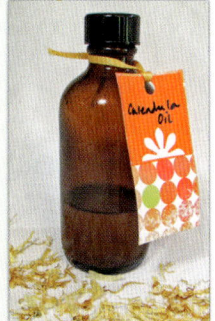

A jarful of calendula flowers
300ml sunflower oil

MAKE Fill your jar with calendula petals and pour over as much sunflower oil as needed to cover them. Pop on a windowsill – somewhere you're going to notice it daily – and give it a shake each day, being careful to always keep the petals submerged. After about three weeks, strain the petals and you have your infused calendula oil.

USE Either apply directly as needed to soothe skin, or use your oil to create a healing salve.

STORE Store sealed in a cool, dark place. It will keep for up to two years.

CALENDULA SALVE

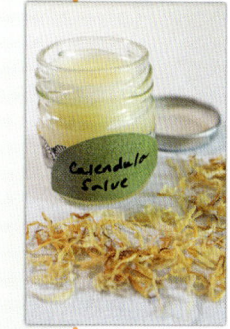

⅓ cup (78ml) calendula oil
15g beeswax
0.25g vitamin E (optional)

MAKE Put the calendula oil and beeswax into the top of a double boiler and heat until the beeswax melts, stirring to combine well. Replace the water in the bottom of the double boiler with cold water and keep stirring as the salve cools. Add the vitamin E (if using). Pour into a jar before it cools completely.

USE Apply to soothe skin and to gradually reduce the presence of scars.

STORE Store sealed in a cool, dark place. It will keep for up to two years.

GENTLE EYE MAKEUP REMOVER OIL

1g dried calendula flowers
1g dried eyebright
2 tbsp (30ml) sunflower oil
2 tsp (10ml) thistle oil

MAKE Macerate the herbs in the sunflower oil using the sun method (see Chapter 14). When ready, strain the macerated oil and combine with the thistle oil. Pour into a bottle.

USE Put 3-4 drops onto a wetted cotton wool pad and sweep across the eye. Use a clean pad for each application.

STORE Will keep for 12 months in a dark bottle.

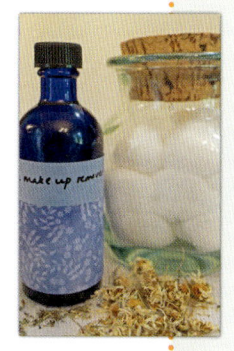

COMPRESS FOR DRY OR TIRED EYES

1g calendula flowers
1g lavender flowers
1g marshmallow leaves
1g walnut leaves

MAKE Put the herbs into a bowl and pour over ½ cup (118ml) of boiling water. Leave to infuse for 10 minutes.

USE Soak cotton wool pads in the infusion and apply to eyes. Lie back and relax for 10 minutes.

STORE Prepare fresh for each application.

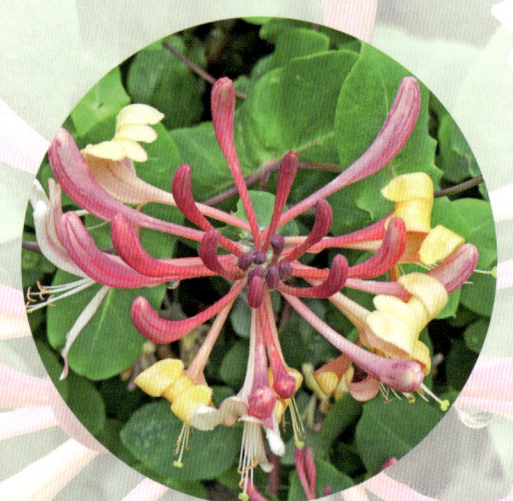

Honeysuckle *Lonicera caprifolium*

Also known as woodbine. The Latin *caprifolium* means 'goat's leaf', as honeysuckle was believed to be a favourite food of goats. It certainly romps like a goat over the hedgerows. Its evocative scent and wildly rambling flowers are enchanting. Traditionally, honeysuckle is a sign of true devotion. In Bach flower remedies, honeysuckle helps integrate past experiences by recognising that the past is the foundation for the present, giving us strength to face the challenges of the new.

Benefits
Honeysuckle is useful for skin inflammations, infectious rashes, sores and sunburn, as well as treating skin blemishes and restoring complexion. In homeopathy, honeysuckle tea is particularly used to treat asthma. Nicholas Culpeper tells us honeysuckles are 'cleansing, consuming and digesting, and therefore fit for inflammations'.

Parts to use
Flowers (much more effective than the leaves)

How to find, grow, harvest
Honeysuckle has strong sweet-smelling flowers. You can often catch its scent on the air before you identify the plant, which may be a few metres away. Oval leaves grow on short stalks, but the plant is characterised by its long winding stems that wrap around the other hedgerow plants. Harvest flowers when they are fully open. They can be used straight away or carefully dried and stored.

HONEYSUCKLE BATH

a fragrant way to keep skin soft

3 tbsp honeysuckle flowers

MAKE Put the flowers in a muslin bag. Alternatively, make a strong infusion from the flowers.

USE Hang the muslin bag from the tap to allow the bath water to run through. Or add the infusion to the bath water.

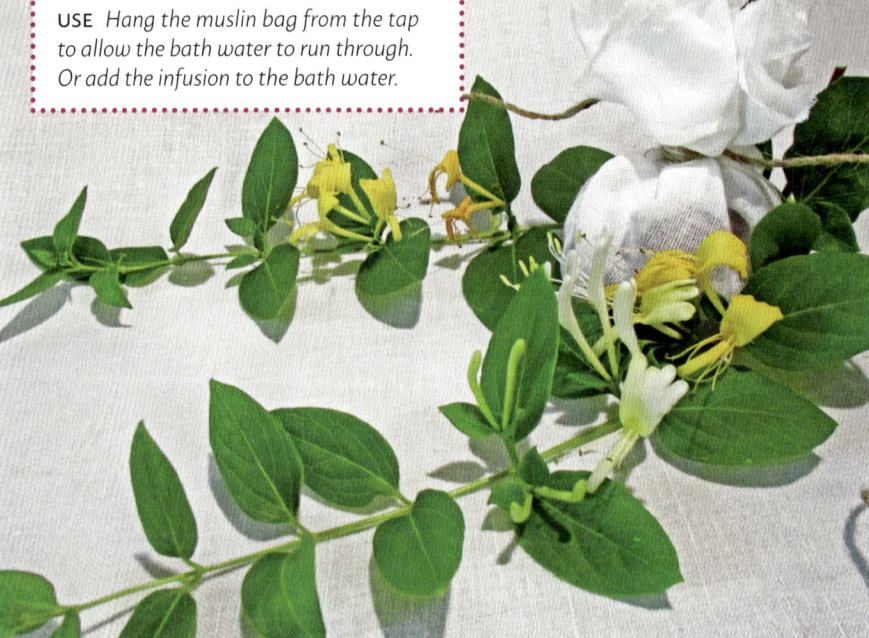

Lavender *Lavandula augustifolia / Lavandula hybrida / Lavandula intermedia*

Lavender has been used so widely, and as such a staple for so long that it's easy to become dismissive about it. If you've ever been a bit sniffy about lavender, I'd urge you to give it another go in a more natural, fresh form. English lavender farms are experiencing a resurgence and creating a new visitor experience, from the highly efficient agribusinesses to the charming pick-your-owns. Following a peak production in Victorian times, most lavender-growing land, being close to London, was built upon. There was only one commercial lavender grower in the UK in the 1980s, but that's changing. The cooler British climate creates sweeter flowers with a higher ketone proportion (which contributes to lavender's calming benefits) so UK growers even export to France. The name derives from Latin *lavare* 'to wash' and since Greek and Roman times it has been added to bath water for its cleansing properties.

Benefits
A widely used cosmetic plant due to its wonderful aromatics and highly volatile, healing oils. Good for acne (because it is antiseptic) and great for oily skin and hair. Lavender is both refreshingly reviving and soothingly sedative. It can be added to a warm bath, to perfumes, herbal oils, creams, lotions, toners, powders, deodorants and hair products. It helps lift moods, soothe burns and speed cell replacement.

Parts to use
The fresh or dried flowers can be used in macerations and infusions. Dried flowers can be used in sleep pillows, potpourri and deodorants, facial scrubs and soaps.

How to find, grow, harvest
Gather the flowering heads as they open (generally in July) and hang to dry before stripping the flower buds from their stems.

Special care
In large doses lavender is a narcotic poison.

How to use
- Add an infusion to the bath for relaxation
- Put flowers into facial steams for cleansing
- Use flower water in a lotion for cleansing
- Use an infusion to rinse greasy hair
- Add flowers to hand creams and lotions
- Use the flower water with witch hazel as a toner

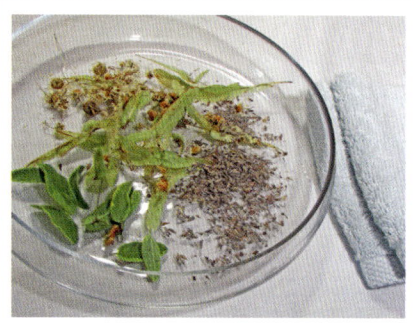

TONING FACIAL STEAM

1 tbsp lavender flowers
1 tbsp limeflowers
1 tbsp chamomile flowers
1 tsp sage leaves

MAKE Put the herbs into a bowl and pour over 2 pints (1 litre) of boiling water.

USE Hold your face over the steam, covering your head with a towel and steam for 10 minutes. Wipe your face thoroughly with cotton wool pads and splash with cold water then apply moisturiser.

LAVENDER SUGAR SCRUB

4 tbsp (60g) sugar
2 tbsp (30ml) rapeseed oil
2g lavender flowers

MAKE Mix the sugar and oil in a bowl then stir in the lavender flowers. Transfer to a small jar.

USE Rub in small circular motions all over your body and rinse off in the shower.

STORE Keeps for six months.

Pelargonium *Pelargonium graveolens*

Pelargonium is a cultivated species of geranium. The geraniums we find growing wild in temperate climates are cranesbill geraniums. They have been associated with storks or cranes since Greek times when the seed head was compared to the bird's beak. They are beautiful and plentiful, with many colours and varieties, but often have an unattractive scent. The cultivated pelargoniums are coveted for skincare use, and have wonderfully scented leaves (including rose, lemon, balsam and peppermint). The seeds were brought back from the Cape of Good Hope (South Africa) by renowned gardener John Tradescant in the 1630s, and have been valued in gardens and greenhouses ever since.

Benefits
Pelargonium balances sebum of oily and dry or inflamed skin and helps clean and improve circulation of pale, sluggish complexions. It is also used for skin eruptions and wounds.

Parts to use
The leaves can be used in cleansers and in treating damaged skin or bruising. They contain geraniol, the oil that is extracted as geranium essential oil, a valuable ingredient in many perfumes and creams.

How to find, grow, harvest
For skincare look for the scented leaved varieties of pelargonium which will impart their special fragrance into your products – rose, orange, lemon, pine or spicier, apply or minty varieties. These are often better grown as pot plants than in garden beds. They can be sensitive to frost so best given shelter in winter.

How to use
Add scented pelargonium leaves to bathwater.

GERANIUM CLEANSING BALM

- 12 fresh-scented pelargonium leaves
- 75ml thistle oil
- 2 tsp (10g) beeswax
- 10 drops geranium essential oil

MAKE Place the leaves in a sterilised heatproof jar. Heat the oil and beeswax in the top of a double boiler, when melted, stir well to combine and then pour over the leaves, ensuring all is fully covered. Seal the jar and leave to infuse for 3 weeks. Scoop everything out into the top of the double boiler and reheat. Strain to remove the leaves then add the essential oil and stir well before transferring to a wide-necked jar.

USE Massage thoroughly into your face, then soak a washcloth in hot water and place across your face. Leave for one minute before using to wipe completely clean.

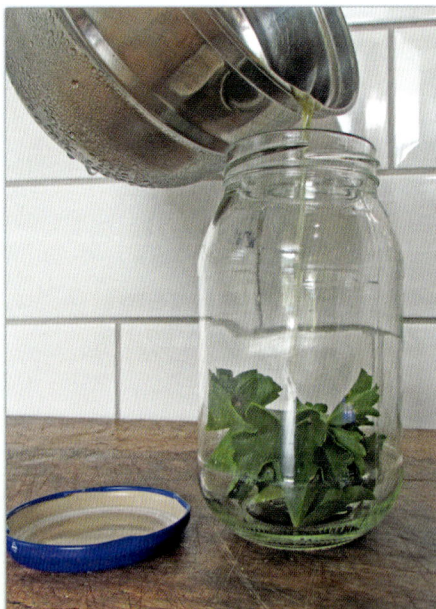

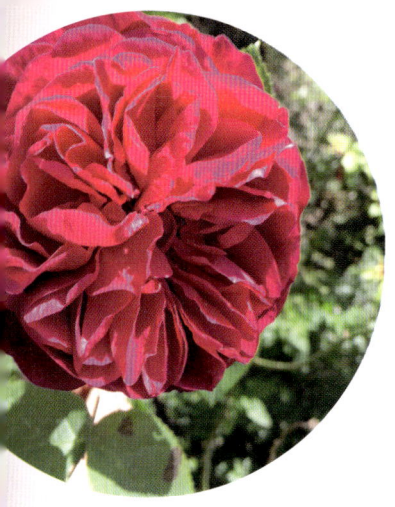

Rose *Rosa gallica var. officinalis*

Rosa gallica (the classic red rose of Lancaster) is known as the apothecary's rose with its wonderful scent. Rose is included in 96% of women's perfumes and 42% of men's fragrances. So fundamental to skincare, cold cream was originally known as 'ointment of rosewater' as both rosewater and rose oil were ingredients. Wilder roses such as sweet briar and eglantine (*Rosa rubiginosa* and *Rosa eglanteria*) are used in making rosehip oil. Roses originated in the Middle East (*Rosa damascena*) and were introduced to Europe by the Crusaders returning from the Holy Land. Most of the world's rosewater still comes mainly from Turkey and Iran.

Benefits

Roses are aromatic, astringent and able to control bacterial infections, promote healing and improve morale. John Gerard (English herbalist in the 16th Century) recommended rosewater as 'good for strengthening of the hart and refreshing of the spirits and likewise in all things that require gentle cooling'. When the temperature rises, dab some rosewater on your forehead and rest for 10 minutes in a darkened room. The combination of rosewater and peace will help you emerge feeling fragrant, refreshed and soothed.

Parts to use

Use the petals either fresh or dried.

How to find, grow, harvest

Look for traditional, highly fragranced roses, not modern hybrids. Damask roses, especially the apothecary's rose, are ideal.

ROSE INFUSED SENSUAL BATH

A handful of rose petals
A handful of lavender flowers
A handful of nasturtium leaves
A handful of rosemary
A handful of honeysuckle flowers
A handful of carnation flowers
A handful of jasmine flowers
A handful of bay leaves
1 tsp (5ml) apple cider vinegar
1 tsp (5g) salt
4 drops rose geranium essential oil (optional)

MAKE *Gather together as many of the flowers and leaves as you have available to you. Put them in a saucepan with 3½ pints (2 litres) of water. Bring to the boil and then simmer for 15 minutes. Strain and add the vinegar, salt and essential oil. Check it is at a suitable temperature, and then add to your bath.*

USE *The infusion turns the bathwater rosy pink and smells divine.*

great for dry and sensitive skin

Yarrow *Achillea millefolium*

One of the most common wild flowers, yarrow has many names, including herba militaris, the military herb, knights' milfoil, bloodwort, staunchweed, soldier's woundwort and carpenter's weed and nosebleed, all drawing on its ability to staunch blood. The botanical name derives from the Greek hero Achilles who is said to have used it to heal his soldiers' wounds during the Trojan war. While the common name derives from the Greek *hiera*, or holy herb, referencing its medicinal properties. Yarrow is a curious plant in that it will help other plants growing nearby to resist disease, and when added to skincare, it will increase the potency of other herbal ingredients. There is much folklore associated with yarrow; in Gloucestershire a sprig will be included in the bridal bouquet under the name 'seven-year's-love'.

Benefits
Yarrow is astringent, so great for greasy, oily or problem skin. Include it in facial steams, deep cleansing face packs and treatments for itchy scalps or oily hair. Use in creams and lotions for cleansing and use an infusion of yarrow with witch hazel as a toner. Yarrow can help darken grey hair and restore a youthful appearance. It will also help with wounds, nosebleeds and inflamed eyes. Kept in the bathroom, it can be a quick remedy to apply to shaving cuts.

Parts to use
Flowers, stems and leaves.

How to find, grow, harvest
Yarrow is a fragile-looking delicate plant, with flat clusters of cream and yellow flowers held up on strong, slender stems. It flowers from early summer through to late autumn, and is best collected in August when it is in full flower. A common roadside plant, it has tough, creeping roots that allow it to spread steadily in most soils. But it doesn't like shady areas and is at its best in open meadows. You might find its feathery, aromatic foliage in lawns, but it's more identifiable when allowed to grow to its full height of about 60cm. Once established in your garden it should thrive and may even need to be kept in check.

Special care
Prolonged use of yarrow may cause allergic rashes and make the skin more sensitive to sunlight.

YARROW LOTION

30g yarrow leaves

MAKE Put the yarrow leaves in a bowl and pour over 2/3 cup (158ml) of boiling water. Leave to get quite cold, then strain and bottle.

USE Wipe on and off as a cleanser.

FACIAL STEAM FOR BLACKHEADS AND OILY SKIN

2 handfuls of yarrow

MAKE Put the yarrow into a bowl and cover with 2 pints (1.1 litre) of boiling water. Cover the head and bowl with a towel and allow to steam for 10 minutes to cleanse and soften the skin. Wipe your face and splash with cold water to close the pores. Can also add chamomile, nettle, limeflower or salad burnet.

How could such sweet and wholesome hours, be reckoned but with herbs and flowers

ANDREW MARVELL, ENGLISH POET, 1621-1678

CHAPTER 16

little rituals – reflecting on your skincare

Skincare is something you do every day, whether you think about it or not, it is part of who you are. So your few moments of self-care each day are the perfect time to think about you, i.e. what you want to achieve that day and how you present yourself to the world. Use it as focused time to know what you're giving out. The beauty you see reflected back in the mirror is a direct manifestation of how you feel.

Mirror, mirror on the wall …

Much of your skincare practice takes place in front of the mirror. They say the mirror never lies, it's your honest friend. Your mirror gives you reflection: a chance to see again, to see more clearly, to think.

By making your daily routine a point of reflection in your day you can avoid the habitual. Thoughtful practice makes the experience refreshing and new each day. This does require dedicating a few moments, rather than multitasking or auto-piloting. Squeezing our necessary grooming into life – brushing our teeth while we scan through messages on our phone, even applying makeup in traffic light breaks while driving – makes it feel like a chore, another thing on the 'to do' list.

There are some beautiful words from the German storyteller Hermann Hesse. This master of allegorical truth-telling conjures up all manner of colourful, grotesque, wonderful, inspiring landscapes and characters within his fairytales, but among all this wild fantasy he knows that:

> 'within you there is a stillness and a sanctity
> to which you can retreat at anytime and be yourself'.

Find that simple, uncomplicated part of you for a few moments at the beginning and end of each day – while preparing yourself to face the world, and when preparing yourself for sleep – and it will resonate through you in the following hours. A simple, uncomplicated skincare practice, rooted in nature, reinforces this connection to your calm inner self.

Your daily 'me' time

Caring for our skin, at the very least keeping it clean, is an essential part of our daily lives. Each one of us spends anything from a few moments to a few hours each day in this activity. It is typically a very personal experience, and one of the very few things in life that is, of necessity, all about you.

For this reason, your approach to looking after your skin and your cleanliness is a vital space in life to tune into who you are. How you treat those moments each day can, over time, change how you think about yourself and your connection with the world. The drip, drip, drip of conscious or unconscious behaviour shapes who you are.

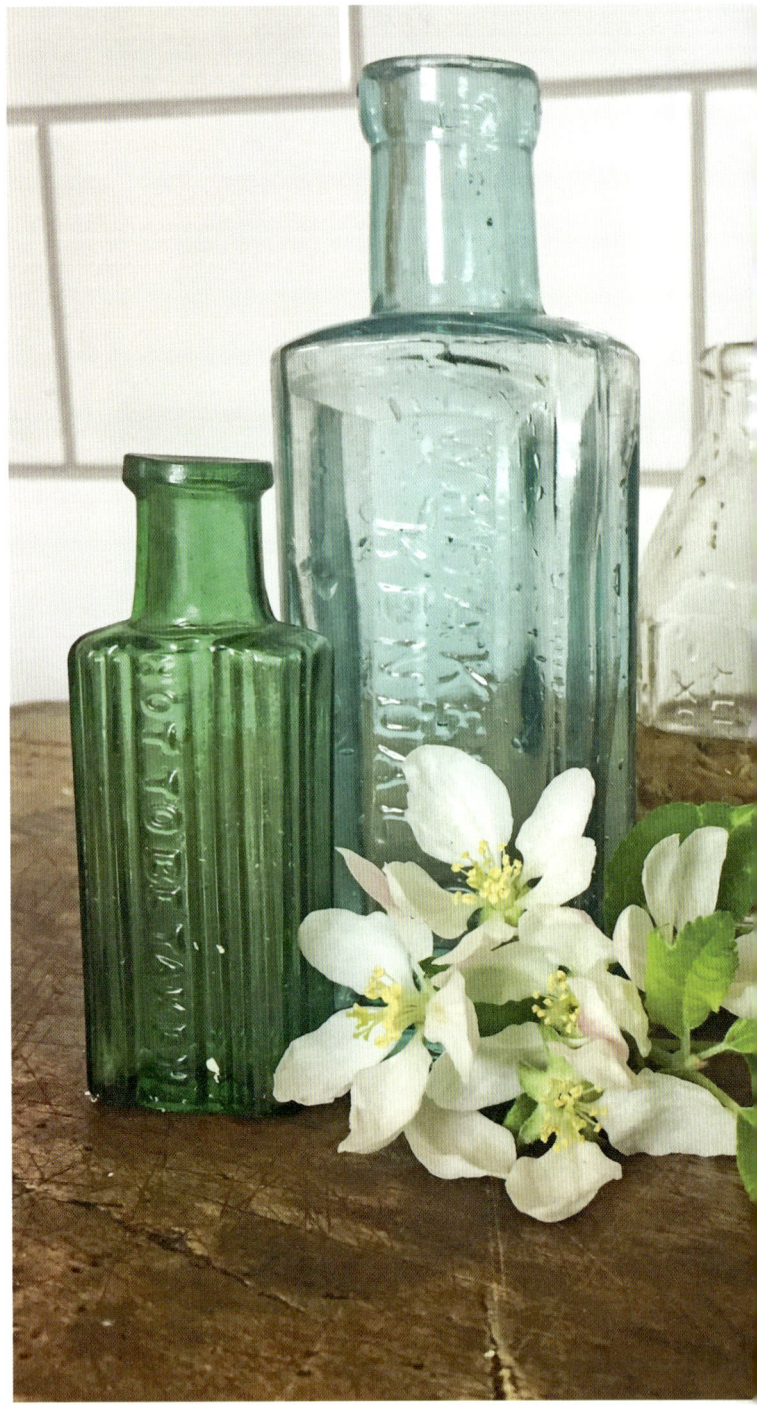

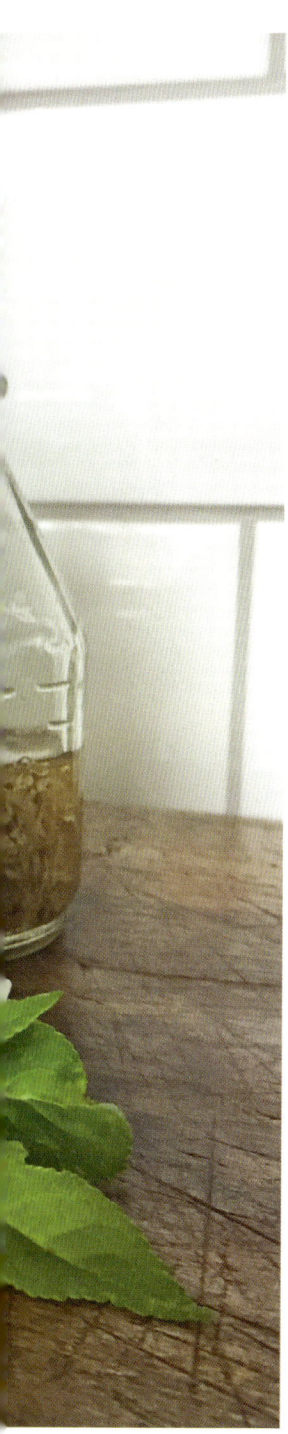

You are what you use

The products we turn to on a daily basis form us. To some extent, this is literally true as we absorb their contents, but it is also true at a psychological level. Each time we buy a product off the shelf, admire the shiny packaging and believe the advertising, we are opting into a particular way of life and of being. Our skincare choices are typically so ingrained, and so commonplace, that we rarely notice them. But they affect us all the same, unknowingly.

Making more conscious decisions about your skincare – what you want to do, what products to use, how or where to source them – can provide a subtle daily reminder (even if unconscious) of the person you want to be and the beliefs you have. It's precisely because our skincare is a regular, daily occurrence and because it is a private occasion about us alone, that it is an ideal space in which to reinforce who we are to ourselves. It can be the pacemaker in our lives.

When you're confident of the ingredients in your skincare; when you know what they are doing for you and where they have come from, it is grounding. Knowing the connection between your skincare and the plants around you connects you to that world; it's a little bit of nature in your life every day. Consciously choosing skincare products that connect you to nature and being aware of that each time you use them can, bit by bit, impact your whole psyche. You can feel good about yourself, you can feel connected to the natural world and the seasons, and you can feel positive about your role in your environment.

Finding the ritual in your routine

Some people are creatures of habit, finding comfort and stability in the cyclical nature of tasks and experiences that come round in a regular pattern. Others are energised by a linear focus, wanting to get things ticked off the list and move on. But cycles are there in all our lives, it's up to us whether we choose to be uplifted or weighed down by them.

Cycles, or routines, make life simpler and easier – things happen 'as matter of routine'; we don't need to think about them. We might rush through them, getting the chores done, multitasking in our attempts to be efficient. With any routine, there are ways to personalise, that it, to ensure that the reinforcing that is naturally happening is shaping you in the way you choose.

For example, you probably use a password most days, likely multiple times a day, to access a computer or other device. Why not make that password something that you know you want to focus on, a characteristic that you'd like others to notice in you, a reminder-to-self of who you want to be? It requires no extra effort on your behalf but gives a regular reinforcement and reminder just for you.

We can make these adjustments in all our routines. They take on a different nature when we personalise them, acknowledge the comfort they bring and honour their role of simple achievement and the satisfaction of doing things our way. Being aware of this impact and consciously choosing to use our routines as a way to connect us to the things that are special to us in life, can turn a regular routine into a life-affirming, soul-strengthening ritual.

You can bring the processes involved in gathering, storing and preparing the herbs you use in your skincare into your cycle of activity, connecting you to your environment, the seasons and nature. Making these vital, natural sources of energy part of your everyday existence.

If you're looking to build new routines, start with the sequence of things you do each morning. The time you get up in the morning may be one of the few times you can choose and control yourself. It's much easier to focus creative energy and willpower when you have the day ahead of you, and you can carry the beneficial results through the day with you. Night time routines are equally beneficial, but may be harder to establish as we come to them from the irregularities of whatever occurs each day.

A cycle of regular activity can be a source of stability and strength. When life is going well it's all too easy to forget these cycles, maybe even dismis them. But it's when we hit difficult times that the cycles and routines can save us. They can remind us of who we are, as an individual or as a community or society, and give us a basis on which to build. Maintaining these routines is like an insurance policy against bad times.

The natural cycles of days, months, seasons and years can be a gift to us of strength and stability. The more we align our rhythms and routines to these, the more powerful they can become in grounding and connecting us with life forces and the spiritual depth of nature.

Your regular skincare routine, aligned with nature (through using natural ingredients and responding to the seasons) can provide a constant source of stability and connection with nature in your daily life.

Balance

A good routine has balance, just as perfect skin has balance. Balance and harmony are the goals and underlying principles of much self-care wisdom and ancient practices. To achieve these, we need to know ourselves inside out, and be happy we know what's right for us; not jumping on every fad, not leaping to change, but steadily learning and growing.

Balance comes through vitality: when we are energised and yet relaxed, fired with enthusiasm while inwardly at peace; when we participate in living everywhere (not just in the living room).

It shows in radiant, glowing skin and age-defying beauty.

Look up, laugh loud, talk big, keep the colour in your cheek and the fire in your eye, adorn your person, maintain your health, your beauty and your animal spirits

WILLIAM HAZLITT, ENGLISH CRITIC, 1778-1830

Ingredients Suppliers

HERBS

Baldwin Herbs	www.baldwins.co.uk
Neal's Yard Remedies	www.nealsyardremedies.co.uk
Woodland Herbs	www.woodlandherbs.co.uk

ESSENTIAL OILS AND PLANT SEED OILS AND SPECIALIST SKINCARE INGREDIENTS

Aromantic	www.aromantic.co.uk
AquaOleum	www.aqua-oleum.co.uk
Naissance	www.discoveringbetter.com/uk
Naturally Thinking	www.naturallythinking.co.uk

POTS, JARS, BOTTLES AND DISPENSERS

Naturally Thinking	www.naturallythinking.co.uk
Ampulla	www.ampulla.co.uk

KITS

Field Fresh Skincare	www.fieldfreshskincare.co.uk
Aromantic	www.aromantic.co.uk

COURSES

Field Fresh Skincare	www.fieldfreshskincare.co.uk
Karen Gilbert	www.karengilbert.co.uk
Aromantic	www.aromantic.co.uk

References

Soap Calculator, www.soapcalc.net
Packaging ideas, http://tiny.cc/FieldFreshSkincare
Skin assessment tools, www.fieldfreshskincare.co.uk
A Country Herbal, Lesley Gordon, 1980
A Modern Herbal, Mrs M Grieve 1931 (revised 1973, republished 1992)
Beauty Oils and Butters, Elaine Stavert, 2010
Complete Herbal, Nicholas Culpeper, 1653 (Wordsworth Edition, 1995)
Cosmetics from the Earth, Roy Genders, 1985
Discovering Hedgerows, David Streeter and Rosamond Richardson, 1982
Hatfield's Herbal, Gabrielle Hatfield, 2007
Herbal Cosmetics, Camilla Hepper, 1987
Herbs, the Herb Society Journal
Herbs for Clearing the Skin, Sarah Beckett, 1973
Homemade Apothecary, Vicky Chown and Kim Walker, 2017
Kitchen Pharmacy, Rose Elliot and Carlo de Paoli, 1991
Kitty Little's Book of Herbal Beauty, 1980
Natural Beauty, Aldo Facetti, 1991
Neals Yard, Natural Health and Body Care, 2008
New Herb Bible, Caroline Foley, Jill Nice and Marcus A. Webb 2002
New Vital Oils, Liz Earle, 2002
Perfect Skin, Amanda Cochrane, 2000
RHS Encyclopedia of Herbs and Their Uses, Deni Bown 1995
Secrets of Natural Beauty, Virginia Castleton Thomas, 1973
Skin Secrets, Liz Earle, 2009
The Aromantic Guide to Unlocking the Powerful Health and Rejuvenation Benefits of Vegetable Oils, Kolbjørn Borseth, 2008
The Complete Book of Herbs, Lesley Bremness, 1988
The Complete New Herbal, Ed, Richard Mabey, 1988
The Encyclopedia of Essential Oils, Julia Lawless, 1992
The Fragrant Pharmacy, Valerie Ann Worwood, 1990
The Herb Bible, Peter McHoy and Pamela Westland, 2005
The Herbal Health and Beauty Book, Hilary Boddie, 1994
The Illustrated Herbal, Philippa Back, 1987
The Ultimate Natural Beauty Book, Josephine Fairley, 2008
Traditional Herbal Remedies, Jenny Plucknett, 1996

Skincare Recipes: Summary and Index

CLEANSERS

Category	Recipe	Page	Area of body	Skin type	Benefit	Product type
CLEANSING OILS	Make every day special face oil	63	Face	All	Circulation, nourishing and reduce pores and fine lines	Cleanser
	Skin balancing face oil	63	Face	Oily	Circulation, nourishing and reduce pores, balance and tone	Cleanser
	Pore reducing face oil	63	Face	All	Balance, tone, good for eczema, psoriasis and acne	Cleanser
	Face oil for troubled skin	63	Face	Troubled	Softening, toning, firming, encourages cell regeneration, good for eczema, psoriasis and acne	Cleanser
	Forever young face oil	63	Face	Mature	Moisturising, soothing, regenerating, revitalising, defends against wrinkles and the elements	Cleanser
	Wrinkle-fighting face oil	63	Face	All	Hydrating and moisturising so good for wrinkles and skin elasticity, helps with regeneration	Cleanser
	Pre Makeup face oil	63	Face	All	Hydrating and moisturising, gives luminescence and glow	Cleanser
CLEANSING MILKS & LOTIONS	Basic cleansing milk	65	Face	All	Cleansing, maintains pH	Cleanser
	Almond milk cleanser for tired skin	66	Face	Tired	Cleansing	Cleanser
	Buttermilk cleanser for oily skin	66	Face	Oily	Cleansing	Cleanser
	Rice milk cleanser for dry skin	66	Face	Dry	Emollient and nourishing	Cleanser
	Oat milk cleanser for sensitive skin	66	Face	Sensitive	Softening	Cleanser
	Cows milk cleanser for all skins	66	Face	All	Nourishes	Cleanser
	Cucumber skin brightening milk	97	Face	Mature	Exfoliating and skin brightening	Mask
	Lady's mantle and buttermilk lotion	160	Face	Spotty	Cleansing	Lotion
	Yarrow lotion	182	Face	Oily	Cleansing	Lotion
CLEANSING CREAMS & BARS	Houseleek facial cleanser	67	Face	All	Cleansing	Cleanser
	Lavender cleansing cream – for feeding and replenishing dry skin	68	Face	Dry	Nourishing	Cleanser
	Geranium cleansing balm	180	Face	Oily, dry or inflamed	Cleansing	Cleansing balm
	Calendula cleansing cream - for sensitive skin	68	Face	Sensitive	Gentle	Cleanser
	Gentle foaming cleanser	70	Face	All	Nourishing and moisturising	Cleanser
	Skin-smoothing clay cleansing bar	74	Body	All	Cleansing	Cleanser
CLEANSING MASKS	Basic face mask	73	Face	All	Cleansing, refreshing	Cleanser
	Cleansing face mask for oily or acne-prone skin	73	Face	Oily	Softening	Cleanser
	Cleansing face mask for mature skin	73	Face	Mature	Soothing	Cleanser
	Cleansing face mask for all skins	73	Face	All	Cleansing	Cleanser
	Cleansing face mask for dry skin	73	Face	Dry	Cleansing	Cleanser
	Herbal Health Mask	75	Face	All	Refreshing	Cleanser
	Sweet Leaf Mask	75	Face	All	Reduces fine lines	Cleanser
	Seaweed Cleansing Mask	75	Face	All	Opens pores	Cleanser

	Recipe	Page	Area of body	Skin type	Benefit	Product type
CLEANSERS (contd)						
CLEANSING SCRUBS	Oats So Simple Cleanser	75	Face	Dry	Anti-inflammatory	Cleanser
	Three in One Cleanser	75	Face	Dry	Anti-inflammatory	Cleanser
	Cleansing water	76	Face	All	Cleansing	Cleanser
CLEANSING WATERS	Dandelion skin tonic	153	Face	Normal	Refreshing	Cleanser
	Raspberry leaf skin cleanser	163	Body	All	Cleansing	Cleanser
MAKEUP REMOVER	Thistle Clean Up Makeup Removal oil	63	Face	All	Restorative	Makeup remover
EYE MAKEUP REMOVER	Gentle eye makeup remover oil	177	Eyes	All	Cleansing	Eye makeup remover
	Herbal skin tonic	80	Body	All	Fresh and supple skin	Toner
	Chickweed lotion to clear and refine skin	150	Face	All	Cleansing and clarifying	Toner
TONERS	Horsetail skin tonic	154	Body	All	Toning	Toner
	Rosemary face rinse	165	Face	All	Refreshing	Toner
	Skin freshener	160	Face	Tired	Toning	Mask
SPRITZ	Refreshing body spritz	79	Body	All	Refreshing	Toner
	Universal flower refresher	80	Face	All	Softening	Toner
STEAM	Toning facial steam	179	Face		Toning	Toner
EXFOLIATORS						
	Salt body scrub	87	Body	All	Exfoliating	Scrub
	Quick exfoliator for hands, feet or lips	87	Hands	All	Smoothing	Scrub
BODY SCRUBS	Herbal body scrub	90	Body	All	Restorative	Scrub
	Sweet mud flower scrub	90	Body	All	Cellulite fighter	Scrub
	Lavender sugar scrub	179	Body	All	Exfoliating	Scrub
	Me Thyme face mask	88	Face	Oily	Softening	Mask
	Green clay mask	88	Face	Oily	Rejuvenating and soothing	Mask
	Honey salt mask	88	Face	Acne-prone	Pore cleansing	Mask
	Strawberry skin food	89	Face	Dry	Firming and clarifying	Mask
	Elderflower earth mask	89	Face	Dry	Soothing and nourishing	Mask
FACIAL MASKS	Almond, rose and marshmallow mask	89	Face	Dry	Gentle, emollient and rejuvenating	Mask
	Apple mask	95	Face	All	Exfoliating	Mask
	Honey clay mask	95	Face	All	Exfoliating	Mask
	Mint leaf face mask	96	Face	Oily	Exfoliating	Mask
	Honey nut face mask	96	Face	Acne-prone	Humectant, helps skin regeneration and protects	Mask
	Cherry ripe summer face mask	97	Face	Mature	Exfoliating	Mask
	Chamomile and honey face scrub	86	Face	All	Exfoliating	Scrub
FACIAL SCRUBS	Oatmeal, witch hazel and thistle face scrub	86	Face	All	Exfoliating	Scrub
	Rose milk scrub	97	Face	Mature	Softening	Scrub

	Recipe	Page	Area of body	Skin type	Benefit	Product type
MOISTURISERS						
BODY CREAMS	Lavender body protecting cream	105	Body	All	Occlusive	Moisturiser
	Flower filled body butter	114	Body	Mature	Moisturising	Body butter
	Bay, chamomile and marshmallow nourishing body cream	112	Body	Mature	Nourishing	Body cream
	Basic body butter	118	Body	All	Moisturising	Body cream
	Marshmallow and Chamomile Lotion	103	Body	All	Humectant	Moisturiser
	Herby post-shower toning and firming body lotion	111	Body	Mature	Moisturising	Moisturiser
BODY LOTIONS	Restorative lotion	106	Body	Damaged	Emollient	Moisturiser
	Blackberry and honeysuckle lotion	107	Body	Oily	Non-oily	Moisturiser
	Basic lotion bar	119	Body	All	Moisturising	Body lotion
BODY OILS	Toning body oil	114	Body	Mature	Toning and moisturising	Body oil
	Floral body spritz	105	Body	All	Hydrating	Moisturiser
BODY SPRAYS	Spray of roses and violets	103	Body	All	Hydrating	Spray
	Lemon, lavender and chamomile hydrating spray	112	Body	All	Hydrating, soothing, restorative and conditioning	Spray
EYE CREAM	Eye cream	110	Eyes	All	Moisturising	Eye cream
FACE CREAMS	Calendula and rose every day cream for face and neck	111	Face	Mature	Nourishing	Face cream
	Lavender and hops night cream	115	Face	Mature	Moisturising	Night cream
	Hedgerow brightening serum	106	Body	Dull skin	Brightening	Moisturiser
	Serum for sensitive skin	107	Body	Sensitive	Moisturising	Moisturiser
FACIAL SERUMS	Calming serum	115	Face	Sensitive	Moisturising	Face serum
	Rejuvenating serum	115	Face	Mature	Moisturising	Face serum
	Night time oils	109	Face	Oil	Moisturising	Night oil
MOISTURISING MASKS	Moisturising face mask	109	Face	All	Moisturising	Mask
HANDS						
HAND CREAM & LOTION	Hand spa 3: Elderflower and comfrey nourishing hand cream	113	Hands	Mature	Nourishing	Hand cream
	Marshmallow hand cream	172	Hands	All	Soothing	Hand cream
	Elderflower lotion for rough, chapped hands	168	Hands	Chapped	Soothing and softening	Hand lotion
HAND MASK	Hand spa 1: Intensive hand treatment	113	Hands	Mature	Softening	Mask
HAND SANITISER	Houseleek hand sanitiser	159	Hands	All	Cleansing	Hand sanitiser
DEODORANT	Herbal spray deodorant	157	Body	All	Deodorising	Deodorant
	Herbal cream deodorant	157	Body	All	Deodorising	Deodorant
	Hungary water	161	Body	All	Refreshing	Cologne

	Recipe	Page	Area of body	Skin type	Benefit	Product type
HAIR						
HAIR MASK	Rosemary hair care for dry hair	165	Hair	Dry	Stimulates scalp	Hair mask
	Cleavers hair tonic	151	Hair	All	Improve texture	Hair rinse
HAIR RINSE	Nettle hair tonic	155	Hair	All	Prevent hair loss	Hair rinse
	Rosemary hair care for greasy hair	165	Hair	Greasy	Astringent	Hair rinse
	Golden hair rinse	167	Hair	Fair	Lightening	Hair rinse
SHAMPOO	Horsetail shampoo	154	Hair	All	Cleansing	Shampoo
BATHTIME						
BATH OILS & SPLASHES	Floating oil bath	109	Body	All	Softening	Bath
	Dispersing oil bath	109	Body	All	Softening	Bath
	Blackberry bath splash	149	Body	All	Brightening	Bath
	Herbal bath bag	90	Body	All	Rejuvenate, stimulate and soothe	Cologne
	Nettle and dandelion bath	155	Body	All	Refreshing	Bath
INFUSIONS	Duchess and Dairymaid skin softening bath	173	Body	All	Soothing	Bath
	Honeysuckle bath	178	Body	All	Softening	Bath
	Rose infused sensual bath	181	Body	Dry	Soothing	Bath
SPONGES & RUBS	Milk sponge bath	95	Body	All	Exfoliating	Bath
	Herbal wine rub	96	Body	Oily	Exfoliating	Bath
TREATMENTS						
COMPRESS FOR EYES	Compress for dry or tired eyes	177	Eyes	Dry	Soothing	Compress
FACIAL STEAM	Facial steam for blackheads and oily skin	182	Face	Oily	Cleansing	Facial steam
FOOT BATH	Soothing foot bath	171	Feet	Aching	Soothing and restorative	Foot bath
MASKS	Green healing face pack	162	Face	All	Toning	Mask
	Carrot and marshmallow mask	172	Face	Dry and sensitive	Soothing	Mask
MOUTHWASH	Rosemary and mint mouthwash	165	Mouth		Refreshing	Mouthwash
NAIL TREATMENTS	Hand spa 2: Nail soak	113	Nails	All	Softening	Nail oil
	Horsetail nail bath	154	Nails		Strengthening	Nail soak
	Nail strengthening balm	108			Protective and strengthening	Nails cream
SALVES & OINTMENTS	Chickweed ointment	150		Irritated	Healing	Ointment
	St John's Wort Oil	173		Damaged	Healing	Ointment
	Comfrey ointment	152		Damaged	Healing	Ointment
	Oil of swallows	169		Damaged	Healing	Ointment
	Elderflower ointment	169		Damaged	Healing	Ointment
	Horse chestnut oil	170		Damaged, bruised or aching	Healing	Ointment
	Calendula salve	177		Damaged	Healing	Salve
SPOTS	Spot treatment lotion	175		Spotty	Spot treatment	Lotion
	Lady's mantle juice for acne	160	Face	Acne-prone	Spot treatment	
SUNBURN	Sunburn lotion	167		Wind or sunburnt	Soothing	Lotion

General Index

A
Abrasive 84, 89, 93, 154
Achillea millefolium 182
Aches 91, 150, 157, 164
Acid mantle 2, 12, 77, 92
Acne 49, 55, 61, 63, 66, 70, 72-73, 75, 80, 82, 86, 88, 92, 94, 96, 108, 135-137, 152, 160, 179, 188-189, 191
Adsorption 72
Aescin 170
Aesculus hippocastanum 170
Aftershave 9, 40, 45, 77
Age spots 173
Ageing 53, 61, 63, 110, 137-138
Alchemilla vulgaris 160
Alcohol 9, 53, 77, 124, 140, 142
Alkaloids 153-154, 175
All Heal (see St John's wort)
Allatonin 152
Allergens 6, 43
Almond milk 65-66, 188
Almonds 89, 92
Aloe 74, 158-159
Alpha Hydroxy Acids (AHAs) 91-95, 97
Alpha-linoleic acid 172
Althaea officinalis 172
Anglo Saxon 151, 159, 167
Anthemis nobilis (see chamomile)
Anti-inflammatory 53, 73, 75, 77, 96, 134, 167, 189
Antioxidant 16, 53-54, 61, 70, 94, 100, 131, 134, 164
Antibacterial 56, 70, 72, 77, 81, 92, 96, 124, 158
Anxiety 5
Apocrine glands 5, 14
Apothecary's Rose 181
Apple 92, 94-95, 167, 189
Apple Cider Vinegar (ACV) 77, 105, 165, 171, 181
Apricot kernel 84-85
Aqua Sambuci 79, 169,
Arrowroot 118, 120, 158, 171
Astringent 77-78, 86, 96, 155, 158, 160-162, 167, 169, 176

B
Bach flower remedies 178
Bacteria 2, 6, 12, 14, 56, 64, 70, 72, 76-77, 81, 92, 96, 124, 130-131, 158
Bain-marie 127, 141
Baking soda 92, 148
Balance 8, 14, 16, 27, 47-48, 52, 58-59, 61, 63-64, 70-71, 77, 81, 107-108, 118, 136-137, 142, 180, 186, 188
Balm 3, 21, 40, 42, 44-45, 57, 108, 116-119, 128, 142, 180, 188, 191
Bamboo cloth 84
Bancke's Herball 164
Basal cells 13
Bath 13, 44-46, 56, 66, 74, 80, 86, 90, 95, 96, 100, 102-104, 107-110, 142, 145, 149, 150, 152-155, 157, 161, 164, 167, 169, 171, 173, 176, 178-182, 191
Bay leaves 143, 157-158, 181
Bear's foot (see lady's mantle)
Bedtime 88, 171
Bees 116, 161, 170-171
Beeswax 68, 101, 105, 108, 111-113, 115-119, 129, 150, 152, 158, 177, 180
Bentonite 72-73, 158
Bergamot essential oil 109, 115
Beta-Carotene 54, 155
Beta Hydroxy Acids (BHAs) 92-93
Bicarbonate of soda 55, 157-158
Birch leaves 141,
Blackberry leaves 79, 106-107, 149
Blackheads 54, 182, 191
Blemishes 3, 53, 70, 144-145, 152, 178
Blend-it-yourself 32, 91, 119
Blonde hair 169
Blushing 5
Body 1-3, 5-6, 9-10, 13-16, 22, 29, 30, 32, 34-35, 39-40, 45-46, 48, 52, 54, 55-56, 58, 72, 74, 79, 82, 84-85, 87, 90, 92, 94-96, 98, 100-102, 105, 107-108, 110-112, 114, 117-119, 128-129, 135-136, 149-150, 158, 164, 169, 172, 179, 188-191
Body brushing 15, 84
Body butters 114, 118
Boils 149, 172
Borage 45, 90, 135, 141-142, 144, 174-175
Borage oil 16, 53, 63, 73, 102-103, 106, 110-112, 114-115, 134, 136
Borago officinalis 175
Bottle-brush (see horsetail)
Bran 90
Breakouts 61, 83
Breasts 160, 162
Brighten 61, 83
Broccoli seed oil 63, 106, 113, 134, 136,
Bruises 162, 169, 173
Brush 81, 85
Burdock root 141
Burns 6, 71, 149-151, 151, 159, 172-173, 179
Buttermilk 65, 66, 94, 119, 160, 188
Butters 57, 62, 71, 114, 117-118, 125, 129-131
Butyric acid 92

C
Calendula 66, 68-69, 73, 75, 78-79, 82, 86, 106, 111, 114-115, 141-144, 158, 174, 176-177, 188-191
Calendula water 141
Calm 5, 33-34, 54, 56, 62, 64, 70-71, 76, 88, 96, 107-108, 115, 167, 171, 173, 179, 184, 190
Camelina oil 63, 106-107, 111-113, 115, 134, 136
Camphor essential oil 96
Candelilla wax 101
Carmelite water 161
Carnation flowers 181
Carnuba wax 101
Carrot 172, 191
Carrot seed oil 61, 110
Castile soap 70, 149
Castor oil 62, 101, 109
Catchweed (see cleavers)
Caustic soda 71
Cedarwood essential oil 103, 106, 111
Cell renewal 53, 56, 83, 92
Cellulite 15, 85, 97, 90, 189
Cetearyl alcohol 129
149-150, 158, 164, 169, 172, 179, 188-191
Cetyl alcohol 101, 103, 105-107, 110-113, 115, 129
Chamomile essential oil 106, 112, 115
Chamomile flowers 86, 90, 103, 105, 107, 110, 112, 115, 167, 179
Chapped hands 168-169, 190
Chapped lips 176
Charcoal 84
Chemical exfoliation 84, 91-95
Cherries 94, 97
Chervil 78
Chickweed 144, 148, 150, 173, 189, 191
Chilblains 169
Cholesterol 16, 101
Circulation 16, 63, 72, 87, 96, 138, 155, 164, 170-171, 180, 188
Citric acid 92
Clary sage essential oil 105-107, 112-113, 158
Clay 56, 72-75, 84, 88-90, 95, 109, 142, 158, 188-189
Cleansing 3, 9, 14, 56-57, 59-65, 67-82, 84-85, 88, 91, 97, 102, 110, 153-153, 160, 162-163, 176, 178-180, 182, 188-191
Cleansing brush 81
Cleansing lotion 65, 188
Cleansing milks 65, 67
Cleansing powders 72, 74
Cleansing wipes 76
Cleavers 141-142, 144, 148, 151
Climate 5, 12, 14, 54, 56-57, 62, 134, 140, 146, 155, 179, 190
Clover 144, 166, 173
Cocoa butter 68, 74, 117-118, 129
Coconut oil 43, 62
Coffee grounds 84
Cold sores 161
Collagen 14, 92
Combination skin 52
Comfrey leaves 113
Comfrey oil 63, 86
Common Balm (see lemon balm)
Complexion 54, 56, 65-66, 151, 162, 169, 178, 180

Conditioning 53, 77-78, 90, 112, 151, 154, 162, 169, 171-172, 176, 190
Connection iii, ix, 2, 5, 21, 23, 33-35, 37, 184-186,
Cornflour 118
Cornflowers 110
Cotton pad 62, 65, 81-82, 89
Cow's milk 66, 95
Cowslip 173
Cracked skin 9, 152, 176
Cream of tartar 158
Creams 3, 9, 13, 20-22, 27, 35, 40, 42, 45, 55-57, 60, 62, 64-66, 68-69, 82, 85-86, 92-94, 98, 100-102, 105-106, 110-120, 123, 127-128, 130, 142, 146, 150, 152, 155, 157-158, 162, 167, 169, 172-173, 176, 179-183, 188-191
Cucumber 67, 78, 97
Culpeper, Nicholas 131, 149-150, 155, 157, 169, 172-173, 178, 187

D
Damaged skin 53, 79, 86, 106, 129, 136-137, 180
Dandelion 141, 144, 148, 153-155, 162, 175, 189, 191
Dandruff 23, 151, 157, 162
Dark circles under eyes 3, 53
Decoction 77, 140-141, 152, 154-155, 164, 172
Dehydrated skin 102, 119
Delicate skin 63, 85, 101, 137
Deodorant 9, 40, 45, 60, 151, 157-158, 179, 190
Dermis 13-14, 17, 29
Diatomaceous earth 89
Dill 79
Double boiler 36, 68, 74, 103, 105-108, 110-115, 118-119, 127, 129, 150, 152, 158-159, 170, 177, 180
Dr Fernie 150
Dried milk powder 173
Dry hair 165, 172, 191
Dry skin viii, 46, 61, 63, 66-68, 73, 75, 86-90, 92, 96, 98, 102, 107, 119,

136-137, 152, 167, 175-176, 188
Dull skin 78-79, 83, 153, 190

E
Eccrine glands 14,
Echinacea 141
Eczema 16, 27, 63, 135-138, 151-152, 188
Egg yolk 129, 172
Egyptians 167
Elastin 14, 63, 86,
Elderflower water 53, 79, 112, 169
Elderflower 53, 66, 75, 78-79, 89-90, 106, 113, 141-142, 144, 166, 168-169, 173, 189-191
Elements 2, 9, 16, 54, 57, 63, 98, 102, 188
Emollient 42-43, 62, 72-73, 89, 101-103, 106-108, 112, 136-138, 169, 188-190
Emperor Charlemagne 159
Emulsifier L 103, 106-107, 110-111, 129
Emulsion 10, 14, 64-65, 67, 119, 127, 129-130
Emulsifier 129
Energy 9, 16, 37, 52-53, 133, 149, 185
Environment iv, vii, ix, x, 2-3, 5, 8-9, 12, 14, 16, 20-21, 25, 28-30, 32-35, 42, 47, 52-56, 60, 77, 82, 100, 107-108, 110, 116, 144, 146, 185
Enzymes 9, 86, 92, 94
Epidermis 13-14, 17,
Equipment 36, 124-127
Equisetum arvense 154
Essential Fatty Acids (EFAs) 16, 53-54, 102, 134-135, 138,
Essential oils 16, 55, 58, 70-71, 73, 78, 87, 103, 105-107, 109, 111-115, 117-119, 126, 146, 157-159, 165, 187
Eucalyptus essential oil 159
Evening primrose 66, 114
Evening primrose oil 16, 61, 102, 136
Evelyn, John 161
Exfoliating gloves 93
Exfoliation 13, 57, 74, 84-87, 91-96, 98
Eye makeup remover 177, 189
Eyebright 177
Eyes 3, 22, 53, 71, 73, 75, 81-82, 88-89, 110, 150, 160, 162-164, 169, 177, 182, 189-191

F
Face 5, 14, 20, 22, 27, 40, 45, 49, 53, 54, 58, 62-63, 65-66, 69-70, 72-76, 78-79, 81-82, 84-86, 88-89, 92, 95-98, 101, 108-111, 114 115, 118, 120, 128, 135-137, 150-153, 160, 162, 164-165, 167, 169, 172, 175-176, 178-180, 182, 184, 188-191
Face cloth 81, 88, 160
Feet 13-14, 45, 84 87, 108, 169-171, 189, 191
Fennel 73, 78, 114, 141, 144, 154
Fennel essential oil 114
Fibroblasts 14
Fine lines 63, 66, 75, 137, 160, 188
Flannel 62, 81, 84, 97
Flare-ups 5, 53
Flax 15, 134, 136, 155
Flow x, 15, 37, 54, 56, 87, 98, 126, 142
Flower waters 67, 78, 80, 140-141, 169
Foot balm 45
Fragrance 43, 48, 55, 109, 161, 169, 171-173, 180-181
Frankincense essential oil 109, 115
Freckles 65, 79, 169, 171,
French green clay 72
Fresh 6, 10, 13-16, 22, 30, 32, 41, 43, 47, 53, 55-58, 62, 64, 66-67, 69-72, 74-87, 89, 92-94, 98, 106-107, 109, 119, 125, 130-131, 140-145, 149, 151, 153-155, 157, 160-163, 165, 167, 169, 175, 179-181, 184, 189
Funnel 127

G
Galium aparine 151
Gamma-linolenic Acid (GLA) 16, 53, 136
Garlic 141
Gel 87, 93, 103, 107, 111, 115, 158
Geranium 73, 79, 141, 144, 180, 188
Geranium essential oil 103, 105, 106, 112, 114, 180-181
Gerard, John 175, 181
German 167, 184
Gloves 13, 55, 93, 110, 113, 152, 175
Glow 3, 10, 13, 16, 47, 63, 88, 94, 98-99, 137, 186, 188
Glycerine 76, 80, 95, 101, 103, 106, 111-113, 129, 131, 157-158, 165, 168
Glycolic acid 92
Goat milk 66
Gommages 87
Goosegrass 151
Grapefruit essential oil 158
Greasy hair 161, 165, 179, 191
Greek 13, 24, 157, 161-162, 167-168, 172-173, 176, 179-180, 182
Green clay 72, 88, 90, 95, 109, 189
Green-herb rate 153
Greying hair 149, 169
Ground almonds 66, 172,
Ground ivy 169

H
Hair 9, 14, 23, 40, 44-45, 79, 81-82, 85, 117, 120, 124, 149, 151-152, 154-155, 161, 161-165, 167, 169, 171-172, 175, 179, 182, 191
Hands 5, 13-14, 28, 45, 54, 77, 81-82, 87, 93, 101, 108, 110, 113, 124, 130, 135-136, 159, 168-169, 172-173, 189-190
Hazelnut oil 61, 63, 68, 73, 86, 95-96, 103, 107, 109, 111, 113-114, 134, 136, 158
Healing 45, 63, 71-72, 88, 94, 118, 152, 157, 162, 167, 176-177, 179, 181, 191
Health viii, ix, 4-5, 8-10, 12, 15-16, 22, 27, 30, 34-35, 38, 41, 47, 51, 53, 55, 60, 75, 83, 88, 94, 98, 108, 137, 144, 154, 162, 171, 186, 188
Hedgerow vii, 20-21, 35, 106, 140, 149, 168, 173, 178, 187, 190
Hemp seed oil 63, 86, 105, 109, 112-113, 115, 134, 136-137
Herba militaris 182
Herbal vinegar 80, 142
Herbalism 140
Herbs 15-16, 35, 48-49, 58, 62, 65-66, 71-80, 88, 90, 96, 105-108, 110-112, 117, 125, 127, 131, 139-151, 153-159, 161-162, 164-167, 169, 171, 173-155, 177, 179, 182, 185, 187
Hindberry 163
Hips 87
Honey 70, 73, 75, 78-79, 86, 88-89, 95-96, 101, 103, 107, 116, 161, 171, 189
Honeysuckle 78-79, 105, 107, 143-144, 174, 178, 181, 190-191
Hops 115, 191
Hormones ix, 14, 83, 108
Horse chestnut 170
Horsetail 108, 144, 148, 154, 189, 191
Houseleek 67, 88, 109-110, 144, 156, 158-159, 188, 191-191
Humectant 42-43, 70, 87, 95-96, 101-103, 105, 107
Hungary Water 142, 161, 164
Hyaluronic acid 53, 101, 103, 107, 111, 115, 172
Hydration 46, 78, 102-103, 107
Hydrolipid 12, 99, 102
Hydrosols 78
Hypericum perforatum 173
Hyssop 90

I
Icing sugar 158
Inflamed skin 79, 88, 135, 160, 169
Infusion 67, 71-73, 76, 78, 88-89, 97, 103-105, 107, 109-113, 115, 127, 130, 140-142, 145, 151-155, 160-162, 164, 167, 169, 172-173, 175-179, 181-182, 191
Insects (and stings) 37, 150, 155, 161-162, 169
Invigorating 149
Irritated skin 150, 167
Itchy skin 6, 159
Ivy 78, 103

J
Jasmine flowers 181
Jojoba beads 84-85
Jojoba oil 61, 85, 101
Jug 126-127, 151, 155, 157

K
Kaolin 72, 74, 89, 158
Keratin 13
Keratosis pilaris (KP) 94
Ketone 179
Kits 85, 124, 187
Konjac sponge 84

L
Labelling 68, 128, 145
Lactic acid 65, 92, 94-95
Lady's mantle 55, 75, 78, 96, 113, 143-144, 156, 160, 188, 191
Lanolin 101, 129-130
Lard 20, 169
Laurus nobilis 143, 157
Lavandula augustifolia 179
Lavender 68-70, 73, 78-80, 86, 88, 90, 105, 107, 112, 115, 141-144, 157, 159, 173-174, 177, 179, 181, 188-190
Lavender essential oil 68, 73, 88, 103, 105, 107, 109, 111, 115, 124, 158-159
Lavender water 68-69, 78, 80
Lecithin 67, 76, 101, 129, 138
Legs 170
Lemon balm 66, 78, 112, 141-142, 144, 156, 171
Lemon essential oil 103, 114, 158
Lemon juice 57, 77, 158
Lemon rind 161
Lemon verbena 78, 144
Lifestyle iv, ix, 23, 37, 47, 52-53, 55, 116
Limeflowers 47, 171, 179
Linden 171
Lines 54, 63, 66, 75, 92, 137, 160, 188

193

Linoleic acid 16, 61, 63, 135, 136, 138
Linseed 16, 169
Lip balm 40, 45, 118, 128
Lips 9, 57, 86-87, 176, 189
Local ix, 3, 5, 21, 24, 30, 32, 35, 58, 72, 116, 139, 144, 146-147, 171,
Lonicera caprifolium 179
Loofah 84
Lord Bacon 150
Lotion 3, 27, 35, 42, 57, 64-67, 70, 93-94, 98, 102-103, 106-107, 110-111, 116-117, 119-120, 123, 129, 149-150, 152, 155, 160, 162, 167-169, 173, 175-176, 179, 182, 188-191
Lovage 90
Lye 71
Lymph 3, 14-15, 84, 87
Lymphatic system 3, 84

M
Maceration 77, 90, 117, 140-142, 151, 161, 164, 167, 172, 175, 179
Makeup viii, 28, 40, 42, 56, 60, 63, 67, 76-77, 79, 82, 121, 177, 184, 188-189
Makeup remover 67, 76, 177, 189
Malic acid 92
Mandarin essential oil 106, 114
Mandelic acid 92
Marigold 176
Marjoram 111, 114, 141
Marshmallow 40, 73, 79, 89, 90, 103, 105, 112, 141, 144, 166, 171-173, 177, 189-191
Marshmallow root 141, 172
Mask 6, 45, 54, 72-73, 75, 88-89, 92, 94-98, 108-109, 123, 142, 162, 172, 181, 188-191
Massage 45, 62, 82, 87, 89, 93, 106-109, 115, 135, 170, 173, 176, 180
Mature skin 72-73, 79, 136, 188
Measuring 71, 126
Medieval 152
Melanin 2
Melissa officinalis 161

Menopause 49
Micro scales 36, 49, 126
Microbeads 32, 85
Microcloth 81
Microdermabrasion 85
Middle Ages 154, 160, 164, 173
Milk 65-67, 71, 75, 92, 94-95, 97, 119, 167, 172-173, 188-189, 191
Minerals 63, 66, 86, 134, 154-155
Mint 78-79, 96, 109, 143, 155, 161-162, 165, 180, 189, 191
Moisturiser 14, 16, 40, 44-45, 54, 60, 73, 76-77, 81, 91, 97-102, 104-105, 107, 116, 119-120, 165, 179, 190
Molecules 1, 67, 93, 120, 127, 130
Moon 37, 82, 100, 140
Morning 14, 34, 46, 64, 81, 110, 120, 150, 153-154, 160, 164-165, 169, 185
Mouthwash 165, 191
Mucilage 150, 155, 159, 172
Mullein 63, 86, 141
Mullein oil 63, 86
Muslin 65, 66, 84, 89-90, 127, 141-142, 145, 160, 173, 178
Myrrh essential oil 165
Myrtle 78

N
Nails 27, 108, 110, 113, 154, 191
Nasturtium leaves 181
Natural
Natural oils 46, 55, 61, 71, 101, 106, 110, 125
Nature 14-15, 33, 35, 37, 52, 54, 56, 65, 71, 75, 78, 82, 98, 150, 184-186
Neck 49, 69, 75, 81, 86, 101, 110-111, 114-115, 128, 136, 190
Neroli essential oil 111
Nettles 141-144, 148, 155
Night 14, 40, 53-54, 66-67, 81-82, 90, 92, 100, 108-109, 114-115, 119-120, 135, 141, 150, 154-155, 165, 169, 172-173, 186, 190
Normal skin 153, 167

Nourishing 10, 30, 53, 62-63, 68, 70, 80-81, 98, 110, 112-113, 135-136, 138, 188-190

O
Oat milk 66, 188
Oatmeal 74, 85-88, 113, 162, 167, 189
Oats 65-66, 75, 84, 90, 97, 173, 189
Occlusive 42-43, 101-102, 104-105, 107, 110, 120, 135, 137, 190
Oil cleansing 61-63
Oil of swallows 169, 191
Oils 12-13, 16, 42-43, 46, 49, 52, 55-58, 60-63, 67-68, 70-73, 78, 81-82, 85-87, 98, 100-103, 105-115, 117-120, 124-127, 129-131, 133-135, 137-138, 140-141, 143, 146, 149, 154, 157-159, 164-165, 167, 176, 179, 187-191
Oily hair 182
Oily skin 1, 52, 61, 63, 65-66, 72, 78, 86, 88, 90, 92, 107, 152, 160, 162, 176, 179, 182, 188, 191
Ointment 3, 45, 150-152, 169, 181, 191
Older skin 86, 97, 172
Oleic acid 61, 136
Olive oil 49, 62, 67, 70, 87, 98, 101, 141
Orange 78, 95, 113, 129, 180
Orange flower water 78, 157, 161
Orange rind 157, 173
Outbreaks viii, 3
Oxidation 53, 140,
Oxygen 14, 16, 54, 136

P
Packaging 22-23, 32, 41-42, 92, 143, 185, 187
Pale skin 16, 54, 180
Paracelsus 161
Parsley 75, 78-79, 90, 144, 156, 162
Patch test 46, 48-49, 58, 98, 152, 175
Peeling gels 87
Peppermint 66, 75, 96, 109, 141, 144, 180
Peppermint essential oil 165

Perfume 5-6, 40, 45, 54, 124, 135, 161, 171, 171, 180-181
Perspiration 3, 171
Pestle and mortar 88, 109, 127, 142
Petroleum oils 134
Petroselinum crispum 162
pH (hydrogen potential) 12
Pheromones 5
Physical exfoliation 84-87, 91, 98
Physicians of Myddfai 164
Phytohormones ix
Piloerection 5
Pine needles 157
Plant seed oils 58, 61, 73, 131, 133, 146, 187
Plantain 93, 103, 169
Pliny the Elder 162, 173, 175
Pollutants 2, 9, 16, 101, 110
Pollution 16, 56
Poly Hydroxy Acids (PHAs) 92
Poppy seed oil 61
Pores 9, 14, 49, 56-57, 59-60, 62-63, 66, 72, 75-76, 78, 81, 83, 88, 92-93, 101, 107-108, 118, 120, 124, 135-138, 160, 162, 182, 188
Post-sport 90
Pregnancy 6, 49, 92, 163
Preservative Eco 103, 105-107, 110-113, 115, 131
Preservatives 9-10, 30, 42-43, 48, 68, 77, 107, 130-131
Priest's Crown (see dandelion)
Prostaglandins 16, 136
Psoriasis 63, 135, 137, 151, 155, 188
Puberty 14, 49
Puffy 14, 53
Pumice 84
Pumpkin 16, 92, 94, 135
Pumpkin seed oil 74, 86, 111, 113, 115, 134, 137

R
Radiance ix, 16
Rapeseed oil 61, 66, 74, 105, 111, 141, 179
Raspberry leaf 114, 144, 156, 163, 189

Red clover 144, 166, 173
Red wine 96, 171
Redness 15, 49, 75, 92, 98, 136-137, 150
Refreshing 64, 72, 75, 78-79, 109, 149, 153, 155, 179, 181, 184, 188-191
Regeneration 6, 52-54, 63, 96, 98, 136-138, 188-189
Rehydrate 101-102
Rejuvenating 53-54, 63, 88-90, 98, 115, 136, 172, 189-191
Renewal 6, 13, 53, 56, 83, 92
Replenishing 13, 68, 102, 145, 188
Restorative 53, 63, 82, 88, 98, 100, 106, 112, 189-191
Retinoid (Retinol, Retinol A) 53, 92, 95-98, 100
Rice bran 74
Rice bran wax 117
Rice flour 118
Rice milk 65-66, 188
Ritual 62, 183, 185
Roman 155, 157, 159, 162, 167-168, 172-173, 179
Rosa gallica var. *officinalis* 181
Rose 66, 78, 86, 89, 143-144, 174, 180, 189-191
Rose de Mal essential oil 111, 115
Rose petals 67, 97, 103, 105, 111, 115, 140-142, 181
Rosewater 67, 71, 75-76, 78, 80, 89, 97, 105, 109, 141, 161, 181
Rosehip oil 63, 103, 105-107, 110, 115, 134, 136-137, 181
Rosemary 70, 79, 80, 88, 90, 96, 111, 141, 143-144, 155-156, 161, 164, 165, 181, 189, 191
Rosemary essential oil 113, 131, 140, 158
Rosmarinus officinalis 164
Rough skin 13, 86, 118
Routine viii, ix, 27-28, 32, 34, 46, 55, 58, 67, 76-77, 86, 91, 93, 98, 108, 184-186
Rubichloric acid 151

Rubus fruticosus 149
Rubus idaeus 163

S
Sage 66, 75, 78, 108, 141-142, 144, 155, 158, 179
Saggy skin 110
Salicylic acid 92-93, 96, 131
Salt 3, 45, 56, 60, 66, 73-74, 80-81, 84-88, 90, 96, 145, 157-158, 169, 181, 189
Salve 177, 191
Sambucus nigra 168
Saponification 71
Saponins 150
Saucepan 36, 65, 95-97, 111-113, 115, 127
Scalp 14, 152, 155, 157, 164-165, 182, 191
Scars 6, 27, 66, 157, 176-177
Scent 5-6, 14, 16, 32, 34, 41-43, 55, 62, 67, 73, 82, 116, 145-146, 161, 167-168, 171, 173, 178, 180-181
Scented leaf pelargonium 180
Scrub 55, 66, 85-87, 90-92, 94, 97, 123, 142, 173, 179, 189
Seasons 8, 37, 47, 52, 57, 82, 98, 100, 114, 140, 147, 185-186
Seaweed 75, 184, 188
Sebaceous glands 2, 14, 54
Sebum 2, 13-14, 60, 77-78, 129, 180
Sempervivum 159
Sensitive skin 66, 68, 72, 78, 84-86, 92, 98, 107, 115, 135-136, 172, 176, 181, 188, 190
Sensitivities 19, 46, 48-49, 119
Serum 57, 77, 91-93, 98, 106-107, 114-117, 119-120, 123, 128, 137, 190
Sesame oil 62
Shakespeare 167, 176
Shampoo 10, 42, 45, 72, 151, 154-155, 157, 161, 167
Shaving 22, 44-45, 87
Shea butter 42, 118-119
Sheep milk 94

Shower 13, 28, 54, 56, 74, 86-87, 90, 92, 95-96, 100, 102-104, 107, 110-111, 149
Silica 108, 154
Skin hunger 5
Skin types 52, 63, 86
Sleep 8, 10, 29, 53, 108, 150, 173, 179, 184
Sleep of Plants 150
Soap 13, 22, 40, 42, 61, 67, 70-72, 74-76, 110, 124-125, 128, 143, 149-150, 154, 179, 187
Soapwort 154
Social media 21, 23, 54
Sodium lauryl sulphate (SLS) 43
Soften 46, 63, 72-73, 78, 80-81, 85, 88, 95, 97, 101, 108, 117-118, 136-138, 141, 152, 167, 169, 172-173, 176, 182, 188-191
Soothing 49, 63, 72, 88-89, 97-98, 102, 112, 118, 136-137, 150, 158, 162, 167, 169, 171, 176, 179, 188-191
Soreness viii, 13, 27, 150, 160
Spatula 124-125, 127
Spearmint 66, 90, 144, 179
SPF 45, 91, 98
Spike (see lavender)
Spinach 75, 162
Splashes 94, 191
Sponge 84-85, 94, 191
Spots 3, 12, 14, 27, 53, 56, 66, 78, 108, 154, 173, 191
Spritz 40, 72-73, 76, 79-80, 88, 104-105, 109, 161, 189-191
St John's Wort 90, 113, 140-141, 144, 166, 173, 191
Stability 9, 71, 185-186
Starweed (see chickweed)
Staunchweed 182
Stearic acid 101, 129
Stellaria media 150
Sterilising 124
Stinging nettle (see nettles)
Stratum basale 13
Stratum corneum 13
Strawberries 89
Stress 5, 10, 26, 53-54, 57, 100, 107-108, 110
Sugar 75, 84-87, 90, 92
Sun 128, 136, 140-142, 149-152, 158-159, 165, 167-169, 175-178, 182, 191

Sun protection 60, 77, 120
Sunburn 151, 159, 167, 169, 176, 178, 191
Sunflower oil 61, 63, 68, 70, 88, 90, 105-106, 109, 113-114, 119, 134, 138, 141, 150, 152, 159, 165, 170, 173, 177
Supple 12, 14, 54, 56-57, 63, 80, 99, 101, 114, 136, 138, 168, 173, 189
Surfactants 42-43
Sustainable iv, 23, 43, 146
Sweat 5, 14, 60, 82
Sweet almond oil 49, 62, 67, 129, 136, 141
Sweet bay (see bay)
Sweet marjoram essential oil 111, 114
Symphytum officinale 152

T
Tannic acid 151
Tannins 63, 86, 96, 159,
Taraxacum officinale 153
Tartaric acid 92, 94
Teenagers ix, 13
Teeth 23, 153-154, 165, 184
Temperate vii, ix, 5, 12, 54, 62, 134, 136, 146, 180
Terpene 167
Thighs 87
Thirties 110
Thistle (safflower) oil 61, 63, 67, 76, 86, 103, 107-109, 112, 115, 134, 138,
Thread veins 76, 162
Thyme 78, 80, 88, 96, 111, 141-144, 153, 157, 159, 173, 189
Thyme tincture 159
Tilleul 171
Tincture 78, 142, 142, 159
Tired skin 66, 188
Tomatoes 94
Tone 54, 61, 63, 71-72, 75-76, 86, 89, 92-93, 95-97, 108, 137, 154, 188
Toner 9, 45, 72, 76-80, 93, 97, 142, 160, 169, 179, 182, 189
Toothpaste 22, 42, 45
Toxins 3, 9, 14-15, 17, 54, 56, 72, 78, 107
Tradescant, John 180
Transepidermal water loss (TEWL) 102, 136

Transition 46, 58, 72
Travel 13, 15, 32, 57, 74, 76, 119, 150, 157
Trefoil (see clover)
Trifolium pratense 173
Triglyceride 133
Turkey Red Oil 109
Twenties 108

U
Urtication 155
Urtica dioica 155
UV 2, 16, 54, 92, 98, 110, 120, 145,

V
Valerian 115
Vinegar 55, 80, 124, 140, 142, 157
Violet leaves 103
Vitamin A 53-54, 92, 106, 115, 137,
Vitamin B 53
Vitamin C 53, 94
Vitamin D 2, 3
Vitamin E 53, 101, 103, 105-105, 108, 110-113, 115, 118, 136-138, 140, 152, 177
Vitamin F 63, 135, 138
Vitamins 16, 53, 54, 61, 63, 66, 86, 94, 134, 155
Vodka 124, 142, 157, 161

W
Walnut butter 105, 111-115, 117, 150, 158
Walnut leaf 78
Walnut oil 61, 63, 106, 114, 134, 138
Walnuts 16
Washcloth 65, 69, 81, 96, 173, 180
Watercress 21, 75, 175
Waxes 27, 43, 57, 62, 103, 116-117, 125, 129-131
Wellbeing iv, 4, 27, 30, 38, 40-41
Wheatgerm oil 140
Whisk 66, 68, 74, 124, 127, 130, 149, 159
White wine 96, 164
White wine vinegar 80
Wine 92, 94, 96, 164, 171, 175, 191
Witch hazel 68, 73, 77-80, 86, 88, 96, 107, 140, 153, 158, 160, 179, 182, 189

Woodbine 178
Workshops 124, 187
Wormwood 169
Wounds 6, 27, 163-164, 169, 172-173, 180, 182
Wrinkles 14, 53, 63, 66, 83, 92, 102, 110, 118, 136, 152, 171, 188

Y
Yarrow 66, 73, 75, 78-79, 90, 96, 106, 141-142, 144, 174, 182, 188
Yoghurt 75, 94, 162

Z
Zinc 94, 137

Praise for this book

A fascinating and informative book with ravishing photographs and careful instructions; this is how the natural world can help us to look fabulous and be philosophical all at once.

Joanna Lumley

If you are looking to make the move to natural skincare or want to start making your own products then this book is an absolute must. Informative, inspiring and empowering. Go the green beauty revolution!

Rachel Whittaker
beauty brand mentor and logistics expert at Indie Beauty Delivers

Vital Skincare is a beautiful book, with easy to follow, inspirational recipes to enthuse everyone to make their own natural beauty and skincare products in harmony with their own skin. Most of the ingredients can be grown at home or foraged locally – I love that I already have so many of the ingredients close to hand at home for truly personal skincare.

Stephanie Hafferty,
no dig gardener and author of *The Creative Kitchen*

Vital Skincare is a beautifully put together publication, bright pages with plenty of colourful pictures, clear text and comprehensive information on the structure of skin, and the practical recipe section is especially useful. This book is a great resource to keeping your skin in optimum health.

Karen Lawton
herbalist

Exposed to so many pollutants and toxins, going back to nature with our skincare is one of the most vital changes we can make. Not just our skin, but for our hormones and overall health too. *Vital Skincare* is an extensive guide to every single step of an effective green beauty ritual. Whether you're battling acne, eczema or just want a bit of extra glow, this book is ideal for anyone wanting to deeply explore natural beauty.

Amy Saunders
natural acne coach, www.skyntherapy.com

A bible about an alternative to shop shelf cosmetics. Harnessing the power of plants can and will make you feel happy and revitalised. A modern book inspired by ancient practices and healing traditions, Laura's knowledge of botanical sciences and the relationship with skin is truly inspiring and interesting.

Tess O'Shea,
founder of Seatox Seaweed, www.seatoxseaweed.com

Enjoyed this book? You might like these

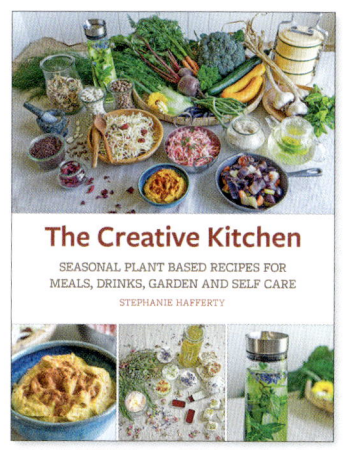 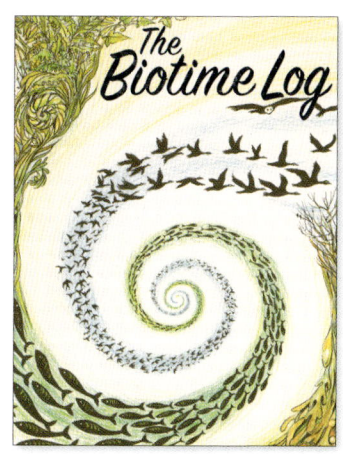 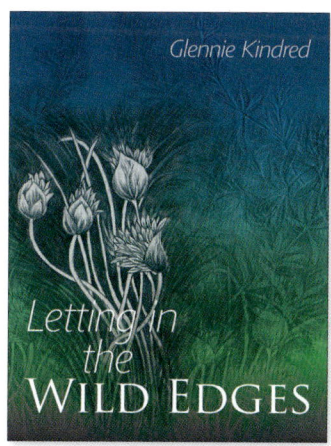

Get 15% off these three books with discount code: **SKINCARE**

Just visit:

https://shop.permaculture.co.uk

Our titles cover: permaculture, home and garden, green building, food and drink, sustainable technology, woodlands, community, wellbeing and so much more

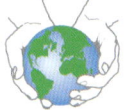

See our full range of books here:

www.permanentpublications.co.uk

Subscribe to a better world

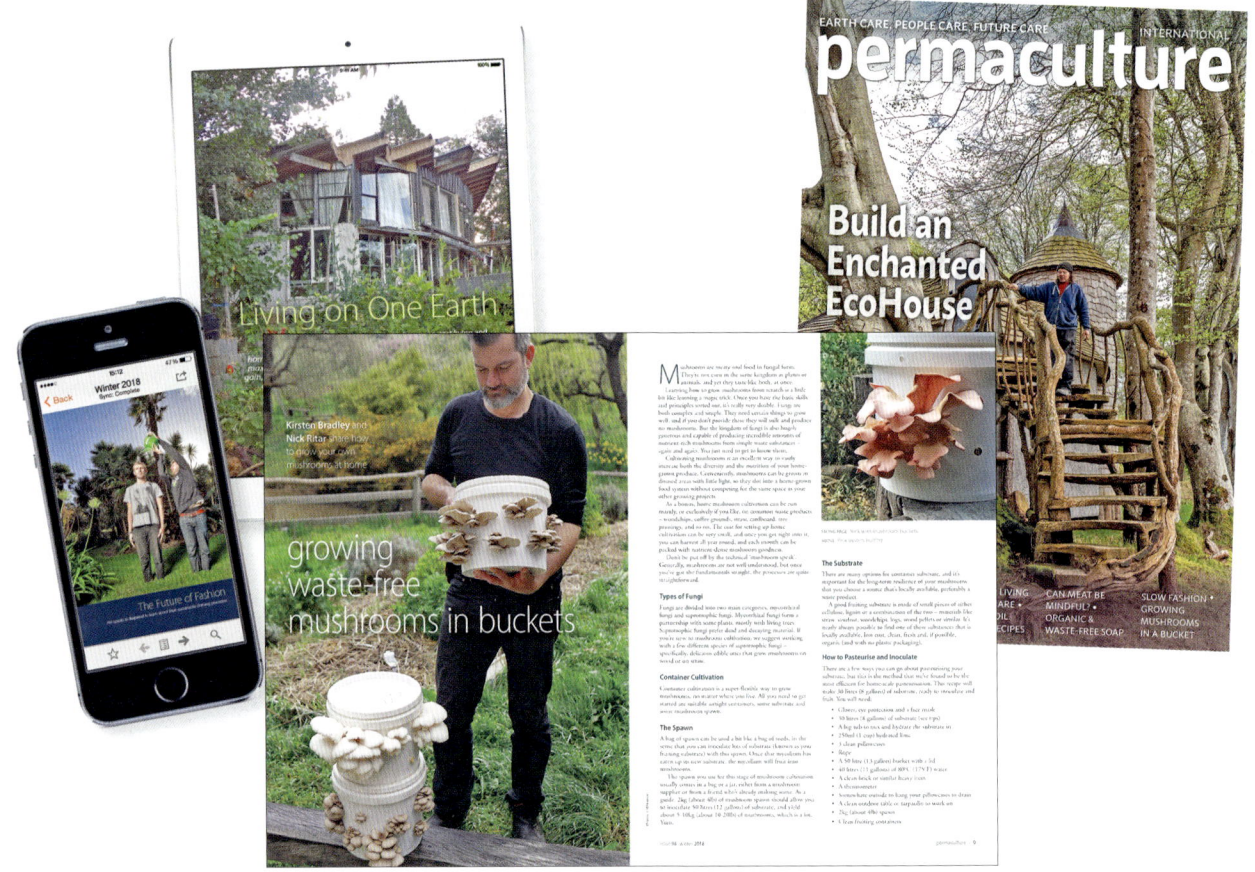

Each issue of *Permaculture Magazine International* is hand crafted, sharing practical, innovative solutions, money saving ideas and global perspectives from a grassroots movement in over 170 countries

Print subscribers receive FREE digital access to our complete 26 years of back issues plus bonus content

To subscribe call 01730 823 311 or visit:

www.permaculture.co.uk